One Man Alone:

An Investigation of Nutrition, Cancer and

William Donald Kelley

NICHOLAS J. GONZALEZ, M.D.

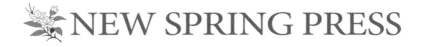
NEW SPRING PRESS

Dedication

To the hundreds and hundreds of Dr. Kelley's patients who more than 25 years ago let me into their lives and showed me there might be a better way, with nutrition, diet, enzymes, and even coffee enemas, to treat the worst of cancers. Each one of you had a story to tell of personal courage against overwhelming odds, of terrible disease conquered. You were and are an inspiration to me, and will be for the duration of my life.

Notice

This book is intended for general informational purposes only, not as a medical manual. The materials presented in no way are meant to be a substitute for professional medical care or attention by a qualified practitioner, nor should they be construed as such. Always check with your doctor if you have any questions or concerns about your condition or before starting or modifying a program of treatment. New Spring Press LLC and the author(s) are not responsible or liable, directly or indirectly, for any form of damages whatsoever resulting from the use (or misuse) of information contained in or implied by this book.

Book design by Anne M. Landgraf, Brooklyn BookWorks LLC.

Publisher's Cataloging-in-Publication
(Provided by Quality Books, Inc.)

Gonzalez, Nicholas J.
    One man alone : an investigation of nutrition, cancer,
and William Donald Kelley / Nicholas J. Gonzalez.
        p. cm.
    Includes bibliographical references.
    LCCN 2009936519
    ISBN-13: 978-0-9821965-1-9
    ISBN-10: 0-9821965-1-2
    1. Kelley, William Donald.   2. Cancer--Diet therapy.   3. Cancer--Alternative treatment.
  4. Digestive enzymes.   5. Dietary supplements.   I. Title.

RC271.D52G66 2010   616.99'406

                                        QBI09-600171

Contents

⁓

Part I: Dr. Kelley in Theory and Practice

Part II: The Data

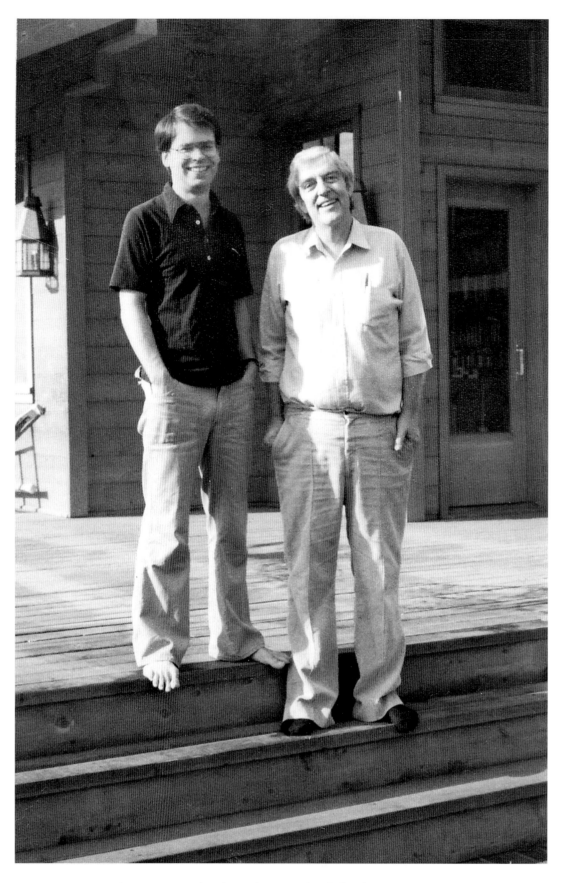

Dr. Gonzalez (as a medical student in the fall of 1982) and Dr. Kelley,
on the porch of Dr. Kelley's Winthrop, Washington home.

Acknowledgements

It's been a long time coming, but finally, 23 years after its completion, I am grateful for the opportunity to present *One Man Alone* to the world. Over the years since I completed the original manuscript back in 1986, my respect for the subject of this book, the late William Donald Kelley, D.D.S, has only grown. As eccentric as he may have been, I appreciate now more than ever his years of dedication, his unappreciated efforts, his many successes with those diagnosed with cancer, this most terrible disease. It surely wasn't easy for Dr. Kelley, his life a series of seemingly insurmountable obstacles beginning with his own terrifying bout with advanced cancer, continuing with the endless assaults against him orchestrated by the conventional medical world and the media. Ultimately, in his lifetime the recognition and respect I believe he deserved eluded him.

I once again want to express my gratitude to my wife Mary Beth, who has been a loyal support through thick and thin, through some past dark days with my research and more recent happier days, as interest in what we do continues to grow and stimulate much needed discussion. She's endured endless long weekends while I was away in the office writing, and rewriting, and rewriting yet again, this book and the others in various stages of completion. She believed in the work from the beginning, and continues to be a vocal champion—thanks, for all your help over the years.

I especially wanted to thank my colleague and scientific sounding board, Linda Isaacs, M.D., a devoted physician and scientist who has nurtured and grown this work with me. She has been an instrumental part of the effort, helping me complete my original Kelley research back in the 1980s, then working with me, side by side, as we started the practice in late 1987, never hesitating over the years to take on the administrative responsibilities of managing our busy practice. She put our websites together, takes care of the details of running a medical office that would otherwise drive me crazy, and has helped over the past two decades to fine-tune the therapy. She is a superb editor as well, who has with great insight refined each of my books including this one, investing considerable time and effort turning my writing into something better. She is a skilled physician who cares enormously for her patients, as well as a loyal and devoted friend who has helped me keep this treatment alive for future generations of scientists and patients. For your unswerving dedication over the years, I thank you.

I also want to thank my dear friend Julian Hyman, M.D., an oncologist and member of an esteemed family of physicians, as well as a wonderful photographer, naturalist, and art student. During the first round of political battles earlier in my career, Julian became a strong supporter and friend, convinced of the value of my therapy, and he proved instrumental in bringing that phase of the warfare to an end. You have been a wonderful light through some difficult times, and I cherish our friendship—may it continue for many more years.

Finally, my loyal, hardworking office staff, Chelsea Leinberger and Angela Rios, deserve thanks for their assistance with our various book projects, including this one. It's been quite a gift, to have employees like these two, who answer the phones, deal with all manner of requests from active patients, potential patients, interested parties from all over the world, and manage my schedule—all the while remaining centered and calm. You're both wonderful assets in our lives.

Nicholas J. Gonzalez, M.D.

Introduction 2010

It is hard sometimes to believe that 28 years have now passed since I first began my investigations of the controversial alternative cancer therapist and dentist William Donald Kelley. In July of 1981, after my second year of medical school at Cornell, a good friend and successful writer called me one afternoon asking if I knew anything about Dr. Kelley and his strange nutritional treatment for cancer. I had certainly heard of Kelley by that point. His name had been splashed across all the major and minor newspapers and TV news shows some eight months earlier, vilified as the practitioner supervising the treatment of the actor Steve McQueen who in November 1980 lost his battle with advanced mesothelioma in a Mexican clinic. The stories had continued for many months even after McQueen's death, and though I hadn't followed the case too closely and knew little about Kelley, I thought the vicious attacks against him somewhat peculiar. After all, McQueen suffered a malignancy that was—and still is—incurable in the conventional world. Kelley had tried, I thought, when I first read articles about him and McQueen, and hadn't succeeded—hardly some grievous sin, since all practicing oncologists try and fail, with many if not most of their patients.

My friend, always looking for a hot new book to write, thought Kelley might make a good subject for a potboiler, given that he had for months been the subject of national and international press attention. She had been in touch with Kelley, and to her surprise, in her conversations she found him to be quite the opposite of what she expected: the celebrity chasing, money driven, greedy "quack" as he had been portrayed in the press and on TV, trolling for dollars among the most vulnerable, those diagnosed with incurable cancer. She instead found him very shy, painfully so, convinced his therapy had value and devastated by the mocking and relentless media assaults.

Apparently, my friend told me, Kelley himself had survived terminal pancreatic cancer in the early 1960s when he still practiced conventional orthodontics. With four young children to worry about and facing an early death, Kelley desperately sought some way to beat the disease. Through a trial and error process, using himself essentially as a guinea pig, he serendipitously put together the therapy that saved his own life. Once recovered, he began to apply what he had learned on others facing equally catastrophic fates with terrible cancer. The rest, she said, with some irony, was history.

At this point in his life, Kelley said he only wanted the chance to have his regimen appropriately and fairly evaluated in clinical trials. When she asked him to explain his treatment, a very complicated approach involving individualized diets, individualized supplement protocols, large doses of pancreatic enzymes, and coffee enemas, she said his comments about the biochemistry of nutrition went far above her head, non-scientist that she was. As she told me, she couldn't be sure if Kelley was truly a genius onto something extraordinary, or simply an inarticulate peddler of snake oil.

At the time, Kelley maintained an office in Dallas, but in recent weeks had sequestered himself at an organic farm he owned in the middle of nowhere in Washington State. There he hoped to avoid the media, but some enterprising reporter had managed to track him down. In some frustration, Kelley had taken a long train ride across Canada to escape the press and a failed romantic relationship, the victim, apparently, of his new-found notoriety. He was scheduled to arrive in New York, where he intended to stay for several days before flying back to Dallas. My friend wanted to meet with him face-to-face during his stay in town, to explore further the possibility of a book, but wanted me to meet with him as well, to size him up, to help her determine if he was simply crazy, or brilliant, or perhaps crazy and brilliant. I had seven years of journalism experience under my belt before going to medical school, including stints under some legendary editors, so she thought my unusual combination of reporting and scientific training might help her sort through Kelley's level of authenticity.

Initially, I balked at the suggestion, having little interest in meeting some controversial alternative cancer therapist. But she persevered, even offering to pay me for my time. Finally, after considerable prodding I agreed to meet with him—for no charge, I might add. I was, in fact, pretty bored, spending the summer in the research lab of one of the professors who had taken me under his wing, the late Walter Riker, for years Chairman of Pharmacology at Cornell. Though Dr. Riker was a wonderful mentor, I felt restless, finding the laboratory work somewhat tedious. Journalist that I was at heart, I was looking for an adventure, even if only a minor one, and Kelley might just fit the bill. So several days later, I trudged out to the Forest Hills offices of a chiropractor known to my writer friend who had agreed to set up a lunch so we might all get together somewhat informally.

I remember so well my first glimpse of Kelley: he was tall, six foot two or three, with blue eyes, a narrow, haggard pale face topped by a mop of unruly thick gray hair. He wore a gray suit, white shirt and blue tie, and walked with a distinctive limp—the result, as I would learn, of the metastatic cancer that 20 years earlier had ravaged his body.

At our first meeting, Kelley was indeed very shy, appearing very uncomfortable, so soft-spoken that initially I had trouble hearing him. We sat together awkwardly in the chiropractor's consulting office, as I tried to get the conversation going. We talked about his trip across Canada, his recent romantic breakup, and the harassment he had endured over Steve McQueen. When I then asked him about his treatment, very quickly his face became animated, his voice strengthened and the words began to flow. He became a totally different person than the bumbling, nervous man he had been only a minute previously. With great authority he discussed his concepts of autonomic physiology, the use of diet and supplements to manipulate the nervous system, the British embryologist and researcher John Beard who had first used pancreatic enzymes to treat cancer some 80 years earlier. The ideas came fast and furious, somewhat overwhelming my two years of medical school knowledge. I tried to hold my own, but quickly realized that whatever the press or the world thought about Kelley, he was one smart man.

Further along into our conversation, I asked him what he wanted, and he answered without hesitation; as he had told my writer friend, he believed this therapy had value, but it needed to be evaluated in appropriate clinical studies in an academic medical setting. If after such testing the regimen proved to be of benefit against cancer, he said it needed to be in the hands of the conventional medical world, where it might be properly studied and made available to those patients who wanted an effective nutritional approach. And if it turned out the therapy had no value, he needed to know that, so he could close his office down and "go fishing."

I thought his answer a far cry from what would be expected from an alternative practitioner—usually portrayed by the conventional medical world as unwilling to accept the challenge of rigorous clinical and laboratory scrutiny. Here, Kelley told me that's just what he wanted—and apparently for all the right reasons.

Fortunately, I had as one of my Cornell mentors Robert A. Good, M.D., Ph.D., at the time Director of Sloan-Kettering, the "founder of modern immunology," as the press called him, and the most published author in the history of medicine. He was a man of many interests and of great accomplishments; though he originally trained in pediatrics, he also earned a Ph.D. in physiology and had been, prior to arriving at Sloan-Kettering, Head of the Department of Pathology at the University of Minnesota. As a pathologist, internationally known as he might have been, he was essentially self-taught—a very unusual circumstance, for such an expert in the field. He once told me how odd it seemed at times for him to have supervised a department in a field in which he had not one hour of formal residency training.

However, his fame—including a *Time Magazine* cover in 1973—came because of his pioneering work in immunology. He helped unravel the workings of the thymus gland, previously considered a vestigial organ but which Dr. Good demonstrated to be the ultimate regulator of immune function. He also, along the way, supervised the first bone marrow transplant in history in 1969, opening up a whole field of high tech therapeutics. To round out the picture, he had developed a strong interest in nutrition, particularly in terms of how diet and specific nutrients influence immune activity.

I had begun meeting with Dr. Good regularly at his invitation to discuss my interest in cancer research, an interest he encouraged enthusiastically. Whatever might be said of Dr. Good, and indeed he was a most controversial man in his lifetime, and whatever his responsibilities at Sloan-Kettering, he always took time to meet with students, to discuss their scientific interests, as if he had no more pressing business. I once read—and I must admit I've never had the statement verified— that more of his fellows have gone on to professorships at U.S. medical schools than from any other research group in history.

As I sat across from a now enlivened Dr. Kelley, sitting in this chiropractor's office in Queens, I mentioned that I knew Dr. Good, the Director of Sloan-Kettering, and might approach him to ask the best way to proceed with an evaluation. Dr. Kelley seemed to stop cold midsentence, before explaining that for years, Dr. Good had been his hero, the one person in the conventional medical world he believed had a mind open enough to allow an investigation of a treatment method such as his. I nodded, in total agreement—Dr. Good did have an insatiable curiosity that at times could lead to dead ends, or even to spectacular controversy. Nonetheless, he had told me in conversation that as a scientist, one must always look beyond the tried and true for the next new advance.

After several hours talking, Kelley explained that he was leaving for Dallas the following day, and wanted me to come with him, so I could start evaluating his treatment and his records. I told him I was in the middle of a commitment to Dr. Riker, and I couldn't be sure Dr. Good would even be interested in such a project, particularly one that Kelley wanted to begin so soon. But frankly, I admired Kelley's no-nonsense approach, and agreed I would try and speak with Dr. Good that afternoon.

After the subway ride back to Manhattan, and my return to the Cornell medical campus on the Upper East Side, I immediately went to Dr. Good's office atop the main Sloan-Kettering building. When I arrived, I heard his typically enthusiastic booming voice talking to someone over the phone about some scientific conference. I asked Dr. Good's secretary at the time, who already had gotten to know me, if it would be possible for me to see him, even if for five minutes. She told me to have a seat, and when he was off the phone, went in to tell him I was there, without an appointment. I heard him say, "Send Nick in, always happy to see him."

My five minutes turned out to be an hour. I reviewed in great detail my meeting earlier that day with Dr. Kelley, and my belief that despite the controversy swirling about his methods, he seemed to be serious about his work, perhaps even truly on to something. Dr. Good, who like me knew of the McQueen controversy, listened very attentively, periodically interjecting comments or asking pertinent questions. He seemed genuinely intrigued by my conversation with Kelley. When I broached Kelley's suggestion that I accompany him back to Dallas the following day, Dr. Good immediately told me I should go, and not think twice about it. He was sure Dr. Riker would understand. And Dr. Good then said what has remained with me for all the many years since that fateful meeting, that even if Dr. Kelley turned out to be a total charlatan, I would learn a lot of medicine by going down to Dallas to sort out what was going on in his office. A student always learns best, he said, when pursuing a project of his own devising, rather than an assignment picked by someone else. I couldn't have agreed with him more.

Dr. Good did offer some suggestions, in terms of how to proceed with my preliminary review. He asked that I try and locate charts of patients who had been appropriately diagnosed with poor prognosis cancer, and who by the standards of conventional oncology were alive years beyond what would normally be expected. He seemed particularly interested in the records of any survivors of metastatic pancreatic carcinoma that might be in Kelley's files, telling me that if I could find even one patient diagnosed with the disease who had lived five years on this nutritional regimen he would be impressed, since no one else in medicine anywhere to his knowledge had such a case. Though a single example might not prove to everyone's satisfaction that Kelley's therapy had value, it certainly should grab the attention of any fair-minded researcher.

So the following day, I was on a plane with Kelley to Dallas, to begin a search through his charts. Kelley, as promised, opened his patient files to me without hesitation. I spent many hours each succeeding day in Kelley's office, poring over his records, and what I found I thought was quite remarkable—patient after patient with properly diagnosed advanced cancer, including pancreatic carcinoma, who had done well under Kelley's care, either in terms of disease regression or significantly prolonged survival.

After two weeks of non-stop work, I bundled up a bunch of Kelley's charts along with my extensive notes, and returned to New York. Dr. Good and I subsequently spent several hours together, reviewing what I had found, such as a patient with advanced metastatic pancreatic carcinoma, alive seven years after diagnosis, and another patient diagnosed with acute myelocytic leukemia, as deadly as pancreatic cancer, whose disease went into remission within months of beginning the Kelley treatment, after chemotherapy proved ineffective. Dr. Good offered the usual caveats about my most preliminary of findings, but told me nonetheless he was impressed by the cases I had presented, impressed enough to encourage me to continue a formal investigation of Kelley's records.

Over the next few weeks, as summer came to an end, I met a number of times with Dr. Good, as we gradually devised a plan to evaluate Kelley's therapy. Dr. Good and I were on uncharted ground since to our knowledge no academic group had ever attempted an objective, fair-minded evaluation of an unconventional therapy or practitioner.

Dr. Good did warn me, early in our discussions, that a retrospective evaluation of Kelley's files such as he proposed could not be used to "prove" definitively the efficacy, or its lack, of Kelley's approach. Only a prospective controlled clinical study could do that. But Dr. Good insisted the project could yield useful data if done properly. Dr. Good often remarked, not only to me but to others, that carefully documented case reports can teach us much about the potential of a new approach. Great new advances in medicine often begin with observations even of a single patient whose disease might have taken an unusual course while receiving some new treatment.

As the plan took shape, Dr. Good suggested I should become familiar with the details of Kelley's treatment, its theoretical framework, and any evidence from the medical literature to support his methods. That would be a preliminary step. Then, to evaluate Kelley's patients, he recommended a two-pronged approach. First, he proposed that I try and put together a series of 50 patients appropriately diagnosed with a variety of poor prognosis cancers who subsequently did well, either in terms of documented disease regression or unusual long-term survival, that could only be attributed to the nutritional regimen. I was to write up each case at some length, providing along with my report copies of pertinent medical records to substantiate the diagnosis and response. Dr. Good said that if I could find 50 such patients from a single practitioner's files, he would be impressed.

As a second component, Dr. Good requested that I track down every patient diagnosed with pancreatic cancer who had consulted with Kelley during a specific time period and write each of these up as well. Since pancreatic adenocarcinoma represented at the time, as it represents today, one of the most deadly, treatment resistant cancers, Dr. Good believed that if Kelley had any success at all with this particular disease, the academic research world would have to take his treatment seriously.

I began the project in earnest during my third year of medical school, in whatever free time I might have in the evenings and on weekends. Unfortunately, that fall, Dr. Good was unexpectedly and unceremoniously pushed out of Sloan. To my dismay, he rather suddenly departed New York for the University of Oklahoma, far removed from the academic power centers of the East, to set up a cancer research center and bone marrow transplant unit. Before he left, he assured me that he would continue to guide and support my "Kelley study," even long distance. Though I felt relieved the project would continue, my dream of pursuing research under him at Sloan had come to a crashing end.

Despite Dr. Good's absence, my Kelley investigation did progress, though slowly because of the enormous demands of the third year of medical school. But with Dr. Good's help, the Cornell Dean approved a four-month block of time allowing me to continue my investigation as an independent study during the fall of my fourth year. Though Dr. Good had departed from Cornell, he would continue as my research supervisor.

I spent most of the allotted time that autumn of 1982 at Kelley's farm, situated in the Methow Valley of Washington State in the foothills of the high Cascades. There, he had lived from 1976 until 1981, while maintaining an office in the nearby town of Winthrop, population 200. After the McQueen fiasco he had moved back to Dallas where he had practiced for many years, but most of his records remained at his home in Washington.

I accomplished much during my stay in Winthrop, but the rigors of internship essentially put a stop to my efforts. Halfway through the year, Dr. Good invited me to join him in Oklahoma as a full fellow after finishing my internship—a position usually offered only after completion of residency. He wanted me to help man the immunology and bone marrow service, but promised I would have considerable time to continue my Kelley work. I accepted at once, and after completing my internship moved to Oklahoma, to work under Dr. Good.

With his blessing I devoted most of my time in Oklahoma to the "Kelley study" as we came to call it. Then after a year in Oklahoma, I followed Dr. Good to All Children's Hospital and the University of South Florida in Tampa/St. Petersburg, where he moved again to set up a cancer research program and bone marrow transplant unit. After another year of hard work in Florida, I brought my investigation to a close. By that point, I had interviewed and evaluated over 1000 of Kelley's patients, concentrating on a group of some 455 who had done exceptionally well under his care. I then put my findings into monograph form as partial fulfillment for my fellowship training—the book herein presented.

In its writing, I adhered to the format suggested by Dr. Good for my overall approach to the research, with an introductory series of chapters describing in some detail the theory behind Kelley's therapy, with supporting evidence if available. I also included in this first section a history of the trials and tribulations he had endured over the years. I then presented in some detail 50 case reports representing 26 different types of cancer (counting the different subtypes of lymphoma as distinct neoplasms), with accompanying medical records.

The monograph concluded with my evaluation of Kelley's experience with pancreatic carcinoma, which proved to be most revealing. I eventually identified 22 patients with the diagnosis who had consulted Kelley during the period 1974–1982. I had been able to document that ten of the patients, all deceased, had not followed the program for a single day. In my interviews with surviving family members I learned that most had gone off to follow some other treatment largely because of opposition to this unconventional approach expressed by their doctors or family. For these, I determined an average survival of 63 days, quite typical for patients in that era with the inoperable form of the disease. This group, we agreed, could serve as an informal "control."

A second group of seven patients, also all deceased, complied only partially, and for limited periods of time ranging from four weeks to 13 months, before abandoning the therapy. Again, surviving family members I interviewed reported strong opposition from the patient's conventional physicians and/or family members as the most common reasons for discontinuing the regimen. The mean and median survival for this group was 302 days, far longer than would be expected.

Five patients, all alive at the time I completed my research, had complied fully. The median and mean survival for this group exceeded eight years, certainly a remarkable statistic in view of the deadly nature of pancreatic cancer, with an average life expectancy reported in the range of 3–6 months.

When I handed my finished manuscript to Dr. Good in the spring of 1986, I felt a sense of some accomplishment. Five years earlier, Dr. Good had presented me with a challenge, which I thought I had adequately met. And he, after reviewing the text over the following days, felt I had found evidence to support my original belief that Kelley's nutritional regimen might offer some significant benefit to patients with advanced cancer. Unfortunately Dr. Good, by that point banished from the "prestigious" academic centers, no longer had the financing, the resources or the power base that would have allowed for further laboratory and clinical studies under his tutelage.

After several conversations, we agreed as a next step I should try and get the monograph published in its entirety as a freestanding book, with perhaps portions structured in article form suitable for the peer reviewed conventional medical journals. Dr. Good thought that publication was essential to get the data out into the world to stimulate discussion, and hopefully encourage further research funding.

As for my own future, after finishing my fellowship I decided to move back to New York to concentrate on getting the book and/or articles published—an effort that ultimately failed completely. Not that the monograph didn't generate interest, for indeed it did. A top flight New York literary agent agreed to represent the manuscript, which he thought might have an explosive effect in the scientific world. However, over the next year, no publisher, either trade or scientific, agreed to back the book, nor would any medical journal consider excerpting portions, even a case report or two. Some editors just didn't believe the records could be real, that an unconventional nutritional therapy could reverse advanced cancer. Others accepted the data as legitimate, but felt the book would generate so much controversy that their careers might be in jeopardy.

I still have in my possession one letter from that time, written by an editor of a well-known conventional medical journal. When the rejection letters from publishers began piling up, Dr. Good suggested I send a copy of my monograph to this particular editor, a friend he had known for years, for his assessment. Before sending him anything, I first called the man, who seemed nice enough, and who expressed his extraordinary respect for the renowned Dr. Good. I subsequently forwarded a copy of the manuscript off to him, hoping for a fair reading, perhaps even an offer to publish a case report or two. Several weeks later the editor wrote a blistering letter, not to me but to Dr. Good, admitting he had only read a few pages, but that was enough to know what he was dealing with. He warned Dr. Good that he had been "hoodwinked" by a typical "scam artist," meaning me, who was about to drag him into fraud and controversy. Even Dr. Good, who had mailed me a copy of the letter, seemed shaken when we discussed the editor's remarks over the phone.

Meanwhile, Kelley had closed his Dallas office for a variety of reasons, and was himself no longer seeing patients. I think he had reached a point where he was burnt out by years of hard work with the very sick, and by the relentless harassment by regulatory agencies, the conventional medical world at large, and the media. To make matters worse, his practice had never really recovered from the intense attacks brought on by his involvement with McQueen, so financially he was in terrible shape. Completely broke, Kelley moved to Philadelphia during the summer of 1986 to live with a former patient of his, a woman physician who later became his significant other. There he had intended to wait for publication of the book—which he saw as his professional salvation—but as the possibility of this outcome faded, Kelley lapsed into a very severe depression.

We experienced a glimmer of hope in early 1987, while Kelley still lived in Philadelphia. I had learned of a government sponsored investigation into alternative cancer therapies under the auspices of the Office of Technology Assessment, a now defunct Federal agency charged with evaluating controversial scientific issues at the behest of Congress. Word reached Kelley and me that activists within the alternative world hoped this project might be the big breakthrough everyone hoped for, finally bringing recognition to legitimate unconventional approaches. And shortly after learning about the investigation, a representative of the OTA contacted me, having heard of my "Kelley manuscript" as she called it, wishing to see a copy. She explained she had learned about my study from someone who heard about it from someone else who knew Dr. Good.

I dutifully sent a copy of my monograph off, but then heard nothing for months. When I finally called the OTA myself to find out what had happened, a staff scientist who spoke with me seemed vague and noncommittal about the timeline for the project. Subsequently, as the OTA study dragged on with no end in sight,

Kelley became suspicious, even paranoid, at one point accusing me of being part of a CIA plot to steal his therapy for the government, another time angrily telling me I had deliberately sabotaged publication of my own report. As his conversations became increasingly irrational, I finally ended all contact with him in July of 1987, and never would speak to him again. Despite the unpleasant break, I actually felt sorry for him, suspecting that years of stress, the endless attacks, and his many disappointments had finally taken their toll. But still convinced of the value of Kelley's therapy, and with the options dwindling, I decided to begin seeing patients myself, using the enzyme treatment. I felt someone needed to keep the therapy alive, as Kelley himself deteriorated mentally.

By 1988, I had given up any hope of having the monograph published, but still thought the OTA project might get my research—and poor Dr. Kelley—the recognition each deserved. Unfortunately the OTA investigation seemed to be going nowhere, as 1989 came and went. But during that period, as our practice flourished, knowledge of my "Kelley study" began to spread, particularly within the alternative medicine underground, through a word-of-mouth network in those days before the Internet. Well-known activists and practitioners began to inquire about my research, and during the late 1980s, several widely read alternative journals discussed my "Kelley study" favorably. Dr. Robert Atkins, the famed diet doctor, invited me on his popular radio show several times specifically to discuss my investigation. Word even reached abroad; in late 1989, a mainstream journalist from Japan interviewed me for a planned book reporting on promising alternative approaches. I still have a copy, in Japanese, with a photograph of my Kelley monograph prominently displayed. Such exposure helped generate a great deal of enthusiasm for the manuscript, as evidenced by the frequent requests we began receiving for it coming in from all over the country. We complied as best as we could, binding up multiple copies of the typed monograph to meet the demand.

A short time after, in February of 1990, the OTA finally released its preliminary report, running over 500 pages. Despite all the initial hopes that this would be an objective and fair evaluation of promising unconventional methods, the OTA document was little more than an ineptly done boondoggle, considered by many to have been organized for one purpose, to discredit alternative approaches to cancer once and for all. The monograph did include an 11 page section on Kelley, clearly created to portray him in as negative light as possible. Though the OTA writers devoted three pages to discussing Kelley's legal problems over the years, nowhere in the text do they even mention my intensive study of his records— though by that point they had a copy of my monograph in their possession for three years. It was as if my lengthy effort just never happened. One would have thought the OTA, if sincerely interested in an objective scientific assessment, would have featured my monograph and my research project, representing as it did the first attempt by an academic group to evaluate a non-traditional cancer treatment.

The OTA missteps did not go unchallenged. During subsequent hearings in Washington, both members of Congress and activists blasted the OTA for its biased report, which seemed to have deliberately excluded any information that might support the efficacy of any alternative approach. In particular, the exclusion of my monograph, the existence of which by that time was no secret, created quite a stir. Though I didn't attend the hearings, I have been told that at one point, a well-known journalist and alternative medicine proponent waved a copy of my manuscript in front of the assembled Congressional committee and OTA staff, then in a dramatic motion threw the hefty document across the room. Though the OTA was sternly instructed to redo their investigation and rewrite their official review, the final version appearing in late 1990 seemed to me only more of the same. Now forced to include mention of my five-year "Kelley study," the OTA writers appeared to me determined to give it as little credit as humanly possible. Elsewhere, I will address at some length that OTA report, which critics of alternative medicine still reference 18 years later as if it were a legitimate study, instead of what it really was, a badly conceived and ineptly conducted waste of government money.

In the early 1990s, Dr. Kelley actually sued both Dr. Good and me in Pennsylvania, for reasons I still don't understand. From my readings of the court papers, which Kelley apparently wrote himself, he seemed to be accusing Dr. Good and myself of colluding to prevent publication of my own manuscript! The case was quickly thrown out when Kelley, acting as his own lawyer, threatened a judge at a preliminary hearing. He was banned, I have been told, from ever again entering a Pennsylvania court. I am sure that little episode did not endear Dr. Kelley to my former mentor Dr. Good.

In the years since, my practice with my colleague Dr. Linda Isaacs, our reputations, and all too often, the controversy surrounding our work have continued to grow. And along the way, my "Kelley study" remained a lightning rod for both sincere interest, as well as dismissive criticism, the latter usually expressed by those who never have seen the manuscript. The situation reached an odd climax of sorts in 1995, when a frail and somewhat pathetic Dr. Good, long outside the academic mainstream, appeared on a national television show, claiming the patients in my evaluation study didn't have cancer and had been "incorrectly diagnosed." His statement I thought bizarre, since he himself had reviewed all patient records and in many cases the pathology slides, before approving each case included in the monograph. He seemed afraid, I suspect fearful of being dragged into a major controversy about an alternative nutritional treatment for malignant disease. Even if Kelley had turned into a nuisance by that point, and a persistent one at that, Dr. Good still should have told the truth—after all, it's the responsibility of any scientist to do so.

Despite all this, we have fortunately attracted considerable interest and support from both industry and government; over the years, Procter & Gamble and Nestle have invested considerable time, effort and money, to help us develop and research our treatment methods. We have presented at the NIH, before the National Cancer Institute (NCI), before a Congressional hearing, and have completed a pilot study of our treatment, funded by Nestle, in patients with advanced pancreatic cancer. The very positive results from this preliminary clinical trial, which we published in the peer reviewed literature in 1999, led the NCI to approve funding for a large scale investigation of our work, comparing our nutritional approach to the best available chemotherapy in patients diagnosed with advanced pancreatic cancer. This project represented the first effort of the government institutions to test a primary nutritional/alternative treatment in a head to head comparison with a conventional approach against a very deadly disease. This study certainly generated considerable interest and once again controversy, prompting the normally staid *New Yorker Magazine* to publish a lengthy and generally flattering profile of me in February 2001. In that article, the writer, Michael Specter, discussed at some length—and with much appreciated objectivity—my Kelley investigation of years earlier.

Though we initially approached our NCI-NIH project with great enthusiasm, unfortunately, after eight years and thousands of hours of hard work on our part, the trial deteriorated into a morass brought on by poor management on the part of the staff heading the trial. Though the details I will tell elsewhere, overall, we believe the project fell victim to the same biases that infected the OTA investigation of 15 years earlier, biases that we believe ultimately sabotaged the study.

Dr. Good died of esophageal cancer at age 81, in 2003, I suspect still worried he would be dragged into some sort of scandal over his involvement supervising my Kelley study. I hadn't spoken to him since 1987, when I first set up my practice in New York. In January of 2005, Kelley succumbed to congestive heart failure, brought on by damage done by his cancer of 40 years earlier. He died angry and alienated from just about everyone, having for some time used the newfound power of the Internet to spew forth bizarre political ideas, suffused with a strong dollop of anti-Semitism. Often, I seemed to be the target of his venom. But I nonetheless forgave his misguided wrath, brought on by years of rejection by the academic world and the media, and too often their vicious disdain. Despite his eccentric behavior in later years, in his theories of "metabolic typing" and in his use of enzymes and detoxification routines, Kelley was surely on to something. I still think of him as a most brilliant man, perhaps the most brilliant of all the many smart people I have had the good fortune to meet over the years, including more than one Nobel Laureate. But he was so far ahead of his time—perhaps outside of his time is a better way to think of him—he simply fell off the edge of the universe.

With the collapse of our NCI-NIH study, Dr. Isaacs and I have decided to begin publishing a series of books on the history, theory, and application of our nutritional therapy. As part of this effort, we realized that it was time, finally, after all these years, to make my "Kelley study" available for the first time in book form. This project and this monograph started me on my journey, and we feel it appropriate, with all the interest and controversy it has generated, to get the document out into the world so that those who wish to know more about us can review the work and judge it for themselves. I believe readers with an open mind will find the time well spent, and hopefully, will appreciate the effort that went into this five-year project.

Certainly, this monograph has had a most unusual history over the past 22 years, particularly when one considers it has not even been previously formally published. It has been the subject of a misguided Federal review, thrown across a Congressional hearing room, discussed at length in a Japanese book, litigated in a Pennsylvania courtroom, debated on national TV, and described in the pages of the erudite *New Yorker Magazine*. It has been lauded as a major breakthrough against cancer, dismissed as inconsequential, and despised as dangerous quackery.

When I myself look at the monograph, at what I accomplished against all odds beginning nearly three decades ago, I remember so clearly how determined I was to do the job right. My "Kelley study" may ultimately not have been perfectly executed, and it may never satisfy the critics who see nothing good in what we do, but none of that matters to me today. When all is said and done, it was, above all, a most honest effort, pursued with the enthusiasm of a young scientist just feeling the excitement of real discovery, and the memory of that excitement will never be tarnished by any critic, however strong or persistent the criticism might be. Discovery is of course the essence of all scientific inquiry and I am only and forever grateful that I had the opportunity, whatever others might think of me or my journey, and however big or small that discovery ultimately turns out to be, to have been allowed if even for a moment in time to experience that unparalleled joy. In his—or her—lifetime, a scientist could hope for no greater reward than that.

Introduction

───◆───

William Donald Kelley is a dentist, a country orthodontist from Texas who over a 20-year period developed a complex nutritional approach for the treatment of human degenerative diseases including cancer. Though Dr. Kelley's methods have never been previously evaluated, the conventional medical community has nevertheless universally condemned him as an outright charlatan. For many years, Dr. Kelley has been investigated and harassed by numerous government agencies, various medical and dental associations, and the press. Despite all this, thousands of seriously ill patients have sought Dr. Kelley's advice and followed his nutritional programs.

My own evaluation of Dr. Kelley began informally in July 1981 as a student project during the summer preceding my third year at Cornell University Medical College. Eventually, my early efforts developed into a more organized study, despite the enormous time constraints of medical school. At Cornell, Robert A. Good, M.D., Ph.D., for eight years Director of the Sloan-Kettering Institute, served as my faculty advisor as the study evolved and expanded.

I pursued my investigation in earnest as an independent research project during the first four months of my senior year. Dr. Good, who by then had moved to the University of Oklahoma, continued under special arrangement as my sponsor and guide. After December 1982, though I was required to pursue more conventional courses at Cornell, I continued to work on my "Kelley Project" during my free time, as scarce as it was.

Internship put a temporary halt to my work, but at the completion of that year, I joined Dr. Good at his invitation as a Clinical and Research Fellow at Oklahoma. Although I had other assigned duties on the Immunology Service, Dr. Good allowed me considerable time to resume my investigation of Dr. Kelley. When in May 1985 Dr. Good moved to All Children's Hospital, the University of South Florida to establish a cancer research and bone marrow transplant unit, I followed him to Tampa/St. Petersburg. At All Children's, I continued and eventually completed my project.

This study represents, therefore, the end result of five years of intermittent work. I do want to emphasize that from the beginning, Dr. Kelley encouraged this evaluation of his methods and results. He has always been cooperative, completely open and available to answer any questions, however pointed they might be. Furthermore, from day one he allowed me free access to all patient records in his Dallas, Texas and Winthrop, Washington offices.

Dr. Kelley supported this investigation for what appear to be simple reasons. He feels that if his methods do have value, they belong in the hands of the academic medical world, which has the resources to study and refine his techniques properly. If his therapy does not stand up to appropriate scientific scrutiny, Dr. Kelley believes he should be doing something else.

At this point, I must issue a warning. Over the years, I estimate at least a dozen imitations of the Kelley Program have been available in the nutritional underground. I suspect that with the publication of this study, scores of similar regimens will suddenly appear and be aggressively promoted in health magazines, in health food stores, and in the offices of the many holistic practitioners operating throughout the country.

Be aware that none—I repeat, none—of these derivatives, either past, present or future, have been developed under Dr. Kelley's supervision or with his approval. Patients who seek out such options may be placing their health if not their lives in jeopardy.

Finally, although Dr. Good served as my advisor throughout this project, I alone must answer for any flaws or inadequacies in it. I conceived the study, I did the work and I have written this report: consequently, the errors are mine and mine alone. However, I do wish to thank Dr. Good for his continued support of my unusual investigation, and his willingness to share his enormous knowledge of cancer medicine with me.

PART I

Dr. Kelley in Theory and Practice

CHAPTER I

—

Biographical Sketch

Dr. Kelley was born on November 2, 1925 in Arkansas City, Kansas, the first of three children. His parents owned a small farm outside of town that his mother tended largely on her own, since his father worked full-time for the Santa Fe Railroad.

Dr. Kelley attended local public schools, finishing high school in 1943 and subsequently training as a Medical Corpsman after enlisting in the Navy. He served primarily as an operating room technician both in the United States and the Philippines during World War II until his discharge in 1945. After the war, Dr. Kelley married, then pursued a premedical course at Baylor University in Waco, Texas. He received an undergraduate degree in biochemistry in 1950, then attended the Baylor University School of Dentistry in Dallas. While a dental student, he earned a master's degree in education, and first developed an interest in nutrition.

After graduating from dental school in 1954, Dr. Kelley completed training in orthodontics at Washington University, the University of Alabama, and the University of West Virginia. Subsequently, Dr. Kelley practiced conventional orthodontics until 1962, first in Midland, then in Grapevine, Texas, a small suburb of Fort Worth. Gradually, as his interest in nutrition evolved, the nature of his practice inevitably changed. By the mid-sixties, virtually all his patients sought nutritional help for a variety of degenerative diseases ranging from cancer to schizophrenia.

Because of difficulties with the Texas State Medical Board who did not approve of his unconventional practice, in 1976 Dr. Kelley moved to Winthrop, Washington, in the foothills of the Cascade Mountains. He lived and practiced in Winthrop until 1981, when he returned to Texas.

Over the years, Dr. Kelley has designed nutritional programs for, I estimate, more than 15,000 patients, most with severe illness. At least 2500 of these have been diagnosed with cancer. However, due to strong and constant government harassment and media condemnation, Dr. Kelley, at present, in 1987, only rarely sees patients. In fact, he may soon refuse to take on any new cases until the political environment changes and the hostility of the medical community toward him lessens.

CHAPTER II

—◆—

The Metabolic Types

Currently, Dr. Kelley believes the human species can be divided into three genetically determined groups: "sympathetic dominants," "parasympathetic dominants," and "balanced metabolizers." Dr. Kelley recognizes 94 additional subtypes, but for the sake of clarity I will restrict my discussion to the three basic classifications.

The actual nomenclature refers to the sympathetic and parasympathetic branches of the autonomic nervous system. In conventional neurophysiology, these nerves regulate metabolic processes perceived as beyond conscious or voluntary control such as circulation of blood, digestion, respiration, the secretion of enzymes and hormones, sexual reflexes, and the overall rate of body metabolism.

Each division of the autonomic nervous system stimulates certain tissues, organs, and glands, and inhibits others. Furthermore, the two divisions tend to operate in a contrary or antagonistic way. For example, the sympathetic system, when firing, increases heart rate and cardiac output but blocks the production and release of hydrochloric acid in the stomach and pancreatic digestive enzymes. When active, the parasympathetic nerves slow the heart rate and reduce cardiac output, but stimulate the manufacture and secretion of stomach acid and the pancreatic juices.

Dr. Kelley believes in certain humans, his sympathetic dominants, the sympathetic nervous system tends to be chronically hyperactive. In turn, the tissues, organs, and glands normally stimulated by the sympathetic nerves—the heart, for example—will be well developed, even overly developed and very efficient. In contrast, the parasympathetic division functions relatively inefficiently, as do all the tissues and organs normally activated by this system such as the stomach and pancreas.

Parasympathetic dominants, the second major type, possess a highly developed parasympathetic nervous system, and all the tissues normally stimulated by this autonomic branch, such as the stomach and pancreas, will be hyperactive. Correspondingly, the sympathetic nervous system, along with the tissues it activates such as the heart, will be weak and inefficient.

In the third Kelley metabolic type, the balanced metabolizers, both branches of the autonomic nervous system, with all the respective tissues, organs, and glands, are equally developed, equally active, and equally efficient.

Dr. Kelley claims these three groups—the sympathetic dominants, parasympathetic dominants, and balanced metabolizers—represent the end product of environmental selection pressures. Each developed, he says, in a very distinctive ecological niche, with a physiological makeup ideally suited to, and determined primarily by, the available food supply.

Specifically, the sympathetic dominants traditionally inhabited the jungles and grassland savannahs of South America, Africa, Asia, and Australia, the classical tropical and subtropical ecosystems notable for a year-round summer and at times, as in the Amazon, lush vegetation. Groups in these regions survived and thrived on a largely plant-based diet of roots, nuts, seeds, fruits, and herbs. Even today, as anthropologists report, the diet of certain tribes in the Amazon and Australian bush consists of at least 80% plant food.

The parasympathetic dominants lived in the more Northern regions of the Arctic, Subarctic, and the colder regions of Europe, Asia, and the Americas, in ecosystems of at times extreme cold, long winters, and a brief growing season—the higher the latitude, the briefer. These groups survived and thrived on a high-fat, meat-based diet, only occasionally consuming plant foods. The traditional Eskimo, as an example, flourished for generations consuming nearly exclusively meat and fat, and few if any plant products.

The balanced types dominated the middle latitude regions of the continents, in ecosystems distinguished by four seasons and a diversity of both flora and fauna. People of these latitudes, Dr. Kelley says, had access to a great variety of both plant and animal sources of food including nuts, seeds, primitive grains, roots, fruits, fish, poultry, meat, eggs, and at times dairy. In a sense, their available diet fell somewhere between the sympathetic and parasympathetic extremes.

For generations, Dr. Kelley believes, the various metabolic types lived largely in isolation, separated by natural boundaries and great distances, though in today's world, of course, this ecological seclusion no longer holds true. In a country such as the United States, particularly, Dr. Kelley identifies all three groups and the various subtypes living together side by side. Because of such mingling and inevitable interbreeding, a certain mixing of genes has occurred, but for the most part, Dr. Kelley believes we as a nation can still be divided along the three basic autonomic lines.

CHAPTER III

— ⌣ —

Nutrition and the Metabolic Types

Sympathetic dominants, Dr. Kelley says, as they exist today, remain adapted to a largely plant-based diet. Though Dr. Kelley identifies gradations of sympathetic dominance, in general he recommends this group consume 80% of all calories from raw plant products such as unprocessed fresh fruits, vegetables, nuts, sprouts, and seeds such as pumpkin and sunflower seeds.

The remaining 20% of the typical sympathetic diet includes lightly cooked vegetables, cooked whole grain products such as bread, and limited animal products such as lean fish and poultry three to four times a week, but no more frequently than this. Dr. Kelley also permits a daily egg and limited quantities of dairy products, but suggests red meat be consumed only occasionally. For his extreme sympathetic dominant patients, he does restrict animal fat in any form, even limiting certain vegetables with a high lipid content such as avocado.

For his parasympathetic dominants, Dr. Kelley prescribes a diet providing at least 50% of total calories from fatty red meat, such as beef, lamb, or pork eaten at least once a day, and oftentimes more frequently. In addition he suggests poultry

2–3 times a week, preferably chosen from the fatty birds such as duck or goose, and fatty fish such as salmon or mackerel. In contrast, this group should consume leaner cuts of meat, as well as lean fowl and fish, only occasionally. Dr. Kelley also allows for this group frequent servings of dairy products, including cheeses, cream, and even butter despite the general perception of these foods as "unhealthy."

Acceptable plant foods include cooked beans and other legumes, avocados, cooked root vegetables such as carrots, potatoes, sweet potatoes, and yams, and cruciferous vegetables such as broccoli, brussels sprouts, cabbage, and cauliflower. Dr. Kelley recommends multiple servings from this group each day, but leafy green vegetables and most fruits should be eaten only sparingly.

The balanced types thrive on a wide variety of foods, including all vegetables and fruits, grains, legumes, nuts, seeds and most animal products—all types of fish and poultry, both lean and fatty meats, eggs, and dairy. Dr. Kelley does suggest plant foods be fresh and unprocessed, and at least 50% of the balanced diet is best consumed raw. Furthermore, each meat meal should alternate with a more vegetarian course, to provide variety.

In his research papers, Dr. Kelley emphasizes each of the three diets contains different levels of nearly all the various nutrients—the proteins, fats, carbohydrates, fiber, vitamins, minerals, and trace elements. For example, the plant-based sympathetic diet supplies the most natural sugar (from fruit) and complex carbohydrates, while the meat-based parasympathetic diet of the three clearly provides the most protein, saturated fat, and cholesterol.

In terms of other nutrients, fruits and certain vegetables yield the most vitamin C, needed to form collagen, the basic intercellular cement. However, vitamin B12, necessary for normal DNA replication, occurs nearly exclusively in animal products. Consequently, the sympathetic foods yield the most vitamin C but the least B12, while the parasympathetic diet provides the largest quantities of vitamin B12, but the least vitamin C.

Overall, the sympathetic vegetarian diet contains, in addition to carbohydrate, the most abundant amounts of beta carotene, the vitamins thiamin, riboflavin, pyridoxine, biotin, folate, ascorbic acid (vitamin C), D (as its plant precursor), and K; the mineral magnesium; the trace elements chromium and manganese; and the electrolyte potassium. All these nutrients, conversely, will be scarcest in parasympathetic foods.

The parasympathetic diet supplies the largest quantities, in addition to protein and fat, of the vitamins A, pantothenic acid, B12, and E; the minerals calcium and phosphorus; the trace elements iron and selenium; and sodium. These nutrients will be least abundant in sympathetic foods.

In the balanced diet, the proteins, fats, carbohydrates, fiber, the various vitamins, minerals, and trace elements occur in intermediate amounts, approximately an average of the sympathetic and parasympathetic extremes.

Finally, all three diets provide more or less equal amounts of two important nutrients, the B vitamin niacin (or niacinamide) and the trace element zinc.

Dr. Kelley says each of the three metabolic types has adjusted precisely, biologically speaking, to the nutrient levels present in their respective ideal diets. For example, he claims that certain nutrients abundant in vegetarian, sympathetic foods, particularly magnesium, manganese, and the B vitamin folate, suppress the sympathetic nervous system. Other nutrients also well supplied in a plant based diet—such as potassium—stimulate the parasympathetic system. Overall, the sympathetic plant-based diet provides large quantities of those nutrients which support the inefficient branch of the autonomic nervous system and inhibit the strong. The recommended diet, therefore, pushes the autonomic nervous system toward a physiological balance so that in turn, all the various tissues, organs and glands function equally efficiently, none too weak or too dominant.

Certain nutrients plentiful in the parasympathetic diet, such as sodium, suppress the parasympathetic nerves while others amply supplied—the amino acids phenylalanine and tyrosine, the mineral calcium, and B12 for example—activate the sympathetic system. This diet, therefore, contains in abundance those factors which support the weak autonomic division but inhibit the strong, in effect, according to Dr. Kelley, pushing parasympathetic dominants toward metabolic equilibrium, with all their tissues, organs, and glands operating with equivalent efficiency.

In the balanced types, the two divisions of the autonomic nervous system are equally developed, equally active, and equally efficient. Their ideal diet in the Kelley cosmology contains moderate amounts of all nutrients—beta carotene, A, thiamin, riboflavin, niacin, pyridoxine, folate, B12, E, calcium, magnesium, manganese, selenium, zinc, potassium, and sodium—that together equally suppress and stimulate both the sympathetic and parasympathetic autonomic divisions. In effect, this diet helps maintain an already balanced equilibrium.

In essence, the appropriate diet for each type supports a state of neurophysiological balance that, in the Kelley model, translates into superb physical and emotional health, with protection against most degenerative, most psychiatric, and even most infectious disease.

CHAPTER IV

—◆—

Metabolic Decline

The ideal physiological equilibrium proposed by Dr. Kelley can be disrupted in several predictable ways. We can follow the "right" diet for our type but rely on refined, processed, synthetic, or otherwise nutrient depleted foods. A sympathetic dominant might eat vegetarian, but consume vigorously cooked canned vegetables and fruits, refined grains and white sugar, instead of raw, fresh—and organic—produce, and whole grain breads and cereals. A parasympathetic might choose mostly processed, chemically preserved meat from feedlot animals raised on hormones and antibiotics, rather than beef from naturally grazing cattle. A balanced metabolizer might consume a varied selection of plant and animal foods, but again, in less than optimal form and from less than optimal sources. In these cases, the proportions and amounts of many nutrients will differ considerably from the proportions and amounts in the ideal recommended diets. In turn, Dr. Kelley says, the metabolic efficiency of both autonomic branches cannot be sustained; over time, both systems deteriorate, regardless of one's initial state of autonomic dominance. The decline may be gradual, but according to Dr. Kelley, it will inevitably occur.

We might also follow a diet suitable for another type. A sympathetic might eat red meat two or three times a day; a parasympathetic might become a vegetarian. In these situations, the diets provide excess amounts of those nutrients that support the overly strong system and further suppress the weak. Eventually, Dr. Kelley maintains, the dominant system can be driven to extreme hyperactivity, while the inefficient system may simply shut off.

A balanced metabolizer who chooses not to eat a variety of plant and animal foods, but who for whatever reasons adopts a more extreme diet—either largely plant based or largely meat—can push him or herself into either extreme parasympathetic or sympathetic dominance.

The situation becomes even more onerous if we follow the wrong diet for our type, and at the same time consume refined, processed, chemicalized foods, combining the worst of all worlds.

Overall, Dr. Kelley recognizes gradations of "wrong" eating. Many of us follow the right diet for our type some of the time, and alternate "wholesome" with nutrient depleted foods. Overall, Dr. Kelley insists the more we stray from the ideal diet, in terms of both quality and content, the further we move from autonomic equilibrium and metabolic efficiency. If the problems are not corrected with appropriate diet and proper nutrition, overt disease inevitably develops.

Dr. Kelley actually designed a very sophisticated graph, to illustrate his concepts of autonomic imbalance and metabolic inefficiency. In his scheme, the horizontal axis represents autonomic function, with the far left point indicating extreme sympathetic dominance, the far right, extreme parasympathetic dominance, and the middle point on the axis, balanced autonomic activity.

The vertical axis, on the other hand, charts overall efficiency, with the highest point correlating with optimal autonomic balance and ideal physiologic function, the lowest point, catastrophic decline in both autonomic divisions and in the various tissues, organs, and glands.

Patients who follow the "right" diet for their type—plant-based for sympathetics, largely meat for parasympathetics, and varied for the balanced—but who consume nutrient depleted, refined, processed, chemicalized food usually end up at the bottom of the efficiency axis in the Kelley scheme, with both autonomic branches hobbled, and all tissues, organs, and glands functioning poorly. Whether innately sympathetic, parasympathetic, or balanced, all tend to converge at the same low vertical point, plagued with problems such as severe chronic fatigue, depression, exhaustion, glandular dysfunction such as adrenal failure, gonadal inefficiency, hypothyroidism, and poor sleep. Often, such patients bounce

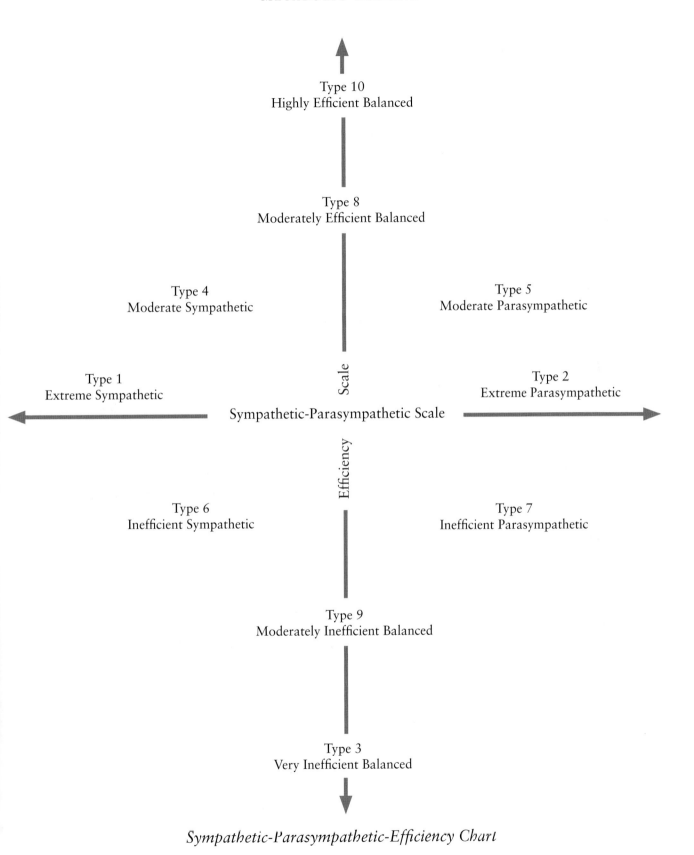

Sympathetic-Parasympathetic-Efficiency Chart

from doctor to doctor, seeking help for their vague but relentless symptoms and chronic ill health.

Those who consume the wrong diet for their type inevitably move to either of the extremes on the horizontal axis. In such cases, Dr. Kelley associates very specific syndromes and illnesses with heightened sympathetic or parasympathetic dominance. For example, a sympathetic on a meat diet might at first experience anxiety, hyperactivity, restlessness, increasing mood swings, and insomnia, as his sympathetic system becomes chronically more active. His—or her—powers of concentration might decline.

As the leftward drift continues, sympathetics can develop chronic problems such as gastroesophageal reflux, colitis, or insulin dependent diabetes, due to the inhibitory effect of the sympathetic nerves on the digestive organs and endocrine pancreas. These patients commonly present with high blood pressure, due to the vasoconstrictive action of the sympathetic neurotransmitters. In extreme imbalance, sympathetic dominants can fall prey to severe, even life-threatening illness, such as congestive heart failure and devastating strokes, as well as psychiatric problems such as hypomania or schizophrenia.

A genetic parasympathetic adhering to a predominantly plant-based diet, as he or she moves further into parasympathetic dominance, might initially require more sleep but never feel rested, and report chronic low grade depression, persistent allergies and hay fever, all due to increased parasympathetic firing. Dr. Kelley identifies most allergies with increasing parasympathetic dominance for several reasons: first of all, in these patients, the immune response in general tends to be exaggerated, leading to excessive reactivity even with mild exposures to offending substances. Then, Dr. Kelley proposes the membranes of parasympathetic dominant cells, including those of the immune system such as mast cells and basophils, tend to be very leaky. The porous membranes easily allow irritating antigens to penetrate, and the mediators of inflammation such as bradykinin, histamine, and serotonin to exit, provoking allergic symptoms.

As the parasympathetic drift continues, this group becomes susceptible to angina, osteoarthritis, asthma—a result of the bronchoconstrictive action of acetylcholine, the main parasympathetic neurotransmitter—and skin disorders such as psoriasis. As they move still further to the right on the horizontal axis, parasympathetics can fall victim to melancholic suicidal depression, severe cardiac arrhythmias, and massive heart attacks.

The balanced metabolizers can experience problems and syndromes associated with either of the other two types, depending again, on their dietary choices. Someone with this genetic inheritance following a meat-based diet can end up with all the symptoms and syndromes brought on by an overly active sympathetic system: on a strict vegetarian diet he or she can experience the various problems associated with parasympathetic dominance.

In his model, Dr. Kelley describes the pathophysiology of cancer in particular detail. In general, for very specific reasons he associates the "hard tumors," the common malignancies of the breast, colon, liver, lung, ovary, pancreas, or prostate with extreme sympathetic dominance.

Most conventional cancer researchers propose that the disease develops from normal cells in any of our various tissues, the end result of defects in the DNA occurring spontaneously due to exposure to environmental toxins or as part of the normal aging process. At times, the thinking goes, these abnormalities or mutations can lead to malignant change. Dr. Kelley believes, however, that cancer forms only from stem cells, undifferentiated precursors located in all our various tissues, that serve as replacements for those cells lost due to normal turnover, disease, injury, or aging. Though they serve a most useful function, without appropriate control of their replicative tendencies, they can form invasive tumors.

Kelley does agree with mainstream scientists that small numbers of cancer cells form in all of us each day, but only rarely do these mutants take hold and lead to clinical disease. Conventional researchers argue that the immune system, especially the natural killer cells, protect us from such malignancies. But Dr. Kelley disagrees: he claims certain pancreatic enzymes, particularly the proteolytic or protein-digesting enzymes—and not the immune system—represent the first line of defense against malignancy.

Dr. Kelley acknowledges that the pancreas releases most of its enzyme supply directly into the small intestine for the purposes of digestion, as has been documented for over 100 years. However, he claims the pancreas also secretes a significant amount of its proteases into the bloodstream, where they circulate and eventually reach all body tissues.

In the blood and in the various tissues and organs, the proteolytic enzymes, Dr. Kelley says, can effectively recognize and digest aged, mutated, and defective cells, including those of cancer. Normal cells, according to Dr. Kelley, manufacture certain membrane proteins (such as analogues of alpha-1-antitrypsin) that protect against the circulating pancreatic enzymes. But cancer cells lack these protective molecules and so remain susceptible to enzymatic destruction.

In the Kelley model, the sympathetic dominant pancreas, of the three types, is the most inefficient, synthesizing the least amount of the various digestive enzymes due to the suppressive action of the sympathetic nerves on the organ. However, a predominantly vegetarian diet will inhibit the overly strong sympathetic division and stimulate the weak parasympathetic nerves, helping in turn to activate the pancreas into greater productive efficiency. Since plant foods can be digested quite effectively with even minimal quantities of most enzymes, as long as a sympathetic dominant follows the appropriate diet, Dr. Kelley claims the pancreas should produce sufficient proteases for both digestion and protection against cancer.

A sympathetic who strays from the recommended diet, consuming fatty meat and other rich foods regularly, stimulates the sympathetic nerves into greater activity, further suppressing the pancreas and its synthesis of the proteolytic enzymes. Ironically, such a diet also requires a significant input of enzymes for its efficient digestion, even as the pancreas grows weaker. The cascade sets the stage for an inevitable systemic enzyme deficiency that allows the cancer cells we all produce daily, no longer kept in check, to grow with impunity.

According to Dr. Kelley, in parasympathetic dominants the pancreas tends to be durable and quite efficient, capable of manufacturing copious amounts of all the various digestive enzymes. Consequently, this metabolic type tends to be protected against the classic hard sympathetic malignancies, such as breast, colon, and lung cancer, which don't stand a chance, surrounded as they take form by large quantities of the pancreatic proteases. However, a parasympathetic following a plant-based diet can develop certain immune-related malignancies despite the usually efficient pancreas. Since the parasympathetic nerves stimulate our various immune cells and organs such as the thymus, eventually, this system can end up in a highly overactive state. Should the extreme parasympathetic drive persist, it will override the protective influence of the circulating enzymes, leading to cancers of the immune cells such as Hodgkin's disease, leukemia, lymphoma, and multiple myeloma.

To make matters worse, Dr. Kelley claims that in the bone marrow and lymphatic organs, phagocytic cells lining the smaller blood vessels filter out circulating pancreatic enzymes. As a result, nests of leukemia or lymphoma cells can thrive in the marrow and in certain organs such as the spleen, largely protected from enzymatic attack.

Sympathetic dominants, Kelley believes, rarely if ever develop Hodgkin's disease, leukemia, lymphoma, and myeloma, due to their inherently weak immune systems. Despite the paucity of pancreatic enzymes, the innate suppression of immunity protects them against such malignancies, even if they should choose the wrong diet for their type.

Balanced metabolizers tend to be innately protected against cancer, as long as they adhere to a varied, high quality diet, consisting of both plant and animal foods. But when they stray off course, adopting a more extreme vegetarian or meat diet, they then become susceptible to either the parasympathetic immune or sympathetic hard cancers, depending on which wrong diet they follow.

As we have seen, sympathetic and parasympathetic dominants and balanced metabolizers who follow the "right" diet for their type, but one consisting of nutrient depleted, processed, and refined foods end up at the bottom of the vertical efficiency axis, with both autonomic branches essentially non-functional along with the tissues, organs, and glands they stimulate. Such unfortunate individuals, regardless of their innate metabolic type, are vulnerable to all manner of illness and can develop malignancies associated with either sympathetic or parasympathetic hyperactivity, or even, in a single patient, multiple tumor types representing each extreme such as breast cancer occurring along with lymphoma.

Our autonomic state, Dr. Kelley claims, even determines how we react to environmental carcinogenic chemicals, such as those found in cigarette smoke. For example, a sympathetic dominant smoker who follows a largely wholesome vegetarian diet might actually be protected against lung cancer, no matter how many cigarettes puffed daily. However, should he or she consume mostly meat and potatoes over the years, lung cancer can easily blossom.

A parasympathetic who smokes, even if heavily, rarely develops lung cancer, whatever diet he or she chooses to follow. The high output of pancreatic proteolytic enzymes protects this group from this particular malignancy under nearly all circumstances. On the other hand, someone with this metabolic inheritance who decides to eat vegetarian and smoke will multiply his or her risk for one of the immune cancers, fed by a combination of parasympathetic hyperactivity coupled with the inflammatory effect of carcinogenic exposure.

Even our resistance to infectious agents—bacteria, fungi, parasites and viruses—depends on our state of autonomic balance. For example, on a molecular level Dr. Kelley believes the membranes of sympathetic dominant cells tend to be very tight, allowing for protection against most viruses which reproduce and work their damage primarily intracellularly. In contrast, bacterial infections can pose a potential threat: such micro-organisms replicate in the extracellular regions, not inside the cells, so that the chronic suppression of immunity by the strong sympathetic nerves enables them to grow with impunity.

The porous membranes of parasympathetic dominant cells, Kelley believes, easily permit invading viruses to penetrate into the cytoplasm and nucleus, where they can replicate protected from the strong immune surveillance characteristic of this group. However, parasympathetics rarely suffer severe bacterial infections, due to their ever efficient immune activity which easily dispenses with extracellular micro-organisms.

Balanced metabolizers, as long as they stick to the appropriate diet, tend to be resistant to both viral and bacterial infection. But should they choose a more extreme way of eating, either vegetarian or largely meat, they can end up victim of infection at either end, viral or bacterial. And sympathetic and parasympathetic dominants, as well as balanced metabolizers who consume nutrient depleted foods, can end up susceptible to both bacterial and viral assault, even at the same time.

Despite what his critics may think, considerable scientific evidence supports Dr. Kelley's claim that autonomic imbalance is the root cause of most disease. The eminent neurophysiologist of the early 20th century, Dr. Francis Pottenger, Sr., attributed much pathology—and most symptoms of disease—to autonomic dysfunction. In his classic text, *Symptoms of Visceral Disease,* Dr. Pottenger in forceful detail presented his case in six editions spanning the years 1919–1944.[1] In his tome, Dr. Pottenger also reported evidence that many nutrients—particularly the minerals calcium, magnesium and potassium—profoundly influence autonomic activity, as Dr. Kelley currently claims. Today, in his Dallas office Dr. Kelley keeps a copy of the latest version of the Pottenger book, which he references frequently.

More recently, Ernst Gellhorn, M.D., Ph.D., for years Professor of Physiology at the University of Minnesota, spent decades documenting his thesis that autonomic imbalance may indeed explain much physical as well as psychiatric illness. In a series of comprehensive texts and over 400 papers published in the mainstream scientific literature, Dr. Gellhorn provided both laboratory and clinical evidence to support his contention, though the medical community at large never seemed to grasp the significance of his findings.[2–4]

In a more unconventional mode, the dentist Royal Lee, active during the first half of the 20th century and best known as the founder of the supplement company

Standard Process, also proposed that autonomic imbalance explains most human disease. Dr. Lee spent years evaluating the influence of diet and specific nutrients on autonomic function, research that provided the basis for much of Dr. Kelley's current therapeutic approach.

REFERENCES

1. Pottenger, FM. *Symptoms of Visceral Disease*. St. Louis; The C.V. Mosby Company, 1944.

2. Gellhorn, E. *Autonomic Imbalance and the Hypothalamus*. Minneapolis; University of Minnesota Press, 1957.

3. Gellhorn, E and Loofbourrow, GN. *Emotions & Emotional Disorders*. New York; Harper & Row, 1963.

4. Gellhorn, E. *Principles of Autonomic-Somatic Integrations*. Minneapolis; University of Minnesota Press, 1967.

CHAPTER V

—❦—

The "Kelley Program" as Therapy

As a dentist, Dr. Kelley cannot legally treat cancer or any other systemic degenerative disease, so he does not, therefore, officially promote his programs as "therapy." In his written materials, Dr. Kelley states clearly to his patients that he provides nutritional guidance for general health purposes only. In fact, all patients must sign a notarized form acknowledging that the Kelley program is not a therapeutic regimen.

Dr. Kelley currently accepts patients only if they have been referred to him by an appropriately licensed physician or other health professional such as a dentist. With patients suffering degenerative disease, the referring physician remains at all times in charge of the patient's primary medical management.

In practice, the Kelley program can be broken down into six basic components:

1. Appropriate diet

2. Intensive nutritional support

3. Protomorphogen support

4. Digestive aids

5. Pancreatic enzyme therapy

6. Detoxification

Any patient wishing to pursue the Kelley program must first complete a questionnaire entitled the "Metabolic Evaluation Survey." Several versions of the questionnaire exist, each printed in book form, the most detailed containing 3200 questions and running 82 pages.

The survey covers a range of subjects including past medical history, current medical problems, and food choices in great detail. Many questions refer to physiological, structural, and psychological traits such as heart rate, pupil size, amount of salivation, skin color, shape of face and fingers, moodiness, sleeping habits, and tendency toward depression or anxiety.

Patients write their answers to each question on cards provided with the survey that when completed, are returned to Dr. Kelley's Dallas office. His rather sophisticated computer then processes the information, and based on answers to the questionnaire, gives a very detailed description of the patient's metabolic type, as well as an analysis of 50 specific tissues, organs, and physiological functions including the autonomic nerves, the cardiovascular, digestive, endocrine, and respiratory systems, and vitamin and mineral metabolism. The printout grades each of these parameters on a scale of 1–1000, with 1000 representing the ideal maximum function, a score of one indicating the tissue or system has essentially shut down. Dr. Kelley explained his scoring as a precise percentage of efficiency; an "adrenal" score of 565, for example, would indicate that the adrenal gland, for the specific patient being tested, operates at 56.5% of its potential capacity.

Dr. Kelley says all this information gives a very detailed sense of each client's current autonomic and metabolic status. The computer program as designed by Dr. Kelley also estimates the actual daily intake for each patient of many nutrients including proteins, fats, carbohydrates, the individual vitamins, minerals, and trace elements. The computer provides this information based on responses to specific dietary questions such as the frequency the patient consumes bananas or whole wheat bread each week. On the printout, this data is then compared to the proposed ideal intake of the various nutrients, based on the patient's autonomic type and level of metabolic efficiency.

Dr. Kelley packages this information in book form for each patient, along with a precise suggested eating plan appropriate for his or her type. The very detailed diets provide actual menus with recipes for three meals a day plus snacks for a full 365 days. Dr. Kelley and his nutritionist designed these meal plans to prove that eating according to his principles need not be dull, regardless of the patient's metabolic type and the actual diet prescribed.

Dr. Kelley says that over the years, he has counseled mostly very ill, nutritionally depleted patients, who have strayed, physiologically speaking, very far from autonomic balance and metabolic efficiency. As a result, he believes that none of them can obtain adequate nourishment from their food alone to rebuild their damaged bodies and regain good health, no matter how well they adhere to the prescribed diet. Therefore, Dr. Kelley prescribes large quantities of nutritional supplements—the vitamins, minerals, etc.—for each patient, depending on the metabolic type, as assessed by the computer, and the efficiency level of each tissue, organ, and gland.

Dr. Kelley insists that the supplements commonly available in health and drug stores are not suited for his particular program, and for nearly a decade he has designed most of the products he recommends, based on his theories of autonomic imbalance and autonomic inefficiency as the root cause of most disease. The various items are available only to his patients through a distributor, and not in health food stores.

The protocols Dr. Kelley prescribes can be quite complex, although each regimen usually includes a basic vitamin and mineral formula which patients ingest three times a day with meals. Dr. Kelley has created ten such supplements: three different sympathetic formulations, three parasympathetic, and four balanced. He developed each with a specific autonomic goal in mind, to stimulate the weak system and inhibit the strong, or in the case of balanced metabolizers, sustain both autonomic divisions equally.

As an example, a full day's dose of the vitamin/mineral complex appropriate for a classic sympathetic dominant provides the following nutrients:

Vitamin D	300 International Units (IU)
Vitamin C	300 milligrams (mg)
Vitamin B1 (thiamin)	200 mg
Vitamin B2 (riboflavin)	100 mg
Vitamin B3 (niacin)	200 mg
Vitamin B6 (pyridoxine)	100 mg
Biotin	150 micrograms (mcg)
Folic acid	800 mcg
Para-aminobenzoic acid	150 mg

Vitamin K-1	1000 mcg
Potassium	90 mg
Magnesium	200 mg
Manganese	30 mg

Three doses of the basic parasympathetic supplement contain:

Vitamin A	7000 IU
Inositol	200 mg
Choline	400 mg
Vitamin E	400 IU
Vitamin B12	300 mcg
Vitamin C	180 mg
Pantothenic acid	300 mg
Niacinamide	300 mg
Calcium	360 mg

The corresponding supplement for balanced types provides:

Vitamin A	10,000 IU
Vitamin D	400 IU
Vitamin B1	110 mg
Vitamin B2	210 mg
Niacinamide	100 mg
Vitamin B6	10 mg
Vitamin B12	225 mcg
Pantothenic acid	20 mg
Folic acid	400 mcg
Vitamin C	200 mg
Vitamin E	30 IU
Calcium	125 mg
Magnesium	62.5 mg
Copper	3 mg
Iron	18 mg
Iodine	150 mcg
Potassium	50 mg
Manganese	2 mg
Zinc	15 mg

Depending on each patient's specific needs and inefficiencies, Dr. Kelley recommends additional doses of particular vitamins, minerals, trace elements, electrolytes, and amino acids.

Dr. Kelley also prescribes for nearly all his patients multiple daily doses of "protomorphogens," concentrates, in pill form, of raw beef organs and glands.

Even mainstream scientists have long recognized that organ meats contain abundant amounts of many essential nutrients, far more so than the standard muscle meats. However, Dr. Kelley and others who prescribe glandular supplements also believe these tissues, when consumed, provide many additional substances such as growth factors, low doses of hormones, natural stimulants, and "protective" molecules, required for optimal efficient metabolism and healing from damage brought on by disease, injury, or aging. These nutrient-like factors are tissue specific, according to Dr. Kelley; for example, the growth factors from the adrenal medulla work only on our adrenal medullary cells, those from beef liver will stimulate healing only in our livers.

Dr. Kelley says when we eat organ meats as food, or take these protomorphogens as supplements, the various "healing" molecules largely survive digestion in the stomach and intestines as do the vitamins and other nutrients, to be absorbed for the most part intact and active into the bloodstream.

The cells of each tissue, organ and gland have specific receptors on their outer membranes which can recognize and combine with these healing molecules from "like" tissues. These various factors then cross into the cell interior, where they assist metabolism in a manner similar to other nutrients.

Each of Dr. Kelley's protomorphogens generally provides only one type of tissue extract. An "adrenal medulla" concentrate provides only beef adrenal medulla; a stomach protomorphogen contains only beef stomach. Dr. Kelley's supplier uses a special freeze-drying process to manufacture the material, which supposedly preserves the nutrients and active molecules.

For each patient, Dr. Kelley usually recommends an array of the protomorphogens to stimulate weak, inefficient tissues, organs, and glands into greater efficiency. Conversely, he avoids glandular supplements that would support tissues, organs, and glands already functioning normally, or at a hyperactive level. In this way, Dr. Kelley employs the tissue concentrates to work synergistically with the vitamins, minerals, and other nutrients to help, at least in his model, bring a damaged, inefficient, diseased body back to autonomic balance, metabolic efficiency, and good health.

Actually, Dr. Royal Lee, who proposed autonomic dysregulation as the root cause of much disease, first recommended protomorphogens during the 1940s

29

and 1950s with reported great success. Not surprisingly, Dr. Lee was a very controversial therapist, thought by medical orthodoxy to be a charlatan.

Most of Dr. Kelley's patients first arrive in his office so physiologically debilitated that few have normal digestive function, whether they be sympathetic or parasympathetic dominant, or inherently balanced. Dr. Kelley claims this to be true even to some extent for his parasympathetic patients, whose digestion under ideal circumstances of appropriate nutrition should be quite efficient. However, parasympathetics eating nutrient depleted, refined, processed, and synthetic foods can end up with compromised digestion, despite their neurophysiological inheritance.

Consequently, Dr. Kelley prescribes for most of his patients supplementary digestive aids with meals including the enzyme pepsin, hydrochloric acid, bile salts, and the various pancreatic enzymes. In general, because of their inherent gastrointestinal inefficiency, sympathetic dominants require the largest quantities, but for virtually all, Dr. Kelley recommends at least some digestive support.

For his cancer patients, Dr. Kelley also suggests frequent oral intake of the proteolytic pancreatic enzymes between meals. The exact dose depends on the extent and type of the tumor, but patients diagnosed with malignancy usually consume the enzymes every two to four hours while awake. When ingested without food, Dr. Kelley believes, these enzymes will be absorbed in an active form directly into the bloodstream, where they then circulate throughout the body, seeking out and destroying cancerous and other defective cells.

Dr. Kelley believes that most early, localized cancer can be gradually eliminated by the enzymes, usually within six months to a year. More widely metastatic disease requires prolonged therapy, from one to two years at least while in cases of very advanced malignancies involving many organs, the tumor may never be completely eradicated. In such patients, Dr. Kelley claims, the enzymes often shrink much of the tumor mass and prevent the cancer from spreading further, even if it is not completely eliminated.

The proteolytic enzymes, if provided in adequate doses, can control even the aggressive leukemias and lymphomas growing in the bone marrow and lymphatic organs. But patients diagnosed with such malignancies must, Dr. Kelley emphasizes, ingest large quantities frequently, to keep the blood concentration of the proteolytic enzymes high enough to penetrate into the protected areas of these tissues.

Conventional physicians have argued that the enzymes, taken orally as Dr. Kelley suggests, could have little systemic effect since they will be destroyed in the gastrointestinal tract as are other proteins. But Dr. Kelley points out that the proteolytic enzymes, as researchers now know, largely resist the digestive effects of acid in the stomach, and when taken without food, for the most part will survive auto-digestion in the intestines, ultimately to be absorbed into the circulation.[1]

Dr. Kelley believes his actual success rate with enzyme therapy varies, depending, not surprisingly, on the patient's predicted life expectancy. For patients given at least three months to live, he says the regimen can control the cancer in 75% or more of cases. For those given less than three months, those diagnosed with very advanced disease, Dr. Kelley claims a success rate between 25–35%.

Other scientists before Dr. Kelley suggested the pancreatic enzymes might be useful against human cancer: Dr. John Beard, a controversial English embryologist working at the turn of the 20th century, seems to have been the first. Dr. Beard developed an elaborate theory proposing that the pancreatic enzyme trypsin, one of the proteolytic enzymes, protected us from malignant disease, a contention he discussed in his 1911 book, *The Enzyme Treatment of Cancer*.

Beard's hypothesis generated considerable interest and controversy for a number of years, particularly from 1906 until 1910. During this period, several prominent specialists, both in Europe and in the United States, used the enzymes to treat selected cases of advanced cancer with some success. In most patients, the enzymes were injected into the buttocks daily—and not into the tumor itself as critics later erroneously claimed.

I have tracked down ten articles and "letters to the editor," recounting the results of enzyme therapy from that era, appearing in respected journals such as the *Medical Record*, *The British Medical Journal*, and *The Journal of the American Medical Association*. In total, the authors describe 11 patients with advanced cancer, including cancers of the breast, colon, and larynx, treated with injectable enzymes. Nine showed remarkable improvement, a number were considered cured.

Despite the documented remissions, the academic research world for the most part condemned the therapy as useless. Then just as the controversy peaked, radiation came into vogue, and the sudden enthusiasm for the X-ray helped push Beard's enzyme therapy into obscurity.

31

Since then, other physicians and scientists have sporadically rediscovered Beard's work. During the 1920s and 1930s, a St. Louis physician, Dr. F.L. Morse, reported that he had successfully treated a number of advanced cancer patients with pancreatic enzymes. When he presented his well-documented findings to the St. Louis Medical Society in 1934—a proceeding published in the *Weekly Bulletin of the St. Louis Medical Society*—his colleagues attacked rather viciously. One physician at the session, a Dr. M.G. Seelig, remarked:

> While I heartily agree with Dr. Allen when he strikes the note of encouragement, I recoil at the idea of witlessly spreading the hope of a cancer cure which is implicit in the remarks of Dr. Morse this evening . . .[2]

A decade later, during the 1940s, Dr. Ernst Krebs, Sr., better known as co-discoverer of Laetrile, tried the enzymes in cancer patients, again with some reported success. In the August 1947 issue of *Medical Record*, Dr. Krebs describes apparent regression of metastatic breast cancer in a single patient. In a later article, appearing in the July 1950 issue of the same journal, Dr. Krebs reaffirms Dr. Beard's hypothesis in great detail.

During the 1950s, Dr. Frank Shively, a Cleveland surgeon, used an intravenous form of the pancreatic enzymes in 192 cases of advanced cancer, describing frequent regression of disease, even 11 long-term survivors. However, in 1966 the Food and Drug Administration issued an injunction forbidding the use of injectable pancreatic enzymes, after which time Dr. Shively resumed a more conventional medical practice.

As the enzymes digest away a tumor, Dr. Kelley says, the dying cells collectively release large quantities of cellular debris into the bloodstream and surrounding tissues, including fragments of membranes, mitochondria, and other organelles; pieces of DNA and RNA; viruses housed in the cell nuclei; proteins, lipids and lipid byproducts, and even enzymes. Some of these molecules are unique to cancer cells, or differ considerably from their equivalents found in our normal, healthy tissues, and can be quite toxic to a patient when released from a dying tumor.

Both the liver and kidney can filter these substances out of the bloodstream with some efficiency, but Dr. Kelley claims the wastes from tumor digestion form so quickly during enzyme therapy that they often overtax our normal detoxification processes. In turn, as the noxious debris accumulates, most patients develop a flu-like syndrome associated with fevers, chills, headaches, severe fatigue, lethargy, and at times, depression. Many suffer muscle cramps and rashes, and lymph nodes may even swell.

All this represents to Dr. Kelley a good sign, an indication of an effective enzyme assault against the patient's cancer. But, since the toxic state can at times become difficult to endure, Dr. Kelley prescribes a series of procedures to help the patient deal more efficiently with these wastes.

First, Dr. Kelley recommends all his patients periodically cycle off the enzymes and other supplements for several days, usually five days at a time after 15–20 days on the pills, to slow down the process of tumor destruction. This respite allows the liver and kidneys to catch up with the body's load of tumor byproducts and when the symptoms diminish, the patients resume their supplement program.

Dr. Kelley also prescribes a number of what he calls "detoxification" procedures, including a strong coffee enema at least once daily. During the procedure, Dr. Kelley claims, caffeine and other substances in coffee, after their absorption, stimulate the sacral parasympathetic nerves that innervate the lower colon. When activated, these neurons send impulses through a spinal reflex directly to the liver and gallbladder, causing contraction of the various hepatic and bile ducts and the release of large amounts of stored wastes into the intestinal tract. At the end of the enema, the debris will be eliminated efficiently via the intestinal tract. In effect, Dr. Kelley says the coffee enemas "clean out" the liver and gallbladder, enhance the efficiency of these organs, and help the body more effectively rid itself of the toxins forming as cancer cells die.

Dr. Kelley didn't "invent" the coffee enemas, which have long been a part of more mainstream medicine, with their first use, according to anecdotal reports I have heard, dating to the Crimean War of the 19th century. During one siege, as the story goes, when pain medication ran out in a front-line field hospital, Florence Nightingale herself administered coffee enemas to her severely wounded soldiers, hoping to relieve their pain—or at least improve their mood. To everyone's surprise, the soldiers reported a reduction in their pain and an increased sense of well-being.

During this century, many nursing texts recommended coffee enemas as a stimulant. In *The Scientific Principles of Nursing,* a respected reference published in 1950, the author, M. Esther McClain, writes:

> Sometimes drugs are given by rectum to be absorbed. Coffee is given by rectum as a stimulant.[3]

33

The esteemed *Merck Manual*, a compendium of conventional medical therapeutics also advocated coffee enemas as a stimulant in all editions from the first in 1899 through 1977. The current editor informed me the section on enemas had been removed from the *Manual* because of space problems, not because of any criticism leveled at the therapy.

Unconventional practitioners other than Dr. Kelley, such as the late Dr. Max Gerson, prescribed coffee enemas as part of a detoxification regimen. During the 1930s and 1940s, Dr. Gerson developed his own nutritional therapy for degenerative diseases including cancer and recommended daily strong coffee enemas for all his patients.[4]

Dr. Kelley first incorporated coffee enemas into his program after reading about them in the *Merck Manual* in 1966. At the time, he was searching the medical literature for some simple method of giving his patients a "boost" during their toxic crises. He found the enemas worked very well, and most of his patients quickly adapted to them.

REFERENCES

1. Liebow, C, and Rothman, SS. "Enteropancreatic Circulation of Digestive Enzymes." *Science* 1975; 189:472–474.

2. Morse, FL. "Treatment of Cancer with Pancreatic Enzymes." *Weekly Bulletin of the St. Louis Medical Society* 1934; 28:599–603.

3. McClain, ME. *Scientific Principles in Nursing*. St. Louis; The C.V. Mosby Company, 1950, page 168.

4. Gerson, M. *A Cancer Therapy: Results of Fifty Cases*. Del Mar, CA; Totality Books, 1959.

ADDITIONAL BIBLIOGRAPHY

Beard, J. *The Enzyme Treatment of Cancer*. London; Chatto and Windus, 1911.

Beard, J. "The Action of Trypsin Upon the Living Cells of Jensen's Mouse-Tumour." *British Medical Journal* Jan 20, 1906; 1(2297):140–141.

Beard, J. "The Scientific Criterion of a Malignant Tumor." *Medical Record* Jan 5, 1907; 71:24–25.

Campbell, JT. "Trypsin Treatment of a Case of Malignant Disease." *Journal of the American Medical Association* Jan 19, 1907; 48:225–226.

Cleaves, M. "Pancreatic Ferments in the Treatment of Cancer and Their Role in Prophylaxis." *Medical Record* Dec 8, 1906; 70:918.

Cutfield, A. "Trypsin Treatment in Malignant Disease." *British Medical Journal* Aug 31, 1907; 2(2435):525.

Goeth, RA. "Pancreatic Treatment of Cancer, With Report of a Cure." *Journal of the American Medical Association* Mar 23, 1907; 48:1030.

Hald, PT. "Comparative Researches on the Tryptic Strength of Different Trypsin Preparations and on Their Action on the Human Body." *Lancet* Nov 16, 1907; 170:1371–1375.

Little, WL. "A Case of Malignant Tumor, with Treatment." *Journal of the American Medical Association* May 23, 1908; 50:1724.

Rice, CC. "Treatment of Cancer of the Larynx by Subcutaneous Injection of Pancreatic Extract (Trypsin)." *Medical Record* Nov 24, 1906; 70:812–816.

Shively, FL. *Multiple Proteolytic Enzyme Therapy of Cancer.* Dayton, OH; Johnson-Watson, 1969.

Wiggin, FH. "Case of Multiple Fibrosarcoma of the Tongue, With Remarks on the Use of Trypsin and Amylopsin in the Treatment of Malignant Disease." *Journal of the American Medical Association* Dec 15, 1906; 47:2003–2008.

CHAPTER VI

—— ⸙ ——

Dr. Kelley and His Critics

Dr. Kelley's problems with the conventional medical world began in earnest in 1969, after his short book *One Answer to Cancer* appeared. In this brief tome, Dr. Kelley presented his thesis that cancer resulted largely from inappropriate nutrition and could, in turn, be treated with diet, intensive nutritional supplementation, large doses of pancreatic enzymes, and detoxification routines such as the coffee enemas.

Dr. Kelley published the book himself, distributing it at a cost of one dollar per copy. Initially, he only hoped this slim volume would aid patients wishing information about his methods, but to his surprise, the book quickly became a best seller in the nutritional underground.

Largely as a result of *One Answer to Cancer*, the Texas State Board of Medical Examiners, in conjunction with the Texas Attorney General's Office, launched an investigation of Dr. Kelley in 1969, complete with undercover agents posing as patients. The Board concluded that Dr. Kelley's practice, whatever he claimed, constituted practicing medicine, forbidden under the scope of his dental license. In the local District Court, the Board obtained a restraining order against Dr. Kelley that forbade him from treating non-dental disease.

In addition, the Court prohibited Dr. Kelley from distributing *One Answer to Cancer*, or any other publication discussing his approach to degenerative illness. The presiding judge stated: "The continued distribution of the book [*One Answer to Cancer*], directly or indirectly by the defendants, would constitute a grave, immediate threat of irreparable harm, a clear and present danger of physical or mental injury or harm to the general public."[1]

Dr. Kelley appealed the decision to the U.S. Supreme Court, claiming the restraining order violated his First Amendment rights. The High Court upheld the ruling and to my knowledge, Dr. Kelley remains the only scientist in this country's history ever forbidden by court decree from publishing his thoughts.

After the final decision in 1971, Dr. Kelley continued seeing patients as before, although he became more cautious. From that point on, Dr. Kelley required all patients to sign a form acknowledging that he was a dentist, not a medical doctor, and that he intended his programs for nutritional support only, not as therapy for any disease. Though his many patients sought him out for treatment of their illness, the forms, at least from a legal perspective, offered some protection against administrative harassment and allowed Kelley to stay in practice as a nutritional counselor.

The American Cancer Society first learned of Dr. Kelley in 1969, as a result of interest generated by *One Answer to Cancer*. That year, according to Dr. Dennis Bertram, Assistant Vice President for Professional Education at the ACS, the Society included a section about Dr. Kelley in their bulletin on controversial cancer therapies. The report essentially summarized information from *One Answer to Cancer*, and mentioned Dr. Kelley's ongoing legal problems. This statement concludes: "The American Cancer Society does not have evidence that treatment with the Kelley Ecology Therapy results in objective benefit in the treatment of cancer."[2]

Today, Dr. Kelley remains on the Society's roster of unproven remedies. To this date, and after sixteen years on the list, no representative of the American Cancer Society has ever spoken directly with Dr. Kelley, communicated with him, attempted to communicate with him or attempted an unbiased evaluation of his methods and results.

The Texas State Board of Dental Examiners began its own investigation of Dr. Kelley in 1973, spurred on by the Medical Board's actions. Because of Dr. Kelley's unusual practice, the Dental Board found him guilty of unprofessional conduct and suspended his license in 1976 for a five-year period, though he continued to consult with patients for purely "nutritional counseling." The Dental Board reinstated Dr. Kelley's license without question or restriction in 1981, giving Dr. Kelley the right once again to practice dentistry in Texas.

Dr. Kelley's most notable—and most publicized—confrontation with the conventional medical world began in 1980, after he agreed to treat actor Steve McQueen.

McQueen had been ill throughout much of 1979 with a variety of misdiagnosed complaints. Finally, in December 1979, after many wrong turns, doctors at Cedars-Sinai Hospital in Los Angeles discovered mesothelioma, an extremely aggressive asbestos-related cancer originating in the lining of the lungs, in McQueen's right chest. For this malignancy, removal of the tumor offers the only hope for prolonged survival, but by the time of diagnosis McQueen's malignancy was already too extensive for surgical cure. At this oncologist's suggestion, the actor did complete a course of radiation treatment to the chest during the early months of 1980, but despite the therapy, the cancer continued to spread.

In the spring of 1980, after reading about Dr. Kelley in a magazine article, McQueen traveled to Winthrop for a consultation. After the session, the actor, thinking the suggested nutritional protocol too rigorous, returned to California to begin a six-week course of experimental immunotherapy. However, the treatment failed to halt the cancer so that by mid-July 1980 the tumor had invaded McQueen's left lung and abdominal cavity. Screenwriter William Nolan reports in his book *McQueen* that with the disease advancing rapidly despite therapy, doctors gave the actor approximately two weeks to live.

McQueen, in the terminal stages of his disease, again called Kelley, this time determined to follow the prescribed regimen. By that point Dr. Kelley thought McQueen too ill to manage the therapy at home, so he recommended the actor be treated at a small, controversial "holistic" hospital on Mexico's West Coast where doctors claimed to use the Kelley regimen. Dr. Kelley never resided at the hospital, nor was he on the staff except as a consultant, but he thought McQueen had no other choice.

At the end of July 1980, McQueen entered the facility in Mexico, though he never did follow the full nutritional regimen as prescribed. According to Dr. Kelley and others on the scene, he refused at times to take his supplements, and smuggled "junk" food into his room, including pints of Häagen-Dazs ice cream. In addition, doctors at the hospital added on a number of unconventional therapies including Laetrile, which Dr. Kelley neither approved of, nor recommended. Yet Dr. Kelley maintains McQueen followed the program sufficiently so that his condition stabilized to the point where, according to those who knew him, he seemed to improve.

Though Kelley tried to keep the actor's treatment in Mexico hidden from the press, in October 1979 reporters from the *National Enquirer* tracked him down and broke the story of the actor's unconventional therapy. Thereafter, Dr. Kelley, his methods, and his life became international front page news.

The relentless publicity in turn brought the American medical establishment into action. Spokesmen from institutions such as the American Cancer Society, the National Cancer Institute, and various academic centers universally condemned Kelley and his methods publicly and repeatedly—though ignoring the fact that the actor had been treated unsuccessfully with both radiation and immunotherapy before beginning his nutritional regimen.

Of all the media reports in my file—and I have scores—one, I believe, best exemplifies the quality of the coverage during that period, Dr. Art Ulene's televised evaluation of Dr. Kelley on NBC's Today Show, at the height of the McQueen controversy. Dr. Ulene, a gynecologist by training, serves as the show's medical correspondent. On the show, Ulene said:

> I don't know exactly what Steve McQueen is getting for treatment, but we have done a lot of research into this so-called Kelley therapy, if you will—the kind of treatments his doctors are talking about in press conferences. And in my opinion, this is not unorthodox, this is common garden variety cancer quackery. We picked up a booklet that talks about the so-called Kelley treatments. You should hear the kinds of things they talk about in it . . .
>
> They have no numbers, they can't produce people. In my opinion this is sheer cancer quackery.
>
> There is a difference between hope and false hope. There is a difference between therapy and deceit. And I think it's important that we make a distinction . . .

At that point, neither Ulene nor anyone else from NBC had spoken to Dr. Kelley, but the following Monday Dr. Kelley himself appeared on the Today Show, along with Dr. Ulene and host Tom Brokaw. This time, Brokaw questioned Dr. Kelley specifically about the lack of data or research studies to substantiate his methods. Kelley agreed this was a problem, but said, in his defense, that he simply lacked the funding to pursue such investigations.

Dr. Ulene, unconvinced, broke in:

> Cancer quackery has no numbers. They have excuses . . . Well, we didn't count . . . we didn't have funding . . .
>
> Last Monday I went on the air and I challenged Dr. Kelley to come with data, to bring in the proof. Dr. Kelley, I repeat that challenge. I will fly anywhere in the world. I am interested. I am willing to look at your data and if you have evidence to prove that your treatment works, I'll read it on the Today Show next week.

Dr. Kelley immediately accepted the challenge, agreeing to open up his patient files to Dr. Ulene. In his comments, he seemed quite reasonable:

> We've always been open, we're not at odds with the medical community. And we're willing to and ready to meet any research challenge on the effect of our program.

In the weeks following the broadcast, Dr. Kelley and his office staff repeatedly tried to contact Ulene by phone at the NBC studios, to arrange his promised visit. The calls were not put through, nor did Ulene ever call back.

I have spoken to a number of Dr. Kelley's patients who wrote to Ulene—I have seen copies of the letters—or called him at NBC; again, according to these patients, Ulene never responded.

McQueen stabilized for a time, but eventually discontinued much if not most of the program. He subsequently suffered a rapid decline while still in Mexico, and died amidst much publicity in early November 1980, only hours after undergoing surgery to remove an apparently dead tumor mass in his abdomen. Officially, McQueen died of a heart attack brought on, Dr. Kelley believes, by the stress of surgery.

The media attacks against Kelley continued after McQueen's death, then gradually tapered off though since 1980, writers have occasionally discussed Dr. Kelley and Steve McQueen in articles and in books. In 1981, a particularly virulent assault against the actor's unconventional treatment appeared in a scientific journal, *Frontiers of Radiation and Oncology,* in a paper entitled "Unorthodox Methods of Treatment for Cancer." Authored by Ms. Helene Brown, a Board member of the American Cancer Society and currently on the staff of the UCLA Comprehensive Cancer Center in Los Angeles, the article describes a trip by Ms. Brown to

41

a health food store. There, the proprietor lectured about the value of Laetrile and diet therapy, but Ms. Brown, unimpressed, mentions Steve McQueen and the Chad Green case. Chad Green was a child diagnosed with leukemia whose parents, in defiance of a court order, took him to Mexico for a course of Laetrile. Dr. Kelley himself doesn't use Laetrile, doesn't recommend it, and had nothing to do with the Chad Green case, but nevertheless, Ms. Brown writes:

> I am not against Laetrile or the metabolic diet if they work. I am against anything wherein a claim is made that is brazenly false and no evidence is offered to indicate otherwise. I think this is enormously wrong and is a new dimension in murder . . .

> This is the very same information that took the lives of both Chad Green and Steve McQueen . . .

> While Steve McQueen's diagnosis of mesothelioma was not as hopeful as the ALL [leukemia] of Chad Green, he undoubtedly died a worse death than necessary. The metabolic diet that he adopted was 180 degrees from being beneficial to a cancer patient and indeed was actually harmful. The diet calls for the following:

> (1) No meat, fish or fowl. These are the major sources of absorbable iron in the American diet. Their lack results in a high frequency of iron deficiency and iron deficiency anemia, *thereby harming cancer patients* [italics Ms. Brown's].

> (2) No dairy products. These are the main sources of calcium in the American diet. Lack of adequate calcium damages bone maintenance, *thereby harming cancer patients.*

> (3) No animal protein. Animal protein is the exclusive source of vitamin B_{12} in the American diet . . . Lack of this vitamin interferes with basic biochemical processes in normal tissue, *thereby harming cancer patients.*

> (4) Increased ingestions of fruits and vegetables. Such a diet is high in bulk and low in calories, just opposite to the needs of cancer patients.[3]

After carefully researching the information Ms. Brown presents, I can only say that I am surprised an official of the American Cancer Society could write such a misinformed article, and that a scientific journal would publish it. Mesothelioma is one of the deadliest of cancers, with a five-year survival rate for patients with unresectable disease reported as 0%. Consequently, anyone with even minimal medical training can only conclude that McQueen's incurable, untreatable cancer, which had been misdiagnosed by the actor's conventional physicians for nearly a year and which failed to respond either to radiation or immunotherapy, claimed his life, not Dr. Kelley. It is ludicrous to imply McQueen had any hope whatsoever by conventional standards; his situation was completely hopeless, from the day his physicians finally diagnosed his condition correctly. And I do not believe Ms. Brown could produce any scientific evidence to support her claim that McQueen, because of the Kelley diet, "undoubtedly died a worse death than necessary."

Ms. Brown's analysis of the McQueen diet is 100% inaccurate. First of all, Dr. Kelley rarely recommends a purely vegetarian diet despite what Ms. Brown implies, and often, for his sympathetic dominants such as McQueen, allows fish, fowl, and some dairy products. In addition, all his patients receive large quantities of nutritional supplements, including amino acids that would compensate for any possible protein deficiency.

The specific diet prescribed for McQueen included a daily egg, a daily serving of fish or fowl, red meat twice weekly and limited quantities of dairy products every day. At no time during McQueen's therapy did Dr. Kelley forbid meat, fish, fowl, animal protein, or milk products.

Dr. Kelley has always made the McQueen protocol, including his recommended diet, available to interested professionals. All one need do is call Dr. Kelley and ask for it.

Drs. Victor Herbert and Stephen Barrett briefly discuss Dr. Kelley in their 1981 book *Vitamins and "Health" Foods: The Great American Hustle*. Dr. Herbert is Professor of Medicine at the Mt. Sinai Medical Center in New York; Dr. Barrett serves as Chairman of the Lehigh Valley Committee Against Health Fraud.

In their section on Kelley, Drs. Herbert and Barrett reference his past legal problems, and the McQueen episode. Like Ms. Brown, they incorrectly describe the actor's diet:

> The much-publicized but futile effort to cure actor Steve McQueen's cancer was conducted under Dr. Kelley's guidance. This 'treatment,' which included a protein-deficient diet, laetrile and coffee enemas, may even have hastened McQueen's death.[4]

My former medical school professor, Dr. Maurice Shils, included a description of Dr. Kelley's methods in an article entitled "Unproved Dietary Claims in the Treatment of Patients with Cancer," which appeared in the April 1982 issue of the *Bulletin of the New York Academy of Medicine*. The references to Dr. Kelley in this report seem largely based on *One Answer to Cancer*. Dr. Shils—for years head of nutrition services at Sloan-Kettering—told me neither he nor his co-author, Mindy Herman, spoke with Dr. Kelley or tried to speak with him, and neither reviewed any of Dr. Kelley's patient records. When I discussed my own "Kelley Project" with Dr. Shils during my senior year in medical school, he appeared genuinely interested, though for some reason surprised Dr. Kelley would talk to me or give me access to his records.

More recently, Dr. Kelley's methods came under scrutiny by the Aging Committee of the United States House of Representatives, which has been investigating health fraud for more than six years. In the Committee's official report, *Quackery A $10 Billion Dollar Scandal,* the authors discuss Dr. Kelley in the section entitled "Clinics—Organized Quackery."[5] I thought Dr. Kelley's inclusion in this chapter peculiar, since he has no "clinic" and never did.

Although no one from the Committee ever called Dr. Kelley, their account does correctly outline Steve McQueen's elusive diet: "McQueen was diagnosed [by Kelley] as a 'Type IV' metabolizer and was placed on a diet of fish, chicken, beef two times a week, and large quantities of raw vegetables."[5] One only wonders if such a diet—similar to those currently recommended by both the American Cancer Society and the National Cancer Institute—warrants a Congressional investigation.

Obviously, the orthodox medical world finds little of value in Dr. Kelley's methods. However, many physicians target one specific aspect of the program, the coffee enemas, for particular ridicule and criticism, and several articles appearing in the medical literature in recent years have specifically questioned their safety. A widely discussed report in the October 30, 1980 issue of the *Journal of the American Medical Association* helped fuel this concern.

In their paper entitled "Deaths Related to Coffee Enemas," two pathologists from the Seattle Medical Examiner's Office, Drs. Eisele and Reay, describe two fatalities they directly attribute to the use of coffee enemas. Neither of the victims, I should add, had ever consulted Dr. Kelley, but followed nutritional programs designed by other unconventional therapists.

44

The first patient discussed, a 46-year-old woman, had not been diagnosed with cancer, but instead had a long history of numerous, chronic digestive problems. In the days prior to her death, she developed acute gastrointestinal distress associated with frequent vomiting, and began, of her own accord, using coffee enemas at the rate of three or four an hour. Subsequently, after more than 30 enemas, she developed an electrolyte (blood salt) imbalance, lapsed into coma and died.

Severe vomiting can itself cause life-threatening fluid and electrolyte loss. In this particular situation, the obvious overuse of coffee enemas may indeed have contributed to the disturbance and her death.

The second example presented, a woman with terminal breast cancer that had metastasized widely, seems far less clear cut. Though this patient did self-administer coffee enemas as prescribed by an alternative practitioner, a postmortem evaluation of her blood revealed "only a small amount of caffeine." Though the authors offer no solid evidence for an electrolyte imbalance, strangely they still try to make a case:

> Using 0.95 L [liter] of this liquid [coffee] three or four times an hour certainly could produce sodium and chloride depletion and fluid overload . . .

This supposed scenario could, of course, lead to death. The writers conclude:

> We are unable to evaluate the prevalence of coffee enemas and are unaware of any other deaths attributed to this treatment. When the second case was publicized by the news media, we received telephone calls and letters from numerous individuals and groups who were using or prescribing coffee enemas. With the current wave of popularity of naturopathic medicine, one would expect an increase in this therapy and consequent morbidity and mortality.[6]

In a "Letter to the Editor" appearing in the March 1984 issue of *Western Journal of Medicine,* two physicians from the University of California, San Diego, describe sepsis—blood-borne bacterial infection—in a 23-year-old woman, diagnosed with widely metastatic breast cancer, who had been self-administering coffee enemas. When chemotherapy failed to halt her disease, she sought an "alternate therapy"—but not the Kelley program—in Mexico. She eventually developed liver failure due directly to her cancer, entered University Hospital in

San Diego, and died. Cultures taken prior to her death confirmed bacterial infection in the blood, attributed to the coffee enemas.

"We believe," the authors write, "that our patient's polymicrobial septicemia from two unusual enteric [intestinal] pathogens was induced by enema therapy in the setting of severely compromised hepatic function and portal hypertension. This complication should be considered an additional potential risk of coffee enema therapy."[7]

I found this article informative, although severely ill, terminal cancer patients can develop sepsis after brushing their teeth.

Finally, Dr. Victor Herbert—who, remember, got the McQueen diet wrong—himself appeared as an "expert witness" before Rep. Claude Pepper's House Committee on Quackery—who, remember, got the McQueen diet right. During his testimony, Dr. Herbert attacked the coffee enemas, stating: "This 100-year-old quack remedy is worthless against cancer but has killed people by producing acute cardiac arrhythmias . . . "[8]

As part of my own research, I have interviewed and evaluated in detail 455 of Dr. Kelley's patients, nearly all of whom have taken daily coffee enemas for prolonged periods, even for five and ten years. Furthermore, I have closely monitored the great majority of these patients, all with cancer and all who employ the enemas daily, over the past four years. Dr. Good and I have examined a number of this group in our own clinic.

I have never been able to document any problem in these patients, from sepsis to electrolyte imbalance to cardiac arrhythmias, that could be attributed to coffee enemas. My experience indicates most of Dr. Kelley's patients with cardiac problems seem to *improve* significantly while on his program.

In the spirit of scientific investigation, I myself took *eight* strong coffee enemas daily for a period of six weeks with no adverse effect and no change in my electrolytes which remained well within the normal range throughout the experiment.

I wrote repeatedly to Dr. Eisele, hoping he might suggest a reason for the discrepancy in our conclusions. However, I have never received a reply.

For the most part, I find Dr. Kelley's critics quite entertaining, though at times I grew dizzy watching the McQueen diet bounce around from those who guessed it right to those who guessed it wrong. But much of the misinformation in the press and in the journals could easily have been prevented, if only the critics had taken a simple, obvious first step—if only they had bothered to call Dr. Kelley.

REFERENCES

1. From transcript of hearing before the Court of Civil Appeals of Forth Worth, Texas: "William Donald Kelley et al. v. Texas State Board of Medical Examiners." May 7, 1971.

2. American Cancer Society. *Unproven Methods of Cancer Management*. New York; American Cancer Society Professional Education Publication, 1982, page 127.

3. Brown, HG. "Unorthodox Methods of Treatment for Cancer." *Frontiers in Radiation Therapy and Oncology* 1981; 16:184–189.

4. Herbert, V and Barrett, S. *Vitamins and "Health" Foods: The Great American Hustle*. Philadelphia; George Stickley, 1981, pages 58–59.

5. Halamandaris, B, et al. *Quackery A $10 Billion Scandal*. U.S. Government Printing Office Publication Number 98-435. Washington, DC; U.S. House of Representatives, 1984, pages 152–153.

6. Eisele, JW and Reay, DT. "Deaths Related to Coffee Enemas." *Journal of the American Medical Association* Oct 3, 1980; 244:1608–1609.

7. Margolin, KA and Green, MR. "Polymicrobial Enteric Septicemia From Coffee Enemas." *The Western Journal of Medicine* Mar 1984; 140:460.

8. Statement before the U.S. House of Representatives' Subcommittee on Health and Long-Term Care, page 95.

PART II

The Data

CHAPTER VII

— ❦ —

Fifty Cases

PURPOSE OF STUDY

As a primary goal in my investigation, Dr. Good suggested I gather together, with supporting medical records, a series of 50 cancer patients who had done well on the Kelley regimen and who met certain prescribed criteria. Dr. Good insisted that each subject included in the group must have been appropriately evaluated by competent specialists so there could be no doubt about the diagnosis. Furthermore, these patients should have been given a terminal or poor prognosis by the standards of conventional oncology. Finally, for each case I was to provide evidence of regression of disease, unusual long-term survival, or both, that might logically be attributed to the Kelley program.

SELECTION OF CASES

I first reviewed the files of all cancer patients who followed the Kelley regimen between 1970 and 1982. I then sent a letter of inquiry, with a questionnaire, to 1306 of this group.

I used the responses to my mailing, along with my own evaluation of Dr. Kelley's records, to create a list of over 1000 patients I thought potentially suitable for my study. Since I worked alone, I knew I could never reasonably expect to interview—and investigate in detail—all these many cancer patients who appeared to have done well over the years. So in essence I began at the top of my list and continued interviewing by phone until I had gathered a sufficient number of cases suitable for my study, with some backup. When I felt I had done enough, I simply stopped calling.

Overall, I interviewed 455 patients at length. I want to emphasize that these people, even the 50 chosen for this study, are not necessarily Dr. Kelley's most "impressive" cases. Instead, I prefer to think of them as "representative." I have on my list hundreds of patients I never called whose clinical histories, at least on cursory examination, seem as unusual as those I did ultimately choose to investigate.

Of the 455 contacted, I eventually rejected 295 patients from further consideration for a variety of reasons. Ninety, though very ill when initially seen by Dr. Kelley, had not been adequately diagnosed. Some of these patients, after re-evaluation by their original physicians, were not thought to have cancer.

Another 100 had been appropriately evaluated and had done well under Dr. Kelley's care; however, these particular patients, while following the Kelley regimen, also pursued intensive conventional therapy such as chemotherapy that might have contributed to their response.

Another 46 patients with a history of well-documented cancer appeared, in my judgement, to have been cured of their disease before they consulted Dr. Kelley. Most of these pursued the Kelley program for preventive, not therapeutic reasons.

Forty-seven, upon careful questioning, admitted they had never followed their nutritional regimen as prescribed, or for any prolonged period of time. I discounted anyone who did not comply with the full program for at least a year, even if he or she had done well.

Fifteen patients on the regimen were doing poorly; another eleven had died since last evaluated by Dr. Kelley.

I finally identified 160 cases that appeared to satisfy Dr. Good's criteria of appropriately diagnosed patients given a poor or terminal prognosis, whose response in terms of disease regression, long-term survival or both, could only logically be attributed to the Kelley regimen. For each of these, I obtained complete medical records, and after reviewing the documentation, ultimately selected the 50 patients for this study. My final choice was really quite arbitrary, determined mostly by Dr. Good's suggestion that I present a wide spectrum of cancer types.

STATISTICAL EVALUATION

These 50 patients presented initially with 25 different types of cancer:

Type of Cancer	# Patients with Each Cancer
Acute Lymphocytic Leukemia	1
Acute Myelocytic Leukemia	1
Bile Duct Carcinoma	1
Brain Cancer	1
Breast	5
Cervical	1
Chronic Myelocytic Leukemia	1
Colon	3
Diffuse Histiocytic Lymphoma	2
Diffuse Poorly Differentiated Lymphocytic Lymphoma	2
Hodgkin's	4
Liver (metastatic to liver, unknown primary)	1
Lung	2
Melanoma (metastatic)	3
Myeloma	1
Nodular Poorly Differentiated Lymphocytic Lymphoma	2
Ovarian	2
Pancreatic, adenocarcinoma	4
Pancreatic, islet cell	1
Prostate	5
Rectosigmoid	2
Renal (kidney)	1
Stomach	1
Testicular	2
Uterine	1

AMOUNT OF CONVENTIONAL THERAPY RECEIVED

Most, though not all, of Dr. Kelley's cancer patients seek him out only after pursuing considerable conventional therapy. In the following table, I summarize, where relevant, the amount of such treatment administered.

Nine patients in the group who refused all standard interventions after their initial diagnostic evaluation pursued the Kelley program as their only treatment.

Type of Therapy	# Patients Receiving
No Conventional Therapy	9
Chemotherapy only	10
Chemotherapy and Radiation	2
Radiation only	5
Surgery only	12
Surgery and Chemotherapy	6
Surgery and Radiation	4
Surgery, Radiation, and Chemotherapy	2

BREAKDOWN OF SURVIVAL

Conventional oncologists consider their patients cured if they are alive and free of disease five years after the initial evaluation confirming cancer. In this series, I include one patient who when last contacted had survived four years from the time of his diagnosis. Although not yet a long term survivor, I chose to discuss this patient because of his unusual clinical history.

In the following list, I group the 50 patients by cancer type and give survivorship (as of May 1987) since diagnosis.

Type of Cancer	Length of Survival Since Diagnosis (in years)
Acute Lymphocytic Leukemia	13
Acute Myelocytic Leukemia	7 (Deceased)
Bile Duct	6 (Deceased)
Brain	5
Breast (5 cases)	11
	13
	13

	14
	17
Cervical	9
Chronic Myelocytic Leukemia	12
Colon (3 cases)	10
	12
	17
Diffuse Histiocytic Lymphoma (2 cases)	6.5 (Deceased)
	10.5
Diffuse Poorly Differentiated Lymphocytic Lymphoma (2 cases)	9
	11
Hodgkin's (4 cases)	5
	9
	15
	23
Liver (metastatic to liver)	6 (Deceased)
Lung (2 cases)	12 (Deceased)
	13
Melanoma (3 cases)	4
	8
	17
Myeloma	11
Nodular Poorly Differentiated Lymphocytic Lymphoma (2 cases)	10
	10
Ovarian (2 cases)	13
	15
Pancreatic, adenocarcinoma (4 cases)	5
	9
	10
	12 (Deceased)
Pancreatic, islet cell	6
Prostate (5 cases)	8
	9
	9 (Deceased)
	9
	11
Rectosigmoid (2 cases)	5
	10
Renal (kidney)	8 (Deceased)

Stomach	10
Testicular (2 cases)	6
	8
Uterine	18

I have also grouped the 50 patients according to length of survival as follows:

Length of Survival	# of Patients
4 Years	1
5 Years	4
6 Years	4
7 Years	2
8 Years	4
9 Years	7
10 Years	6
11 Years	5
12 Years	4
13 Years	5
14 Years	1
15 Years	2
17 Years	3
18 Years	1
23 Years	1

DEMOGRAPHICS

In this series of 50 patients, I have evaluated 28 males and 22 females. Their ages, at the time each began the Kelley program, ranged from 21 to 77, with a current age distribution spanning 33-83 years. In the following chart, I group these patients by age in five year intervals.

Age in years	Patients in This Range
31–35	2
36–40	5
41–45	4
46–50	5
51–55	5
56–60	4

61–65	9
66–70	6
71–75	5
76–80	3
81–85	2

Graphically, the age distribution curve would show a peak at age 61–65.

GEOGRAPHIC DISTRIBUTION

The 50 patients in this study come from 24 states and Canada. Of the states, California is the most highly represented, with a total of six patients.

Home State	# of Patients
Arizona	1
Arkansas	1
California	6
Colorado	2
Florida	3
Georgia	1
Illinois	1
Iowa	3
Louisiana	2
Michigan	2
Minnesota	4
Missouri	2
Montana	1
New York	2
North Carolina	1
Ohio	2
Oklahoma	2
Pennsylvania	2
Texas	2
Utah	1
Vermont	1
Virginia	1
Washington State	4
Wisconsin	1
Canada	2

OCCUPATIONS

These patients pursue a variety of occupations, from dairy farming to law. In the following chart, I list representative fields.

Occupation	# of Patients
Army (career)	1
Artist	1
Business (owns)	5
Chiropractor	1
Construction business (owns)	1
Dairy Farmer	2
Engineer	1
Factory Worker	1
Football Referee	1
Harpist (professional)	1
Health Food Store Owner	2
Housewife	5
Independently Wealthy	2
Lawyer	1
Merchant Marine (sailor)	1
Minister	2
Nurse	2
Photographer (professional)	2
Railroad Worker (freight clerk)	1
Teacher	1

PSYCHOLOGICAL PROFILE

Over the years, a number of "experts" have described the psychological characteristics of cancer patients who seek out unconventional therapies. For the most part, these investigators portray such individuals as gullible, uneducated victims, often suffering some form of personality disorder or overt mental illness.

In a classic article published in the *Journal of the American Dietetic Association* (1970), psychiatrist Hilde Bruch evaluates the psychoanalytical processes—ranging from unhappy childhoods to a distrust of authority—that lead patients to the unorthodox.

Dr Bruch writes:

> If early experiences are unwholesome, instead of developing basic trust, an individual will become deeply mistrusting and will experience many situations in life as threatening. Such people become characterologically rigid, repressing many impulses for experiencing satisfaction, and they show an ever-ready tendency to discharge their repressed hostility or project their repressed sexual strivings, whenever a convenient cultural scapegoat is presented to them. To such individuals, security is equated with purity, and health with naturalness. These are the people who become exceedingly concerned with pure food, pure morals and pure races . . .
>
> When becoming manifestly sick, one of the commonest delusions is the fear of being poisoned . . .
>
> Others on the brink of mental illness hope that they will acquire greater spiritual strength by absorbing the qualities of special food . . . [1]

Although I have read this article several times, I have absolutely no idea what Dr. Bruch is talking about. And, as is so often the case in psychoanalytically-oriented psychiatry, the author includes no data and no statistics to support her theorizing. In fact, I find no evidence in her article that she has ever spoken to a single patient pursuing an unorthodox cancer therapy.

I tried to contact Dr. Bruch at the Department of Psychiatry at Baylor University Medical School, where she taught for many years. I had hoped she might enlighten me, by providing me with appropriate data to substantiate her claims. However, I was disappointed to learn she died several years ago.

I did not pursue a formal psychological evaluation of Dr. Kelley's patients, although I have come to know many of them very well over the years. Contrary to what experts such as Dr. Bruch claim, I found most to be quite sane and sober. They simply believe Dr. Kelley might know more about cancer than anyone else.

REFERENCE

1. Bruch, H. "The Allure of Food Cults and Nutrition Quackery." *Journal of the American Dietetic Association* 1970; 57:316–320.

CHAPTER VIII

——

An Answer to Potential Critics

In this chapter, I anticipate—and answer—potential criticisms that might be raised about my study. I hope such an exercise convinces even Dr. Kelley's staunchest adversaries that these 50 cases are indeed what they appear to be.

1) The patients in this study really did not have cancer in the first place.

All 50 patients selected for review have been extensively evaluated by appropriate specialists at accredited institutions before consulting with Dr. Kelley. Furthermore, 25 were diagnosed at two or more medical centers. For these, we have definitive confirmation of disease by a second group of physicians.

In addition, 23 of these patients, or 46%, were initially diagnosed—or had their diagnosis confirmed—at what I would call major national institutions. In the following table, I list these centers with the number of patients evaluated at each.

Institution	# of Patients Diagnosed at Institution
Mayo Clinic	5
Memorial Sloan-Kettering	4
Stanford	3
UCLA	2

Institution	# of Patients Diagnosed at Institution
Loma Linda	1
M.D. Anderson	1
New York University Medical Center	1
Ochsner Clinic	1
University of Iowa Medical Center	1
University of Michigan	1
University of Utah	1
University of Washington	1
W.W. Cross Cancer Center (Alberta)	1

Twenty-two of the patients seen at one of the above medical centers were also evaluated at a second hospital. Overall, 26 of the 50 patients studied were diagnosed at either a "major" institution, at two or more hospitals, or both.

For 48 cases, I provide biopsy confirmation of cancer but lack such evidence for two patients, one with presumed bile duct carcinoma, the other with pancreatic. Both these patients initially presented with histories consistent with advanced cancer. Both subsequently underwent exploratory surgery, at which time large, inoperable tumors were discovered with clear evidence of metastatic spread. In each case, the attending surgeon, believing the diagnosis obvious, chose not to risk biopsy, fearful of the risks involved with the procedure. Since the clinical histories of each of these two were so unusual, Dr. Good suggested I include them among the 50.

2) **These patients had slow growing tumors usually associated with prolonged survival.**

Most cancers are rapidly fatal if untreated as W.L. Harnett, an English physician, demonstrated in a classic paper entitled "The Relation Between Delay in Treatment of Cancer and Survival Rate" (*British Journal of Cancer*, 1953). In his study, Harnett evaluated 625 patients diagnosed with 28 different types of cancer who for a variety of reasons refused all conventional therapy including surgery. For each of these malignancies, Harnett determined the average length of survival after the initial diagnosis. I enclose his results for selected cancers in table form. The data are indeed sobering; most untreated cancer patients simply do not live very long.[1]

Cancer Site	Average (mean) Survival in Months
Breast	35.9
Rectosigmoid	22.4
Bladder	22.0
Anus and anal canal	21.9
Prostate	19.5
Rectum ampulla	19.0
Cervix	17.5
Uterus (body)	17.4
Stomach (pylorus)	11.5
Ovary	9.6
Larynx	9.0
Colon	8.7
Stomach (mid-gastric)	8.7
Pharynx	8.4
Kidney	7.7
Stomach (upper portion)	5.7

Certain cancers, such as the slow-growing liposarcomas or chronic lymphocytic leukemia, can follow a more prolonged course over many years. For this reason, I have excluded these classically indolent malignancies from my study.

I do discuss two cases of nodular poorly differentiated lymphocytic lymphoma. Several reports in the literature indicate patients diagnosed with this particular malignancy can occasionally live for years, even without treatment. However, the cases I present have most unusual histories, each enjoying documented regression of disease within months of beginning the Kelley regimen.

3) These cases represent spontaneous regressions.

In 1966, Drs. Everson and Cole, then at the University of Illinois, published their classic text *Spontaneous Regression of Cancer*. Today this study remains the most exhaustive investigation of spontaneous remission in the scientific literature.

These two physicians evaluated all reports of spontaneous regression appearing in the world's literature between the years 1900 and 1966, ultimately identifying 176 legitimate cases, described at length in the first edition of their book. In a later printing, Everson and Cole added another six patients. I myself have surveyed the more recent medical literature seeking out additional accounts of spontaneous remission and have uncovered, to date, another 44 cases.

Obviously, spontaneous regressions occur only very rarely. In a 1974 interview, Dr. Cole himself, at one time Chairman of the Department of Surgery at Illinois, described an incidence rate of only one per 100,000 cancer patients.[2] Another investigator, Dr. Solomon Garb of the University of Missouri Medical School, also calculated the frequency of spontaneous regressions, which he describes in his book, *Cure for Cancer: A National Goal* (1968):

> There is less than one chance in 1,000 that any single physician will encounter in his lifetime one true case of spontaneous cure or long-term regression of advanced cancer. The chances against his encountering two would be less than one in a million. The chances against encountering three would be less than one in a billion. The chances of a physician encountering ten such cases are much too small to have any meaning.[3]

4) These patients were cured by their conventional therapy.

Twenty-two of the patients in this series experienced *documented* regression of cancer while pursuing only the Kelley program and no other treatment. For most of these patients, I provide the appropriate supporting evidence in the form of physicians' records and/or radiology reports of CT scan studies, etc.

Another five patients described to me regression of superficial, biopsy-proven malignancies, such as breast tumors or cancerous lymph nodes, while under Dr. Kelley's care. These patients never returned to their conventional physicians for follow-up studies, so I lack formal confirmation of improvement for this group by an outside physician.

Two patients began the Kelley regimen while receiving chemotherapy. In each case, standard treatment alone failed to halt the disease, and for each I provide appropriate documentation demonstrating tumor regression only *after* each began the Kelley regimen.

Six patients were found at surgery to have extensive inoperable abdominal or pelvic disease, such as metastatic pancreatic or metastatic prostate carcinoma.

64

All in this group were given terminal prognoses. None have ever returned to their conventional physicians, so strictly speaking I have no proof of tumor regression in the form of CT scans or other radiographic studies. However, each of these has survived for years with cancer that usually kills within months.

The remaining 15 cases represent a mixed group, although all had been diagnosed with obvious poor prognosis malignancy. Prior to beginning the Kelley program, several of these patients, including one with leukemia, were intensively treated by their conventional physicians. I cannot "prove" that the Kelley regimen cured them, but each has enjoyed a prolonged disease-free survival that is, by the standards of conventional oncology, either rare or previously unknown.

5) **These patients may have improved while following the Kelley program, but this improvement represents a delayed effect of either chemotherapy or radiation.**

Chemotherapeutic agents have only one documented delayed effect; they cause cancer in a significant number of aggressively treated patients. These drugs are, of course, very toxic substances; many, in fact, are carcinogenic. As a result, some patients receiving intensive chemotherapy, if they survive their original disease, develop secondary, treatment-induced malignancies.

Patients given multi-agent regimens incorporating several powerful drugs, such as the "MOPP" protocol for Hodgkin's disease, seem particularly at risk. In a recent study, Dr. C. Norman Coleman and colleagues at Stanford evaluated 1222 Hodgkin's patients treated with MOPP or similar regimens. These investigators report that 9.7% of this group developed leukemia and other malignancies as a result of their prior cancer therapy, usually within five years of treatment.[4]

To this date, I have found no evidence supporting the claim that chemotherapeutic agents produce "delayed" regression of disease. If these drugs work, they work immediately.

After intensive radiation therapy, tumors do at times continue shrinking for a period of up to eight weeks. However, only one patient in my study, a woman with ovarian carcinoma, received radiation therapy that might be defended as partially responsible for the observed response. In the other 49 cases, this argument simply does not apply.

6) **The observed improvement can be attributed to the placebo effect.**

Placebos, of course, are inert substances disguised as active medication. While placebos and the placebo effect can account for diminished pain and symptomatic improvement in cancer patients, these non-drugs do not cure the disease, ever.

7) The records are fake.

I alone chose the patients I wished to evaluate, without input from Dr. Kelley. I interviewed each of them myself, at length, repeatedly. I obtained the medical records for these patients from the respective hospitals, clinics and physicians. Dr. Kelley never handled these documents, which remain in my possession.

Any doubting researcher wishing to invest the time could track down the same patients discussed in my study, and obtain their medical records for additional confirmation.

REFERENCES

1. Harnett, WL. "The Relation Between Delay in Treatment of Cancer and Survival Rate." *British Journal of Cancer* 1953; 7:19–36.

2. Interview with WH Cole. "Spontaneous Regression of Cancer." *Ca—A Cancer Journal for Clinicians* Sep–Oct 1974; 24:274–279.

3. Garb, S. *Cure for Cancer, a National Goal.* New York; Springer Publishing Company, 1968. As quoted in Glassman, J. *The Cancer Survivors and How They Did It.* New York; The Dial Press, 1983, page 324.

4. Coleman, CN. "Hodgkin's Disease; The Risks of Secondary Malignancies." *Primary Care and Cancer* Oct 1985; 15–19.

ADDITIONAL BIBLIOGRAPHY

Cole, WH and Everson, TC. *Spontaneous Regression of Cancer.* Philadelphia; W.B. Saunders Company, 1966.

Glassman, J. *The Cancer Survivors.* New York; The Dial Press, 1983.

CHAPTER IX

—◦◦—

An Overview
of Cancer Statistics

In 1987, approximately 965,000 Americans developed cancer, excluding skin cancer, and 483,000 died from the disease.

Many studies report that overall survival rates for cancer patients have improved in recent years. Enthusiastic medical officials, particularly at the American Cancer Society, claim up to 49% of all cancer patients now live five years, a sign of significant progress.

However, a number of well-respected researchers question the legitimacy of these estimates and the associated optimism. For example, recently a group of epidemiologists at the Yale University School of Medicine reported that the much publicized improvement in survival rates for patients with lung cancer represents little more than a statistical artifact. These investigators discovered, on close examination of case records, that lung cancer patients as a group seem to be living longer only because they are diagnosed at an earlier stage than in previous years as a result of improved imaging studies. But in fact, actual longevity for these patients has not changed in three decades.[1]

In a much publicized statement, Dr. John Bailar, for 25 years with the National Cancer Institute, strongly condemned most official claims of progress against cancer—and the data used to support such arguments. At the annual meeting of the American Association for the Advancement of Science in 1985, Bailar remarked, "My overall assessment is that the national cancer program must be judged a qualified failure."[2] In an article appearing in the *New England Journal of Medicine*, Dr. Bailar emphasized how often academicians manipulate statistics to create the illusion of progress and success.[3]

In the following section, I provide data on projected cancer deaths and five-year survival rates for a variety of malignancies, largely based on the American Cancer Society (ACS) publication *Cancer Facts and Figures—1987*. Keep in mind, when reading these figures, that some experts believe the ACS estimates to be overly optimistic.

REFERENCES

1. Feinstein, AR, et al. "The Will Rogers Phenomenon." *The New England Journal of Medicine* Jun 20, 1985; 312:1604–1608.

2. "Scientist: Cancer Program a Failure." *The Spokesman-Review* (Spokane, Washington) May 30, 1985; B6.

3. Bailar, JC and Smith, EM. "Progress Against Cancer?" *The New England Journal of Medicine* May 8, 1986; 314:1226–1232.

CHAPTER X

———◆———

Presentation of Fifty Case Histories

BILE DUCT CARCINOMA

In 1987, cancer of the liver and gallbladder duct system claimed 10,600 lives.

Few patients with bile duct carcinoma live five years, even with aggressive ther-apy, and experts estimate the average survival at less than one year.

Patient #1

At the time of his death at age 59, Patient #1 had survived nearly six years on the Kelley program after his diagnosis of bile duct carcinoma.

In September 1976, Patient #1 first experienced intermittent episodes of cramping abdominal pain, which his family physician attributed to ulcer disease. On a course of prescribed antacid therapy, Patient #1 did well for about a month, but in mid-October 1976, he suddenly developed severe nausea, associated with bouts of vomiting. With the nausea persistent and his appetite in decline, over a six-week period he lost a total of 28 pounds.

When he subsequently became jaundiced in late November 1976, Patient #1 was admitted to DeKalb General Hospital in Decatur, Georgia, for further evaluation. Laboratory studies revealed elevated liver function tests (bilirubin 9.7, SGOT 324, SGPT 500), indicating possible obstruction of the bile duct system. However, the cause of Patient #1's symptoms could not be determined and when discharged from the hospital in December 1976, his doctors only advised him to continue antacids.

But once home, Patient #1 continued to deteriorate. When his bilirubin level reached 20 (normal values less than 0.7), he was re-admitted to DeKalb on December 15, 1976. Several days later, at exploratory surgery he was found to have a large, inoperable tumor in his bile duct system described in the operative note as "Carcinoma of the right hepatic bile duct with extension into the left and common hepatic ducts with total obstruction." The attending surgeon, believing the disease terminal, chose not to risk biopsy.

Postoperatively, Patient #1 completed a brief (500 rad) course of radiation therapy to his right upper abdomen aimed at relieving the ductal obstruction. Despite the treatment, Patient #1 continued to worsen after leaving the hospital, and in desperation, decided to investigate unorthodox cancer therapies. In early March 1977, he learned of Dr. Kelley, consulted with him and began the full nutritional program.

Only several days after returning home from his meeting with Dr. Kelley, Patient #1 developed an infection of the bile duct system and re-entered DeKalb General on March 20, 1977 in a very weakened state. While hospitalized, he began hemorrhaging profusely along his gastrointestinal tract as a complication of liver failure. His doctors opted *not* to treat the bleeding, since he seemed so close to death but nevertheless, Patient #1 rallied and at his family's insistence, was discharged. Once home, he resumed the Kelley regimen.

Although still extremely ill, Patient #1 improved somewhat over the next three months, then was again admitted to DeKalb in August 1977 after developing ascites (fluid in his abdominal cavity). Eventually, Patient #1 improved to the point he was able to return home and resume his nutritional therapy. The discharge summary reports his diagnosis at that time as "Terminal carcinoma of the bile ducts with ascites." In November 1977, when his ascites worsened, Patient #1 underwent placement of a LaVeen shunt, a tube implanted in the gut to divert abdominal fluid into the venous system.

For the next five years, Patient #1 enjoyed a reasonably good quality of life despite frequent hospitalizations for recurrent gastrointestinal bleeding and problems related to his liver failure. During this time, he faithfully continued his nutritional protocol, except when hospitalized. Finally, in May 1982, after lapsing into hepatic coma, Patient #1 was admitted to Emory University Medical Center in Atlanta and died.

Few patients with inoperable bile duct carcinoma survive one year. As MacDonald writes: "The prognosis of bile duct cancer, like that of hepatocellular and gallbladder carcinoma, is also poor." He describes studies by Warren and colleagues, who report that only one of seven patients diagnosed with the disease survive three years. In Longmire's series of 63 patients with carcinoma of the bile ducts, only four (6%) survived more than four years. In another investigation of patients with surgically unresectable disease, researchers calculated a median survival of five months.[1]

Patient #1's longevity—unusual, given his diagnosis of inoperable bile duct carcinoma with associated liver failure—can only be attributed to the Kelley regimen.

Dr. Kelley believes Patient #1 would have fared even better, had he avoided radiation therapy when initially diagnosed. The treatment only contributed to Patient #1's liver dysfunction, which in turn hampered the effectiveness of the nutritional regimen. According to Dr. Kelley, Patient #1 also lost ground because he was not allowed to continue his regimen while hospitalized.

I have been unable to document in the medical literature additional patients surviving more than five years with unresectable carcinoma of the bile ducts.

REFERENCE

1. DeVita, VT, et al. *Cancer Principles & Practice of Oncology*. Philadelphia; J.B. Lippincott Company, 1982, page 595.

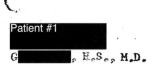

Patient #1

G_____, H.S., M.D.

DATE OF OPERATION: 12-20-76   DATE OF DICTATION: 1-29-77

PREOPERATIVE DIAGNOSIS: Obstruction of common hepatic bile ducts, due to
                           carcinoma of bile duct origin with secondary jaundice.

POSTOPERATIVE DIAGNOSIS: Carcinoma of the right hepatic bile duct with extension
                           into the left and common hepatic ducts with total
                           obstruction.

OPERATION: Exploratory laparotomy
                           Choledochotomy
                           Lymph node biopsy
                           Irrigation of common duct for cell study and
                           T-Tube choledochostomy

ANESTHETIC: General

SURGEON: H. S. G_____, M.D.   ASSISTANT: S. A. W_____, M.D.
                                              Mrs. L_____, CORT.

PROCEDURE: Prep with betadine, routine drape for right subcostal
                           incision. Incision went through all the layers of
the abdominal wall. Bleeding was controlled with electrocoagulation. All tissues were
markedly jaundiced. Upon opening the abdominal cavity, exploration was carried out. The
gallbladder was empty and flat. The common duct was extremely decompressed and very small.
The common duct was dissected out for a distance of about 2.5 inches proximal and distal
to the cystic duct entrance. No abnormalities were found. Dr. W_____ assisted in a further
exploration of the common duct which went through the common hepatic ducts, which were intrahepatic in nature. The junction of the left and right was palpated and extending down into
the common duct, the common hepatic duct, for about 1 cm. from the junction of the right
and left, was a hard mass which was consistent with carcinoma. Attempts were made to do
everything but to biopsy the duct at this particular point, since no improvement in the patient's
condition could be generated by removing the duct, or by attempting any sort of anastomosis.
The common duct was entered and exploration was carried out. Attempts to obtain tissue were
made, none were successful. The lymph node was biopsied in the area which revealed no evidence
of disease. The duct was irrigated and the material sent for cell study. A T-tube was placed
in the common duct and run proximal and distally for about 2.5 inches on each side. It was
perforated to allow for escape of bile, should any be fortunate enough to pass this obstruction
at a later time. All attempts to dilate or enlarge the duct in the site of obstruction were
unsuccessful. There was no signs or stones. The duct was closed around the T-tube and
brought out through a stab wound in the patient's side. Drains were placed in the area and
irrigation followed, this aspirated clear and the abdomen then closed in layers, using chromic
catgut in the peritoneum, #0 dexon in the fascia, #000 plain catgut on the subcutaneous tissue
and 4-0 black silk on the skin. Sterile dressing was applied. Patient tolerated the procedure
well and went to the recovery room in good condition.

2/8/77 lw   SIGNATURE:

DEKALB GENERAL HOSPITAL
Decatur, Georgia

DISCHARGE SUMMARY

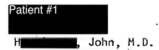

Patient #1

H_____, John, M.D.

DATE OF ADMISSION: 3-20-77   DATE OF DISCHARGE: 4-5-77

ADMISSION DIAGNOSIS: Carcinoma of common hepatic duct, status post T-tube
                        choledochostomy.

DISCHARGE DIAGNOSIS: Primary: Carcinoma of common hepatic duct, status post T-tube
          P 156.1   choledoshostomy.
              569.9   Gastrointestinal hemorrhage.

OPERATIONS, PROCEDURES, TREATMENT: None.

INFECTION: Yes, on admission.
              Site: bile.
              Organism: Pseudomonas aeruginosa

CONDITION ON DISCHARGE: Unchanged.

BRIEF HISTORY AND PHYSICAL: This 54 year old male had undergone exploratory laparotomy
                               12-20-76 and was found to have unresectable carcinoma of
the bile ducts with common hepatic bile duct obstruction. Choledochotomy and T-tube choledo-
chostomy were performed at that time and he was treated with a course of radiotherapy for 8
weeks totalling 500 rads. He had a T-tube cholangiogram at DeKalb General Hospital on 3-14-77
which indicated no essential improvement in his biliary blockage but within 24 hours began
having spiking fevers and severe chills. His T-tube was opened for drainage and treated with
Tylenol sponges, etc. He began vomiting the day prior to admission. He was admitted for
symptomatic relief and palliation of his underlying disease.

Physical exam showed a deeply jaundiced male in slight respiratory distress with minimal
ascites and enlarged liver edge, 4 FB below the right costal margin. There was some tenderness
and secondary skin changes. The patient had the following pertinent lab data:

PERTINENT LAB AND XRAY DATA: The patient had admitting hemogram with Hgb. 11.2; Hcrit.
                                35%; WBC 10,200 with 92% segs and 1 band. Urinalysis was
positive for bile; he had bacteria and trace albumin. Bile cultures were taken serially
during hospitalization and basically they grew out Pseudomonas with varying sensitivities.
He was treated initially with Tetracycline and this was later changed to Gentamicin and later
still, based on repeated re-cultures, to Carbenicillin.

HOSPITAL COURSE: The patient continued to have spike fevers almost throughout
                    his time in the hospital. They were as high as 103-104 on
admission and gradually diminished but he persistently had fevers to 100 degrees by the time
of discharge. His admission bilirubin was 20 and this diminished to 7.6 at the time of
discharge. He did have elevated liver enzymes with SGOT as high as 117; alk. phos. as much as
545; SGPT ranged from 58-72. On the fifth hospital day prolonged discussion was carried out
with the patient's wife and daughter and there was a great deal of denial on the wife's part.
However the patient comprehended his sutuation completely. By the 9th hospital day the patient
was having respiratory distress and his Hgb. was found to be 4.8 with blood pressure in the
80's. He developed melena and after prolonged discussion once more it was decided to treat the

CONTINUED

DEKALB GENERAL HOSPITAL
    Decatur, Georgia

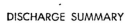

DISCHARGE SUMMARY

DISCHARGE SUMMARY CONTINUED - page 2

Pseudomonas with appropriate antibiotics but the GI bleeding was not treated with any
transfusions. By 4-5-77 the patient was slightly improved; his Hgb. was still only 5.7
but he and his family requested discharge. The ultimate prognosis was repeated and because
both the patient and his wife wished that he spend his remaining time at home, he was
discharged on 4-5-77, taking Carbenicillin per os and Tylenol III p.r.n. pain.

6-6-77 jvj   SIGNATURE: John H_____ MD

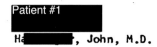

DEKALB GENERAL HOSPITAL
Decatur, Georgia

DISCHARGE SUMMARY

Patient #1

Ha_____, John, M.D.

DATE OF ADMISSION: 8-23-77   DATE OF DISCHARGE: 8-30-77

ADMISSION DIAGNOSIS: Terminal carcinoma of the bile ducts with ascites.
Possible impending hepatic coma.

DISCHARGE DIAGNOSIS: Primary: *P 156.P* Terminal carcinoma of the bile ducts with ascites.

OPERATIONS, PROCEDURES, TREATMENT: Paracentesis, 6,000 cc. 8-26-77.

INFECTION: *P 39.4* None.

CONDITION ON DISCHARGE: Improved.

BRIEF HISTORY AND PHYSICAL: This 54 year old male was diagnosed by laparotomy as
having carcinoma of the bile ducts in November, 1976.
A palliative procedure was performed and he was treated with radiotherapy postoperatively.
He was readmitted to DeKalb General Hospital in March, 1977 with a gastrointestinal
hemorrhage and no heroic treatments were undertaken; in spite of this he eventually improved
and was discharged. During the summer of 1977 he has begun having ascites which has
necessitated paracentesis and for the two nights prior to admission the patient had severe
abdominal pain, restlessness, inability to sleep, constant motor activity and some degree
of mental stupor. Physical exam showed BP 80/60; he was afebrile. He was wasted, slightly
jaundiced, in moderate distress. He was mentally obtunded, confused and required a tremendous
deal effort to speak. Massive ascites as well as slight ankle edema was noted. The patient
was admitted for what was presumed to be terminal care at this point.

PERTINENT LAB AND XRAY DATA: CBC showed Hgb. 9.2; Hcrit. 30.6; WBC 9,100 with 86% segs.
There was a moderate hypochromic and anisocytosis.
Urinalysis was essentially normal. Biochemical profile showed alk. phos. 720; total
bilirubin was normal. Protein was 5.6 and albumin was 1.7. Serum calcium and potassium were
also low. Chest X-ray showed marked elevation of the hemi-diaphragm secondary to the
ascites with some linear atalectatic changes in the lung bases, otherwise unremarkable. EKG
showed non-specific flattening of T-waves.

HOSPITAL COURSE: The patient was treated conservatively with oral liquids,
Tylenol III p.r.n. pain. He had orders for Morphine
Sulfate for ear pain but this was not called for. He had Tigan for nausea and on August 26th
underwent paracentesis of over 6,000 cc. with prompt relief. The patient improved with
bedrest and diet and was discharged on 8-30-77 for followup as an outpatient.

DISCHARGE MEDICATIONS AND
    INSTRUCTIONS: Tylenol III; disposition home.

PROGNOSIS: Poor.

9-27-77 dict
10-12-77 jvj   SIGNATURE: *John H_____ MD*

DEKALB GENERAL HOSPITAL
Decatur, Georgia

DISCHARGE SUMMARY

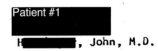

Patient #1

H_____, John, M.D.

DATE OF ADMISSION: 11-28-77   DATE OF DISCHARGE: 12-7-77

ADMISSION DIAGNOSIS: Intractable ascites, secondary to carcinoma of the bile
                              ducts.

DISCHARGE DIAGNOSIS: Primary: *P 197.6* Intractable ascites, secondary to carcinoma of the bile
                              ducts.

OPERATIONS, PROCEDURES, TREATMENT: Insertion of Levin peritoneal venous shunt 11-30-77.

INFECTION: *P 27.7* None.

CONDITION ON DISCHARGE: Improved.

BRIEF HISTORY AND PHYSICAL: This 55 year old white male had undergone exploratory
                              laparotomy in November 1976 with the findings of
carcinoma of the bile ducts. He was treated postop with palliative Cobalt therapy and
approximately 8 months ago had a severe ascending cholangietis, stress ulcers with upper
GI hemorrhage and profound jaundice. He survived this admission at DeKalb General and was
doing fairly well on essentially no treatment until July, 1977 when he began developing
ascites. This was refractory to Lasix and required repeated paracentesis, yielding anywhere
from 4,000-7,000 cc. of fluid weekly. This was performed 24 times since July and he was
admitted for a peritoneal venous shunt to palliate the need for the repeated paracenteses.

Physical exam, showed a wasted, debilitated white male with massive ascites. He had marked
muscle wasting, especially in the upper extremities, was slightly dehydrated.

PERTINENT LAB AND XRAY DATA: Hgb. 12.1; WBC 10,500. Urinalysis demonstrated 69 red
                              cells, trace bacteria, no bile. Clotting studies
were essentially within normal limits. Biochemical profile showed a low serum calcium and
potassium of 3.3; CPK was elevated; alk. phos. was 1,280; SGOT 52; SGPT 33. Albumin was 2.8.
Chest X-ray showed some blunting of both costophrenic angles but no change since August, 1977.
EKG was abnormal and showed low voltage with non-specific T-wave changes but unchanged
since August, 1977. The patient underwent liver scan on 11-28-77 which showed a massive
effect in the region of the porta hepatus, possibly representing recurrent cholangio-carcinoma.
Minimal evidence of hepatocellular dysfunction. No peripheral metastatic disease.

HOSPITAL COURSE: The patient was taken to surgery on 11-30-77 and under-
                              went insertion of a Levin shunt through a peritoneal
incision, implantation of the valve in the right rectus sheath and tunnelling over the right
costal margins to insert the other end of the valve into the internal jugular vein which was
then threaded into the superior vena cava. He tolerated this procedure quite well and his
postop course was marked by profound diuresis. Hcrit. remained stable and he required no
transfusions. His serum potassium improved and at discharge it was 3.3; serum albumin was 2.9;
alk. phos. was 825; CPK slightly elevated. Dermal sutures were removed prior to discharge and
he was sent home.

DISCHARGE MEDICATIONS AND
        INSTRUCTIONS: Lasix, Tylenol III.

DISPOSITION: Home.
                              CONTINUED

FORM # 3-5682 (3/71) - CONTINUOUS FORM   DISCHARGE SUMMARY

79

DEKALB GENERAL HOSPITAL
Decatur, Georgia

DISCHARGE SUMMARY

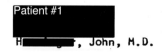

DISCHARGE SUMMARY CONTINUED - page 2

PROGNOSIS: Poor.

12-31-77 dict
1-20-78 jvj   SIGNATURE: John H▇▇▇▇▇▇ MD.

DEKALB GENERAL HOSPITAL
Decatur, Georgia

DISCHARGE SUMMARY

Patient #1

H_____, John, M.D.

ADMITTED: 9-25-78   DISCHARGED: 9-27-78

ADM DX: Status post carcinoma of bile duct with Levin peritoneal venous
                           shunt 11-77.

DISCH DX, Primary: Y/o 3   Status post carcinoma of bile duct with Levin peritoneal venous
                           shunt 11-77.

OP, PROC, TREAT: None.

INFECTION: None.

COND ON DISCH: Improved.

BRIEF H&P: This 56 year old white male was admitted at this time for re-evaluation
                           of his current status, briefly he had undergone laparotomy for
carcinoma of the bile ducts in November, 1976 and had postop radiation. Following this he
had a severe ascending cholangitis, stress ulceration with upper gastrointestinal hemorrhage,
jaundice and hepatorenal syndrome. He had refractory ascites in July, 1977, and was admitted
to DeKalb General in November, 1977 and underwent insertion of Levin shunt. Since then he
has done quite well in that his weight increased from 116 to 134 pounds. His girth measurement
diminished from approximately 37-38 inches to 32 inches and he no longer looks wasted and
debilitated. Physical findings at this time were limited to the abdomen which showed a well
healed right lower quadrant Kocher incision and the neck which showed evidence of a previous
shunt. Liver is palpable 5 cm. below the right costal margin, is non-tender and slightly
irregular. The left lobe is palpable almost at the umbilicus.

PERT LAB & XRAY: Admission urinalysis was within normal limits. Hgb. was 12.3;
                           Hcrit. 38.5; WBC 5,700 with normal differential. PTT was within
normal limits. Protime was 100%. Sed rate was noted to be 53 mm./hour. Platelet count
was 231,000. Biochemical profile was within normal limits except for the alk. phos. which was
1,500, total bilirubin 2.6. Albumin was 3. SGOT was 133, CPK 249 and SGPT 89. The patient
underwent a barium enema which was evident of a persistent deformity of the proximal ascending
colon above the level of the cecum which was concentric and externally circumferential.
On review of these films it was obvious that this was due to the intraperitoneal tubing which
was the inferior aspect of his shunt. Chest X-ray showed some sub-optimal bi-basilar pulmonary
scarring but no change since December, 1977. Minimal ascitic fluid was noted. Upper GI
series showed minimal deformity of the distal gastric antrum, base of the duodenal bulb
consistent with scarring from previous peptic ulcer disease, no active ulcer noted. EKG
was normal. Liver scan showed little change of the liver scan in the past 10 months with a
large left lobe of the liver, prominent porta hepatic area and probable malignancy in the
porta hepatus.

HOSP COURSE: Following completion of his evaluation, and the decision being
                           made not to go any further, the patient was discharged for office
followup.

DISCH MEDS: Lasix, 20 mg. p.o. q.d.; Phenaphen III, p.o. q.3-4 h. p.r.n.pain;
                           medication for nausea; Dalmane, 30 mg. p.o. q.h.s. p.r.n. sleep.

DISP: Home.

PROG: Guarded.
10-30-78 d/dt CONTINUOUS FORM   SIGNATURE: _____   DISCHARGE SUMMARY

81

DEKALB GENERAL HOSPITAL
Decatur, Georgia

DISCHARGE SUMMARY

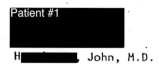

ADMITTED: 3/28/79   DISCHARGED: 3/30/79

ADM DX: Upper gastrointestinal bleeding.

DISCH DX, Prim: 578.9 Upper gastrointestinal bleeding.

    Sec/Compl: 155.1 Terminal carcinoma of bile duct.

OP, PROC, TREAT: None.

INFECTION: No.

COND ON DISCH: Improved.

BRIEF H&P: This 57 yr. old white male with known carcinoma of the bile ducts,
                     first operated on in Nov. 1976. Also has a LeVeen shunt from /N
Nov. 1977. He presented in my office on 3/28/78 with a 2 day history of melena with
passage of multiple black tarry stools. Hemoglobin was 6.7 grams and he was admitted
for palliative treatment involving blood transfusions. Details of H&P are found in
dictated record.

PERT LAB & XRAY: Admitting hemoglobin was 6.7 grams, hematocrit 21.4 percent,
                     white blood cell count and differentials were normal. Protime
and PTT were within normal limits. Urinalysis was grossly unremarkable. Discharge
hemoglobin was 11.5, hematocrit 35.3 percent.

HOSP COURSE: The patient was typed and crossed-matched and transfused with
                     4 units of packed red blood cells over a 36 hr. period. His
hemoglobin responded and he felt fairly well at the time of discharge.

DISCH MEDS: Tagamet 300 mgs. q.i.d.
                     Vicrodin 1 q. 6 h. p.r.n. pain.
                     Gelusil 1 tblsp. q. 2 h. while awake.
                     Torecan 10 mgs. p.o.q. 6 h. p.r.n. nausea and vomiting.
                     Resume previous use of Lasix 20 mgs. p.o.q.a.m.

DISCH INSTRUCTIONS: See me in 3-4 days for recheck of H&H.

DISPO: Home.

PROG: Poor.

3/30/79 dict
4/3/79 ss   SIGNATURE: John H___ MD

BRAIN CANCER

Cancer of the brain and spinal cord killed 10,200 Americans in 1987.

Pathologists recognize several distinct types of brain tumors; some of these, such as the astrocytomas, are deadly. Others, such as meningiomas, are more slow-growing.

The five-year survival rate for all brain cancer considered together falls in the range of 22–25%.

Patient #2

Patient #2 is a 35-year-old man from Michigan, who has survived nearly five years since diagnosed with an inoperable brain tumor.

In early August 1981, Patient #2 first experienced numbness in both legs that worsened over a four-week period. When he became incontinent in October 1981, his local physician referred him to the Ann Arbor Veterans' Administration Hospital for a neurological evaluation. At the VA, Patient #2's doctor assigned to the case noted mild muscle weakness associated with loss of sensation in his legs on physical examination, but all diagnostic tests, including a spinal tap, were inconclusive. When the symptoms spontaneously improved, Patient #2 was discharged on October 23, 1981, with plans for a repeat lumbar puncture in six weeks.

On December 3, 1981, Patient #2 returned to the hospital as scheduled. This time, his spinal fluid revealed an excess number of white blood cells, suggestive of an inflammatory process in the central nervous system such as multiple sclerosis. Although the diagnosis was not certain, Patient #2 began a course of ACTH, an anti-inflammatory pituitary hormone.

Patient #2 did well until June 1982, when, after suddenly losing all sensation in his legs, he was admitted on an emergency basis to Wyandotte Hospital. There, a lumbar puncture demonstrated elevated protein in the spinal fluid—an inconsequential finding—but no other abnormalities. Though the cause of his symptoms remained unclear, Patient #2 improved sufficiently to return home, aided by a walker and with plans to continue ACTH therapy.

Within a week after leaving the hospital, Patient #2 developed daily frontal headaches, usually lasting several hours at a time. Then, in September 1982, after becoming confused, disoriented, and forgetful, he was re-admitted to Wyandotte Hospital. When a CT scan of his head revealed a large mass in the third ventricle of the brain, Patient #2 was transferred to the VA at Ann Arbor on September 14, 1982. Two days later, he underwent exploratory brain surgery, at which time two inoperable tumors were discovered, as reported in the operative note:

> A large bulge was present in the right lateral wall of the third ventricle and smaller bulge present in the left wall of the third ventricle.

The attending surgeon biopsied one of the tumors, but made no attempt at re-section. Initially, the lesion was diagnosed as a "high grade glial tumor," one of the most aggressive nervous system malignancies. After further study, the biopsy specimen was believed to be more consistent with lymphoma, or a combination of glioma and lymphoma.

Several days later, a liver-spleen scan revealed an enlarged liver but no definitive evidence of metastatic disease. A bone marrow biopsy was negative for cancer, but a myelogram, a dye study of the spinal cord, clearly documented a third, large tumor in the thoracic spinal column, in the region of the mid-back.

Patient #2's doctors informed his wife that he had four to six months to live—at most. His physicians recommended a course of radiation for symptomatic relief, but advised no additional treatment.

On September 19, 1982, Patient #2 was transferred to the Allen Park VA Hospital in Michigan, to begin a proposed course of 4,000 rads of cobalt to the brain, and another 3-4,000 rads to the involved areas of the thoracic spine. At the same time, his wife decided to investigate unconventional approaches to cancer, quickly learned of Dr. Kelley, and discussed this option with her husband, who had already begun radiation. Shortly after, Patient #2 chose to discontinue all conventional treatment and pursue the Kelley program. Against his doctors' advice, he left the Allen Park VA on October 13, 1982, having received 2200 rads to the brain and 2277 rads to the dorsal spine, little more than half of the projected course. In the discharge note from the hospitalization, his doctor described the mixed results from his treatment to that point:

> During that time his memory had improved considerably. There was [after radiation] no detectable change in his neurological findings as far as the lower extremities are concerned.

Although confined to a wheelchair, Patient #2 and his wife traveled to Boston in mid-October 1982 to hear Dr. Kelley speak at a convention of cancer patients. After returning to Michigan, Patient #2 then began the full Kelley program.

Patient #2's first months on his nutritional regimen were difficult: at times, he lapsed into such confusion that his wife had to force the supplements into his mouth. Nevertheless, on the therapy he slowly began to improve, to the point his mental status normalized and over a period of a year, he progressed from a wheelchair to a walker to a cane.

On April 7, 1983, his wife called a staff oncologist at the VA to discuss her husband's unexpected progress but was only told that he required immediate, appropriate treatment. Although determined to refuse conventional therapy, Patient #2 did agree to a diagnostic evaluation in June 1983, mostly to satisfy his own curiosity. According to Patient #2, his various physicians were stunned when he walked unaided into the Oncology Clinic. They were further surprised when a CT scan of the brain revealed no evidence of the previously documented tumors, as summarized in the radiology report: "post surgical changes, right frontal region, otherwise grossly negative."

In January 1984, Patient #2 returned to the Oncology Clinic at Allen Park where his physician documented his continuing improvement in the records:

> [Patient #2] Has refused conventional Rx [treatment] & only partially completed R.T. [radiation]. Has had dramatic improvement in neural symptoms.

Today, nearly five years after his terminal diagnosis, Patient #2 still follows the Kelley program. Though he walks with a slight limp, he otherwise reports no residual symptoms and appears to be in excellent health.

In summary, Patient #2 was diagnosed with unresectable cancer of the brain. He did receive a partial course of cobalt therapy, but this treatment was intended only to relieve pressure in the spinal cord and skull, not as his attending physicians warned, as a cure. Most importantly, all of Patient #2's symptoms resolved only after he began the Kelley program.

CLINICAL REPORT	OPERATION REPORT

PREOPERATIVE DIAGNOSIS

Third ventricular tumor.

SURGEON Dr. D█████	FIRST ASSISTANT Dr. C█████	SECOND ASSISTANT		
ANESTHETIST Dr. H███████ m.V██████,CRNA/D.D█████,CRNA	ANESTHETIC General IT		TIME BEGAN 0855 TIME ENDED 1420	
SURGICAL NURSE J.G██,RN/K.M████████,RN	INSTRUMENT NURSE N. G███, NCT	TIME OPERATION BEGAN 1005	TIME OPERATION COMPLETED 1350	
OPERATIVE DIAGNOSES	DRAINS (Kind and number) Foley to O.R.; ICP; #9 Jack- son Pratt to head		SPONGE COUNT VERIFIED Correct	

Third ventricular tumor.

MATERIAL FORWARDED TO LABORATORY FOR EXAMINATION
1. Brain tumor, frozen section.
2. Brain tumor, for permanent.

OPERATION PERFORMED Position: Supine.   Prep: Betadine.

Right subfrontal craniotomy with biopsy of third ventricular tumor.

DESCRIPTION OF OPERATION (Type(s) of suture used, gross findings, etc.) Adm. 9/14/82; EBL - 500 cc.; Complications - none.	MAJOR X	MINOR	DATE OF OPERATION 9/16/82

The patient was taken to the operating room and general endotracheal anesthesia was
instituted. An arterial line was placed, as well as two intravenous lines. The entire head was then shaved and placed in the Mayfield head holder in the face up
position and slightly to the left. The entire scalp area was then prepped and draped
in the routine fashion. Betadine was used for preparation. A standard transcoronal
incision was then fashioned and carried down to the level of the galea. Raney clips
were applied to the skin edges. Using the scalpel, the skin flap was resected in an
anterior direction until the right supraorbital ridge was encountered. Skin flap was
then reflected back on towel clips and rubber bands. The Bovie and bipolar electrocautery devices were used for hemostasis. The paracranium was then incised in a semi-
circular fashion with its base towards the right supraorbital ridge and reflected as
one flap with the skin flap. This exposed the right frontal bone well. Two bur holes
were then drilled with the air powered perforator along the sagittal sinus inferiorly
and approximately 2 inches superiorly. Two more bur holes were then drilled in symmetrical locations in a more lateral position. These bur holes were lined with bone
wax and connected with a Gigli saw guide, and the Gigli saw was used to connect the
bur holes. The region of the right frontal sinus was encountered with the inferior
bur holes, and both the anterior and posterior walls of the sinus were separately incised. The mucosa of the frontal sinuses reflected in an inferior direction, and was

SIGNATURE OF SURGEON	DATE
ROBERT D█████, M.D./WILLIAM C███████, M.D.	9/16/82

PATIENT'S IDENTIFICATION (For typed or written entries give: Name—last, first, middle; grade; date; hospital or medical facility) D: 9/29/82 T: 10/3/82 mer	REGISTER NO.	WARD NO.

Patient #2 ████████

VAMC, Ann Arbor, MI

OCT 7 RECD

General Services Administration and
Interagency Committee on Medical Records
FPMR 101-11.806-8—October 1975
516-109

87

53

Standard Form 507

CLINICAL RECORD

Report on _____
               or
Continuation of S. F. _____

(Strike out one line) (Specify type of examination or data)

(Sign and date)
-2-

felt to be violated in one location. In this manner, the right frontal bone flap
was then removed. It was then realized that adequate lateral exposure with this bone
flap was not obtained, and the craniotome was then used to remove an approximately one
inch farther lateral segment of bone. This gave rise to two free bone flaps therefore.
Then 50 grams of Mannitol were administered, and the dura was then opened in a semi-
circular fashion with its base posteriorly. A large draining vein from the right frontal lobe entering the sagittal sinus was carefully preserved. Using the head light
and SELF RETAINING retractors and protecting the brain at all times with Cottonoid
strips, the right frontal lobe was retracted in a superior direction and the floor
of the frontal fossa was followed until the optic nerve was clearly identified. The
LAYLA self-retaining retractors were then inserted at the wound and used for frontal
lobe superior retraction. The microscope was then brought into the wound and the
optic nerves were clearly visualized. The retractors were set somewhat deeper and
further frontal lobe retraction, then exposed the left optic nerve and the optic
chiasm. In addition, the right internal carotid artery and A-1 segment of the
anterior cerebral artery were clearly identified. Using the Janetta and micro-
dissector and the ball dissector, the arachnoid was removed from around the exposed
arteries and the optic nerve and chiasm. Further dissection in a more posterior
direction then exposed the lamina terminalis immediately behind the optic chiasm.
This area of the lamina terminalis was then open with the Janetta and ball dissectors,
and CSF was seen to issue force. Several small vessels along the lamina
terminalis were bipolared and the micro-scissors were used to further open the lamina
terminalis, thereby giving a good view of the anterior portion of the third ventricle.
A large bulge was present in the right lateral wall of the third ventricle and smaller
bulge present in the left wall of the third ventricle. Using various sized Hartman's
and curettes, several small pieces of tissue were removed from this right lateral wall
bulging area and sent for pathological examination. Frozen section report came back
high grade glioma. It was felt that further operative removal of the tumor was unwarranted. The wound was irrigated and hemostasis was ensured. The retractors and
Cottonoid strips were then removed from the wound and the frontal lobe allowed to return to its more anatomic position, after hemostasis was ensured. The deep dura was
then closed with 4-0 silk running and interrupted sutures. The two free bone fragments were then wired together with two 3-0 wire sutures placed into Hall drill holes.
The bone flap was then wired back into place with multiple 3-0 wire sutures placed
through Hall drill holes also. The twisted ends were buried into the Hall drill holes
themselves. It should be noted that a piece of muscle was inserted into the frontal
sinus defect, and a flap of paracranium tacked down over the opening into the frontal
sinus to the dura. The wound was once again irrigated, and the skin was closed with
one layer of running and interrupted 2-0 and 3-0 nylon vertical mattress sutures. A

(Continue on reverse side)

PATIENT'S IDENTIFICATION (For typed or written entries give: Name—last, first,
middle; grade; date; hospital or medical facility)

Patient #2
VAMC, Ann Arbor, MI

REGISTER NO. | WARD NO.

REPORT ON _____ or CONTINUATION OF _____

STANDARD FORM 507
General Services Administration and
Interagency Committee on Medical Records
FPMR 101-11.80 6-8
October 1975 507-106
☆U.S. G.P.O. 1979-281-629/1364

88

CLINICAL RECORD

Report on _____

or

Continuation of S. F. _____

(Strike out one line) (Specify type of examination or data)

(Sign and date)

-3-

Jackson Pratt drain was left in the subgaleal space and brought out through a separate stab wound. A red rubber Robinson was left in the subdural space to act as an intracranial pressure monitor and also brought out through a separate stab wound. Both drains were anchored with 2-0 silk ligatures. A sterile head dressing was then applied. The patient was awakened and returned to the post-anesthesia recovery room in stable condition.

(Continue on reverse side)

PATIENT'S IDENTIFICATION (For typed or written entries give: Name—last, first, middle; grade; date; hospital or medical facility)

Patient #2

VAMC, Ann Arbor, MI

REGISTER NO.   WARD NO.

REPORT ON _____ or CONTINUATION OF _____

STANDARD FORM 507
General Services Administration and
Interagency Committee on Medical Records
FPMR 101-11.80 6-8
October 1975   507-106
✰U.S. G.P.O. 1979-281-629/1364

55

MEDICAL RECORD	TISSUE EXAMINATION

SPECIMEN SUBMITTED BY	DATE OBTAINED
Dr. D▮▮▮▮▮	9-16-82

SPECIMEN
Brain tumor, frozen section.

BRIEF CLINICAL HISTORY *(Include duration of lesion and rapidity of growth, if a neoplasm)*

PREOPERATIVE DIAGNOSIS

Third ventricular mass

OPERATIVE FINDINGS

POSTOPERATIVE DIAGNOSIS	SIGNATURE AND TITLE

PATHOLOGICAL REPORT

NAME OF LABORATORY		ACCESSION NO(S).
VAMC, ANN ARBOR, MI	mlw/ehs	S-2248-82

(Gross description, histologic examination and diagnoses)

GROSS:
   I. "Brain tumor." Tumor only a piece of soft semitranslucent tissue not in formalin. FROZEN SECTION REPORT: High grade glial tumor. DGR/
   II. "Brain tumor." A 2 mm piece of white to red tissue. 1 cassette ns.
     NOTE: Portion of specimen also taken for electron microscopy.   DGR

MICROSCOPIC:
   Small piece of tissue which consists mostly of small cells which are consistent with lymphoma. The nuclei of several of these cells are convoluted. There are occasional large cells which may represent trapped normal neural cells.

   Since primary lymphomas in the brain are frequently in immuno-compromised patients an immunologic workup is indicated.

DIAGNOSIS:
   Brain, biopsy; small cell neoplasm consistent with lymphoma.

CODE:
   I

(Continue on reverse side)

SIGNATURE OR PATHOLOGIST		DATE
DAN G. R▮ ▮▮▮ M.D./B. S▮▮▮▮▮▮ , M.D.		9.21.82

	AGE	SEX	RACE	IDENTIFICATION NO.
		M		

PATIENT'S IDENTIFICATION *(For typed or written entries give: Name—last, first, middle; grade; date; hospital or medical facility)*	REGISTER NO.	WARD NO.
Patient #2 ▮▮▮▮▮▮	▮▮▮▮▮▮	

TISSUE EXAMINATION

STANDARD FORM 515 (REV. 9–77)
Prescribed by GSA and ICMR, FPMR 101–11.806–8

11⅞

MEDICAL RECORD	PROGRESS NOTES

DATE

TRANSFER SUMMARY

DIAGNOSIS
1. Probable lymphoma of the third ventricle
2. Extradural mass T5 through T8, possibly lymphoma
3. Possible multiple sclerosis
4. History of rheumatic fever

This is the third Ann Arbor VAMC admission for this 31 year old white man with presumed lymphoma of the third ventricle, transferred from Neurosurgery to Medicine for staging evaluation. The patient had an onset of progressive weakness greater on the right than on the left lower extremities and numbness below the T8 dermatome, somewhere approximately 16 months. Work up at that time (10/81) included a physical exam which showed a decreasing sensitivity to pin below T8 and negative Babinskis and mild general lower extremity weakness. Myelogram was officially normal but showed a possible mild lesion at T5. TFT's, VDRL and a rheumatoid factor were all negative. CSF showed mild pleocytosis with 12 lymphocytes, no red blood cells and negative cytology. Protein was 59. Diagnosis at that time was possible demyelinating lesion or a peri-inflammatory myelopathy. Oligoclonal banding and Myelin basic protein were sent but were negative subsequently. Patient was readmitted on December 3, 1981 for repeat LP which was negative except for again a mild white blood cell pleocytosis with 7 white blood cells, all lymphocytes and 0 red blood cells. Repeat EMG was negative. Patient was lost to follow up at that time.

His weakness slowly improved until June of 1982 when his weakness increased again, he became partially paraplegic. During the interim time between his second and third admissions, a possible diagnosis of multiple sclerosis had been offered. Patient was begun on ACTH therapy with what he thought was good effect in October 1981. Patient had improved slowly at that time and was able to walk with a walker but his weakness was exacerbated whenever his ACTH was discontinued. Over the past five months before this admission, the patient had increasing cerebral headaches, particularly frontal headaches, lasting for several hours. These were not claimed to be significantly

(Continue on reverse side)

PATIENT'S IDENTIFICATION (For typed or written entries give: Name—last, first, middle; rate; hospital or medical facility)

Patient #2

VAMC, Ann Arbor, Michigan
dict: 9-29-82 trans: 9-29-82 nl

REGISTER NO.

WARD NO.

PROGRESS NOTES
STANDARD FORM 509 (Rev. 11-77)
Prescribed by GSA/ICMR.
FPMR (41 CFR) 101-11 806-8
509-110

91

-2-

different from his other typical sinus headaches. Over the past two months before admission he was noted to have increasing confusion without other neuro symptoms but noted occasionally he had a temperature as high as 103. Finally in September of 1982 the patient was admitted to Wyandotte Hospital, presumably because of fevers and other symptoms. A CT scan at that time showed a third ventricular cystic mass. He was transferred to the Neurosurgery Service at this hospital, who performed a right subfrontal craniotomy with biopsy of the tumor, which on path exam was felt to be a lymphoma versus small cell metastatic tumor. The patient's post operative recovery was unremarkable except for a recurrence of low-grade fever to 101 or 100.4. This was not different then a fever he had pre-operatively.

The patient had an evidence of urinary tract infection preoperatively which revealed Pseudomonas aeruginosa which was sensitive to amino-glycosides. The patient was begun on Tobra on 8/15 without great effect of this fever and the urine cleared significantly. Patient had no dysuria but has had chronic urinary retention and decreased feeling in the area secondary to his neurologic process. He has been forced to use intermittent self-catheterization.

The patient has had a one to two month history of low grade fevers without obvious etiology. The fever has not been progressive and he had no other symptoms of infection.

The patient was transferred from the Neurosurgery Service to the Medicine Service for further staging and evaluation of the third ventricular tumor.

Past medical history other then above includes a positive history of rheumatic fever times two as a child with rash, carditis, arthritis and possibly chorea. Surgical history includes tonsillectomy and lipoma removal and a craniotomy as noted. At the time of transfer his medications included post operative Decadron 1 mgs q.6, Phenobarb 32mgs p.o. t.i.d., Tobramycin 80mgs I.V. piggyback q.8, Actifed 1 tablet p.o. t.i.d., Cimetadine 300mgs q.6h., Mylanta p.r.n. and Tylenol #3 1-2 tabs q.3-4h.

Physical examination revealed a well developed well nourished white man status post frontal craniotomy with a large scar. Patient was in no acute distress, was moderately cushingoid. His admission vital signs were as follows: Blood pressure was 138/94 without orthostatic changes, pulse was 90 and regular. Respiratory rate was 20 and regular. Patient was afebrile. HEENT exam was normal except for the healing craniotomy scar in the bifrontal areas. Patient did have slight moon facies. Occular exam was normal with flat disks and without hemorrhages. TM's were normal as were lymph and throat. Neck was supple without adenopathy or thyromegaly. Chest was clear to auscultation and percussion. Cardiovascular exam was normal, there was, however, a I/VI systolic murmur heard best at the left lower sternal border going to the apex. Pulses were generally 2+ throughout without bruits. Back and extremities were free of costo-vertebral angle tenderness, clubbing, cyanosis and edema. Skin revealed acne over his chest otherwise normal. There was no detectable adenopathy in the cervical, inguinal or axillary areas. Neurologic exam revealed an alert oriented man who was easily forgetful of details that had just been repeated to him. Cranial nerves II through XII were intact. Motor showed normal strength in the upper extremities, there was marked decrement in the lower extremities, specifically hip flexors on the left were 3-. They were 2+ on the right. The extensors were 3 on the left and 2+ on the right. Dorsiflexors were 4 on the left and 4 on the right. Plantar flexors were 4 on the left and 3 on the right. There was also mild decrement to pin and position in the lower extremities below T10 dermatome. Deep tendon reflexes were 2+ throughout in the upper extremities and 4+ throughout in the lower extremities with plantar responses extensor bilaterally.

It was felt that the patient's most urgent requirement was that of radiation both to his cranial lesion and possibly to an area of blockage in the spinal cord producing the lower extremity findings as noted. Therefore the first effort was to obtain a myelogram which was performed on 9/28/82. This did show partial obstruction to flow of the patopaque dye from T5 to T8 on the left posterior lateral view. This was consistent with a metastatic tumor or lymphoma. Because of that it was felt essential to transfer the patient to the Allen Park VA Medical Center where specific radiation therapy is available. Radiation therapists at the Allen Park VAMC will plan radiation therapy both for the extradural lesion in the spinal cord as well as the intracerebral lesion in the third ventricle. After the patient's received a sufficient radiation course he will be returned to the Ann Arbor VAMC where further staging work up shall proceed.

Laboratory tests done during this admission at the time of transfer to Internal Medicine on 9/27/82 showed a hgb of 13.0, hct 38.5, white count 11.4, platelet count 313,000. Sodium 137, potassium 3.6, chloride 102, bicarbonate 23, BUN 15, creatinine 0.9, glucose 99. Bilirubin 0.3, SGPT and SGOT were mildly elevated as they had been previously to 111 and 94 respectively. Calcium was normal at 8.5, clotting times were normal.

(Continue on reverse side)

93

DATE	
	-4-

Patient did undergo a liver spleen scan on 9/28/82 which showed a slight colloid shift to the spleen and inhomogeneous uptake on the right lobe of the liver, although this was interpreted as showing no definitive metastases.

As noted above, the patient will be sent to Allen Park VAMC as soon as possible to expedite the radiation therapy and perhaps some of his severe ~~paretic~~ symptoms. His discharge medications include Decadron 1 mg p.o. q.6h., Phenobarbital 32 mgs p.o. t.i.d., Cimetadine 300mgs p.o. q.6h, Mylanta 300cc. p.o. p.r.n., Actifed 1 tablet p.o. t.i.d. and Tobramycin 80mgs q.8 I.V. Piggyback.

The patient was ~~transferred~~ discharged to the Allen Park Veterans Administration Medical Center on 9-29-82, regularly.

Addendum: ① IV Tobra was discontinued as a urine culture from 9/25 was negative

② Dr. Bell of Radiology left 3cc of Pantopaque dye within the pt's subarachnoid space to be used if desired as future myelogram dye (without having to do a myelogram)

FRANK B____S, M.D.

MD ___ MD
attending physician

9.29 admission note
3 ___ admitted for radiation therapy
to head & T-spine area for ___
Refd to Memorial ___ for ___

94

DATE	
10-27-82	Patient has not been seen since 10-15-82.
	His wife came in on 10-18-82 and collected all records
	from community hospitals in the area.
	He has received a mid line dose of 2200 rads to the
	cranium and a tissue dose of 2277 rads to the dorsal
	spine canal from 9-30-82 to 10-15-82 in 16 days.
	During that time his memory had improved considerably.
	There was no detectable change in his neurological findings
	as far as the lower extremities are concerned.

J. E. T███████, M.D.

(Continue on reverse side)

PATIENT'S IDENTIFICATION *(For typed or written entries give: Name—last, first, middle; grade; rank; rate; hospital or medical facility)*

REGISTER NO.

WARD NO.

Patient #2

PROGRESS NOTES
STANDARD FORM 509 (Rev. 11-77)
Prescribed by GSA/ICMR.
FPMR (41 CFR) 101-11.806-8
509-110

95

MEDICAL RECORD	CONSULTATION SHEET

REQUEST

TO: *Ann Arbor* | FROM: *(Requesting physician or activity)* *oncology* | DATE OF REQUEST *4/21/83*

REASON FOR REQUEST *(Complaints and findings)*

CAT scan of brain
follow - Craniotomy brain tumor 1982

PROVISIONAL DIAGNOSIS

lymphoma

DOCTOR'S SIGNATURE ███ MD	APPROVED	PLACE OF CONSULTATION	☐ ROUTINE ☐ TODAY
		☐ BEDSIDE ☐ ON CALL	☐ 72 HOURS ☐ EMERGENCY

6/11/83   **CONSULTATION REPORT**

CT BRAIN SCAN:
6/2/83
Routine axial sections were obtained following the uneventful IV administration of
100cc Conray 60.
FINDINGS:
The scan is of poor quality due to the inherent limitations of the EMI scanner.
Post surgical changes are noted in the right frontal region. There are several
dense foci which are presumably attributable to residual pantopaque from a
previous myelogram. The exam is otherwise grossly negative.
IMPRESSION: POST SURGICAL CHANGES, RIGHT FRONTAL REGION; OTHERWISE GROSSLY
NEGATIVE.
R. J█████,MD/T. G█████,M.D. /lra

(Continued on reverse side)

SIGNATURE AND TITLE		DATE
IDENTIFICATION NO.	ORGANIZATION	REGISTER	WARD NO.

PATIENT'S IDENTIFICATION *(For typed or written entries give: Name—last, first,
middle, grade, rank, rate; hospital or medical*

██████████

GOVERNMENT PRINTING OFFICE : 1982 O - 361-495 (2068)

DATE

JAN 1 2 1984

32 yr. WD ♂ w│ hx? Ca of spine + brain
Has refused conventional Rx & only partially
completed R.T. Has had dramatic improvement
in neural symptoms.
Phys Ex: WD & obese.
  Heent: ⊖ adenopathy   Chest: ⊖
  Cor: $S_1 S_2$ ⊖ m   Abd: Liver WNL. no node
  Ext: gross spasms both legs.
  Neuro: ⊖ papilledema   PERRL EOM·WNL

RTC 9-84   DTRs arms 2+= legs 4+ bil Bil Babinski
2 9·84   Impression: Stable Neuro Status
9:30   Plan: report of CT.
          CBC ē diffs platelets ✓
          SMA·17 ✓
          Bun Cal lytes, Triglycerides
          RTC 1 mo.
             Kich

(Continue on reverse side)

BREAST CANCER

In 1987, breast cancer claimed 41,300 lives, with 300 of the victims men.

For diagnostic purposes, physicians usually divide the breast into four quarters, or quadrants. Most breast tumors—in fact, nearly 50%—occur in the upper outer quadrant, the region closest to the shoulder.

If diagnosed early, most women can be cured with surgery, but once metastatic, experts consider the disease incurable.

Today, approximately 75% of women with breast cancer, considering all stages together, live five years.

Patient #3

Patient #3 is a 62-year-old woman from Iowa with a history of metastatic breast carcinoma, now alive more than ten years since her diagnosis.

Prior to developing cancer, Patient #3 had a long history of benign breast disease as confirmed by biopsy in 1973. In June 1976, she noticed a new left breast mass in the region of the old biopsy scar. When a mammogram in late August 1976 revealed a "suspicious" lesion, Patient #3 was admitted to Iowa Methodist Medical Center.

On September 2, 1976, after biopsy studies documented intraductal carcinoma, Patient #3 underwent a left modified radical mastectomy. The tumor was described as 3 cm in diameter, with areas of "comedo type carcinoma" and focal areas of necrosis, both signs of aggressive disease. Ten of 17 axillary lymph nodes examined were positive for cancer, although subsequent bone and liver scans showed no evidence of distant metastases.

After leaving the hospital in mid-September 1976, Patient #3 began a course of the drug 5-fluorouracil as an outpatient. While receiving chemotherapy, she developed severe fatigue, associated with diminished appetite and rapid weight loss. She reported to me that a series of follow-up chest X-rays at that time revealed lesions in her lungs consistent with metastatic malignancy.

As her condition worsened clinically, Patient #3 decided to investigate unconventional approaches to cancer including the Kelley method. In November 1976, after completing only two months of a projected one year regimen, Patient #3 refused further chemotherapy, instead choosing to travel to Washington State and consult with Dr. Kelley. When first seen by Dr. Kelley, she was very ill, in her own words "going down the drain very quickly." In fact, she felt so weak that she could barely walk into Dr. Kelley's office.

After Patient #3 returned home and began her nutritional therapy, over a period of several months her appetite improved, she gained weight, and her many other symptoms resolved. Today, nearly 11 years since beginning the Kelley program, Patient #3 follows a maintenance protocol, is in excellent health, and remains apparently cancer-free.

In summary, Patient #3 was initially diagnosed with breast cancer that had metastasized to multiple regional lymph nodes and possibly the lungs. Even discounting the lung findings, statistically, the number of positive axillary nodes is, as Hellman writes, the "single most important prognostic factor for patients with breast cancer."[1] For aggressively treated patients with four or more cancerous nodes, Valagussa describes a 16% ten-year disease-free survival, Haagensen a 27% ten-year disease-free survival, and Fisher a 14% ten-year disease-free survival.[1]

Although Patient #3 received an abbreviated course of 5-fluorouracil, single drug chemotherapy has never been shown to cure metastatic breast cancer. Carter reports a *response* rate of only 26% in a group of 1263 patients treated with 5-fluorouracil, and no long-term survivors.[2] Here, it's useful to keep in mind the technical National Cancer Institute definition of the term "response," which indicates at least a 50% reduction in tumor size lasting a minimum of four weeks.

I cannot provide definitive evidence of active cancer when this patient began her nutritional protocol. Nonetheless, Patient #3 was in rapid decline at the time, her X-rays had shown possible metastatic disease, and her tenuous condition, coupled with the findings at surgery, make her disease-free survival unusual.

REFERENCES

1. DeVita, VT, et al. *Cancer Principles & Practice of Oncology*. Philadelphia; J.B. Lippincott Company, 1982, page 920.

2. Carter, SK. "Integration of Chemotherapy into Combined Modality Treatment of Solid Tumors." *Cancer Treatment Review* 1976; 3:141-174.

IOWA METHODIST MEDICAL CENTER
· DES·MOINES, IOWA

NAME:	Patient #3	AGE:	51
SPECIMEN NO:	S-7677-76	HOSP. NO.:	▮
DOCTOR:	L. D. R▮▮▮ M.D.	ROOM:	▮
DATE:	9-2-76	REFERRING PHYSICIAN:	

PREVIOUS PATHOLOGY:

FROZEN SECTION DIAGNOSIS:

Dr. B▮▮▮▮: Left breast - infiltrating ductal carcinoma

GROSS DESCRIPTION:

The specimen is a 3 cm. mass of tumor surrounded by a small amount of ✓ adipose tissue. Some of this was sent for estrogen receptor assay.

The second part of the specimen is a left breast measuring 30 x 25 cm. The nipple appears normal. Above and slightly lateral to the nipple there is a curved linear biopsy incision site 7.5 to 8 cm. long with no definite tumor in the base of the biopsy incision site although there is some white fibrous type breast tissue. The breast is mainly adipose tissue and scattered through-out there are white rubbery nodules of fibrosis. There is some pectoralis muscle at the base of the breast and the axillary tail is identified by the fact that there are large firm lymph nodes. The largest lymph node is 2 cm.

MICROSCOPIC EXAMINATION:

The breast neoplasm is an infiltrating ductal carcinoma. The neoplastic cells are fairly uniform and have generous amounts of pink staining cytoplasm. Nuclei are oval to round and somewhat vesicular. There are areas of comedo type carcinoma in the neoplasm. Stroma tends to be moderately fibrous and there are focal areas of necrosis within tumor clumps. There is very little tendency to gland formation. A section of nipple shows no evidence of neoplasia. Additional sections of breast show it to be somewhat atrophic generally. Seventeen axillary lymph nodes are examined microscopically and ten of them contain metastatic deposits.

DIAGNOSIS: Infiltrating ductal carcinoma of the left breast.
Metastases in ten of seventeen axillary lymph nodes.

SNOP 6

RWA:lkb
9-4-76

Richard W. A▮▮▮, M.D.
PATHOLOGIST

IOWA METHODIST MEDICAL CENTER
1200 PLEASANT
DES MOINES, IOWA 50308

ADMISSION DATE: September 1, 1976
DISCHARGE DATE: September 15, 1976

Admitting history revealed a 51-year-old white female who had noticed a lump in her left breast a couple months ago which was present in an old biopsy scar. The patient had had mammograms in March that showed only minimal scar tissue in the area. Repeat mammograms two days prior to admission showed a suspicious growth in the area. The patient had had the original biopsy in May of 1973 which revealed two benign lumps.

PAST MEDICAL HISTORY: Significant in that the patient had a sister and an aunt who both had breast carcinoma. Present medications included Aldactazide 1 p.o. every day and Diuril 500 mg. every day for high blood pressure.

PHYSICAL EXAMINATION showed a blood pressure of 160/100 with a pulse of 80/minute. Breast examination on the left showed a 2 cm. x 2 cm. hard, smooth, mobile mass deep in an old incision from a breast biopsy at about 2 o'clock in the left breast. The axilla was within normal limits, as was the right breast. The lungs were clear and the heart had a normal sinus rhythm without murmur. Abdominal examination was within normal limits.

LABORATORY DATA: Admission CBC was within normal limits, as was the urinalysis. Electrolytes showed a potassium of 3.7 mEq./L.. SMA-12 profile was within normal limits. Bone scan and liver scan were both within normal limits, as was the chest x-ray and EKG.

HOSPITAL COURSE: Admitting diagnosis was (1) suspicious lump in the left breast, and (2) hypertension. The patient was taken to the operating room on September 2, 1976 where a breast biopsy was performed. Frozen section revealed intraductal carcinoma and a modified radical mastectomy was performed. Postoperative pathology diagnosis showed infiltrating ductal carcinoma of the left breast with metastases in 10 of 17 axillary lymph nodes. The patient had an uneventful postoperative course and was discharged on September 15, 1976. She will be followed in the office by Dr. R▮▮▮. Consultation with Dr. H▮▮▮▮▮▮ was also performed and he was planning to start adjuvant chemotherapy on an outpatient basis.

Robert M. K▮▮▮, M. D.
Surgical Resident, for

LOUIS D. R▮▮▮▮ M. D.
RMK:1m
9-26-76 (28)
cc: Richard R. H▮▮▮▮, M. D.

DISCHARGE SUMMARY

0350 6454

103

Patient #4

Patient #4 is a 44-year-old woman from Los Angeles with a history of recurrent breast carcinoma, alive 13 years since her original diagnosis.

Shortly after developing a painful left breast mass in mid-1973, Patient #4 consulted her primary physician, who sent her immediately for mammography. When the study revealed a lesion thought to be benign, no further evaluation was recommended.

However, over a period of a year the mass gradually enlarged. Finally, in June 1974, Patient #4 was referred to the surgery clinic at Century City Hospital in Los Angeles where a needle biopsy confirmed cancer, an adenocystic adenocarcinoma of the left breast.

On July 7, 1974, Patient #4 was admitted to Cedars-Sinai Medical Center in Los Angeles for a modified left radical mastectomy. In the pathology report, the tumor was described as 2 cm in diameter, identified as a "focally mucin secreting adenocarcinoma with focal adenoides cysticum features, infiltrative." Multiple axillary (armpit) lymph nodes removed with the breast were also positive for locally metastatic disease.

After her discharge from the hospital on July 12, 1974, Patient #4 continued her evaluation as an outpatient. X-rays of the chest, a bone scan, and a liver scan showed no evidence of distant disease. Nevertheless, because of the extensive lymph node involvement, Patient #4's doctors recommended a two-year course of chemotherapy with the drug Alkeran, which she began that summer.

In October 1976, only months after completing the regimen, Patient #4 developed a nodule on the left chest wall in the region of her mastectomy scar. Her surgeon removed the lesion, which proved consistent with recurrent carcinoma, although a bone scan and X-ray studies were clear.

At that point, the patient's physicians proposed a course of radiation to the chest wall, followed by another round of aggressive chemotherapy. However, Patient #4 refused the suggested treatment, instead entering a clinic in Tijuana, Mexico where she received Laetrile along with the drug Cytoxan. When Patient #4 reacted badly to the treatment, she left the clinic and returned home to California.

In late 1976, Patient #4 began a series of injections with BCG, a modified tuberculosis vaccine at times used as an experimental cancer therapy. Despite her various treatments, in December 1977 she noted a new nodule in the region of her mastectomy scar. On December 29, 1977, the lesion was removed at Cedars-Sinai, and classified as "Dermal and subcutaneous metastatic breast ductal carcinoma."

At that point, Patient #4 decided to continue her BCG regimen, but less than nine months later a third nodule appeared in her mastectomy scar. This was excised, and identified as "adenocarcinoma, consistent with metastatic carcinoma of mammary gland origin."

Patient #4 had now suffered three recurrences in a two-year period. In addition, throughout the fall of 1978, her general health gradually deteriorated. She experienced bouts of severe fatigue and depression, her appetite decreased, and she began losing weight. But despite warnings from her doctors, Patient #4 refused to proceed with chemotherapy.

In early 1979, Patient #4 learned of Dr. Kelley, consulted with him, and in February 1979 began the full nutritional program. Within months, all her symptoms and problems—her fatigue, depression, weakness, and weight loss—resolved. Today, eight years since beginning the Kelley regimen, Patient #4 still follows her nutritional protocol and is in excellent health. During this time, her once persistent malignancy has not recurred.

In summary, Patient #4 experienced four bouts of breast cancer between 1974 and 1978, despite surgery, two years of chemotherapy, Laetrile along with more chemotherapy, and immunotherapy. Her subsequent long-term disease-free survival can only logically be attributed to the Kelley program.

PATIENT	Patient #4
HOSP. NO.	
ROOM	
AGE	31
DOCTOR	L. MC

See also:
4483-74

DATE RECEIVED: **July 8, 1974**

PATHOLOGY
NUMBER: **4504-74**

SPECIMEN:
Left breast; Left axillary contents; Frozen section, left axillary contents; Highest axillary contents; Tail of breast

GROSS DIAGNOSIS (SURGERY): Extensive fibrocystic disease   (LK)

FROZEN SECTION DIAGNOSIS (SURGERY): Metastatic adenocystic carcinoma, breast to lymph nodes   (LK)

GROSS DESCRIPTION

Labeled "left breast" is a breast that measures 19 x 13.5 x 3 cm. The skin ellipse measures 13.5 x 2.7 cm. The nipple is smooth and measures 1.5 cm. in diameter. In the upper outer quadrant there is an ill defined firm area measuring 2 cm. in diameter. On section this area is granular and mottled pink and grey. There is focal hemorrhage surrounding this area. There is a sutured defect in the hemorrhagic area. Serial sectioning of the remaining breast shows multiple cysts measuring up to 0.2 cm. in diameter and abundant grey-white breast tissue. There is a black suture attached at the axillary margin.

Labeled "axillary contents" is an 8 x 2.6 x 1.5 cm. portion of fat with firm grey lymph nodes ranging from 0.5 cm. up to 2 cm. in diameter. There is a suture attached at one margin.

Labeled "frozen section, axillary contents" is a 1 x 0.7 x 0.2 cm. grey tissue fragment.

Labeled "highest axillary contents" is a 9 x 3 x 1 cm. portion of fat with a blue suture at one end. It contains multiple grey lymph nodes ranging from 0.6 cm. up to 1 cm. in diameter. There are six lower portion lymph nodes and there are six upper portion lymph nodes.

Labeled "tail of breast" is a 10 x 2 x 1.2 cm. portion of fat with a blue suture attached at one end. It is focally hemorrhagic and lobulated.

A. Nipple - 1   )
B. Firm area - 2   )
C. Firm area - 2   )
D. Upper-outer quadrant - 2)"Left breast"
E. Upper-inner quadrant - 2)
F. Lower-outer quadrant - 2)
G. Lower-inner quadrant - 2)

(Cont. on Page 2)

DATE OF REPORT_____   _____M.D., PATHOLOGIST

SURGICAL PATHOLOGY REPORT

FORM 3703-75 3-74

106

CEDARS-SINAI MEDICAL CENTER

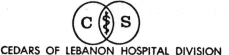

CEDARS OF LEBANON HOSPITAL DIVISION

PATIENT: Patient #4

PATHOLOGY NUMBER: 4504-74

CONTINUATION OF REPORT — PAGE 2

H. One half of lymph node - 2)
I. Other half of lymph node - 2) "Axillary contents"
J. Four lymph nodes - 4
K. "Frozen section, axillary contents" - All embedded
L. Six lower portion lymph nodes - 6) "Highest axillary contents"
M. Six upper portion lymph nodes - 6)
N. "Tail of breast" - 3

WJW:ew/jhc

MICROSCOPIC DESCRIPTION AND DIAGNOSIS

Modified radical resection, left breast, showing:

a) Status following prior biopsy for intraductal papillary
    cribriform and focally mucin secreting adenocarcinoma
    with focal adenoides cysticum features, infiltrative.

b) Multifocal areas of residual papillary cribriform and
    mucin secreting adenocarcinoma adjacent to side of biopsy,
    upper outer quadrant.

c) Diffuse fibrocystic disease of the breast - all quadrants -
    with adenosis, apocrine metaplasia.

d) Metastases to axillary lymph nodes adjacent to breast.

e) Marked lymphoid and reticulum cell hyperplasia midaxillary
    lymph nodes without metastases.

f) Marked lymphoid and reticulum cell hyperplasia, highest
    axillary lymph nodes.

g) Specimen, tail of breast, fibrofatty tissue with recent
    hemorrhage.

LK:ew/jhc

DATE OF REPORT 7-10-74   LEO K█████, M.D. INC.   M.D., PATHOLOGIST

FORM 3703-77   **SURGICAL PATHOLOGY REPORT**

107

CEDARS-SINAI MEDICAL CENTER

SEE ALSO: 4483-74
          4504-74

PATIENT
HOSP. NO.   Patient #4
ROOM
AGE -   34
DOCTOR   L.M

DATE RECEIVED: November 9, 1976

PATHOLOGY   8485-76
NUMBER:

SPECIMEN: Nodule left axilla

GROSS DIAGNOSIS (SURGERY): Deferred, left axilla   (NBF)

GROSS DESCRIPTION

Labeled "nodule left axilla" and received in Bouin's is a previously
bisected soft tissue fragment measuring 1.8 x 1.5 x 0.8 cm.

A. 2)
B. 2) All embedded

                                                        ES:pt

MICROSCOPIC DESCRIPTION

Fibrofatty and muscular tissue infiltrated by mammary carcinoma.
It varies from well differentiated papillary to poorly differentiated
infiltrating.

DIAGNOSIS: Secondary mammary carcinoma, skin, axilla, chest wall

                                                        NBF:cb

11-11-76   NATHAN B. F_____ M.D., PATHOLOGIST
DATE of REPORT   DIV. of ANATOMIC PATHOLOGY • LEO KAPLAN, M.D. DIRECTOR

Form No.: 3980-54 (Rev. 12/75)

108

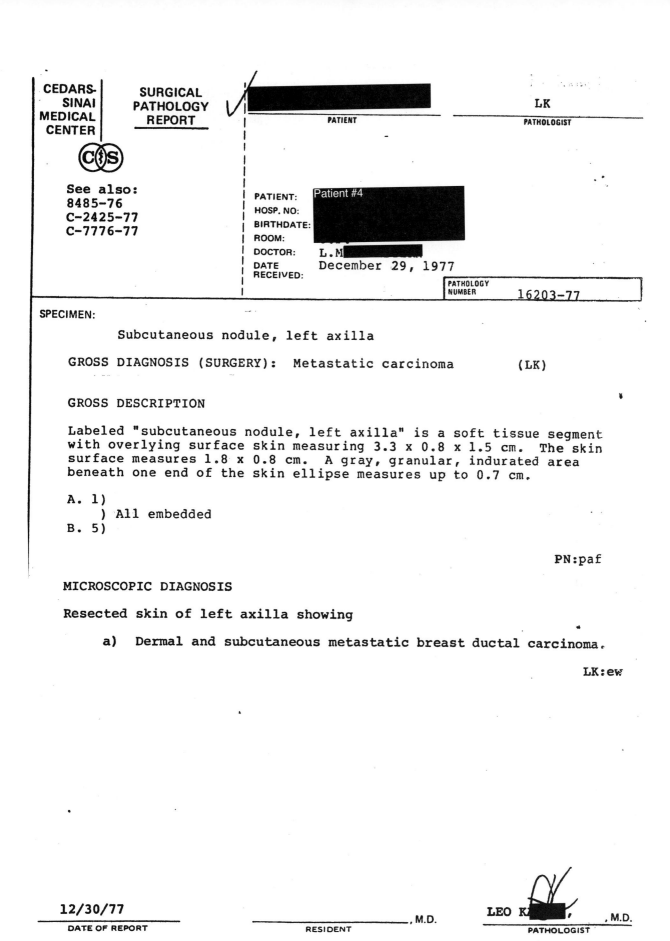

See also:
8485-76
C-2425-77
C-7776-77

PATIENT   LK
                                          PATHOLOGIST

PATIENT: Patient #4
HOSP. NO:
BIRTHDATE:
ROOM:
DOCTOR: L.M
DATE RECEIVED: December 29, 1977

PATHOLOGY NUMBER   16203-77

SPECIMEN:

Subcutaneous nodule, left axilla

GROSS DIAGNOSIS (SURGERY):   Metastatic carcinoma   (LK)

GROSS DESCRIPTION

Labeled "subcutaneous nodule, left axilla" is a soft tissue segment
with overlying surface skin measuring 3.3 x 0.8 x 1.5 cm. The skin
surface measures 1.8 x 0.8 cm. A gray, granular, indurated area
beneath one end of the skin ellipse measures up to 0.7 cm.

A. 1)
) All embedded
B. 5)

PN:paf

MICROSCOPIC DIAGNOSIS

Resected skin of left axilla showing

a)   Dermal and subcutaneous metastatic breast ductal carcinoma.

LK:ew

12/30/77   _____, M.D.   LEO K_____, M.D.
DATE OF REPORT   RESIDENT   PATHOLOGIST

109

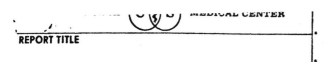
cc
11-9

OPERATION
8/24/78

D. B_____, M.D.
L. M_____, M.D.
J. B_____, M.D.

SURGEON	D. Br_____, M.D.
ASSISTANT	J. He_____, M.D.
ANESTHESIOLOGIST	None
PREOPERATIVE DIAGNOSIS	Left chest wall mass
POSTOPERATIVE DIAGNOSIS	Same
OPERATION	Excisional biopsy of same

INDICATIONS AND FINDINGS: The patient is a 36 y/o female Caucasian
who is four years status post left modified mastectomy for carcinoma.
She has had two occurrences in the past of nodularity in the incision
from her mastectomy. Both of these nodules were excised and were
found to be recurrent carcinoma. She presents at this time with a
one month history of a firm 7 mm. nodule in the lateral portion
of her mastectomy incision. This nodule was firmly attached to
the skin, was not tender and not freely mobile. It was felt at this
time that the nodule should be excised for pathologic examination.

The findings at the time of surgery were a firm 7 mm. nodule in
the lateral portion of the incision, which did not invade the subcutaneous tissue greater than a depth of approximately ½ cm.
The nodule was firmly attached to the overlying skin and was excised
with the overlying skin.

PROCEDURE: With the patient in the supine position and prep'd and
draped in the usual fashion, anesthetic was given by local infiltration of 1% Lidocaine without epinephrine. This local anesthesia
was given in a field fashion for a distance of approximately 1 cm.
in a radial direction around the aforementioned lesion. After
anesthesia had taken place, an elliptical incision was made along
the line of the previous mastectomy incision to include the aforementioned nodule. This incision was approximately 5 cm. in length.

The incision was carried down through the layers of the skin to
the subcutaneous tissue. The elliptical piece of skin was then
grasped at its lateral corner and dissected from the surrounding
tissue and from the subcutaneous tissue by sharp dissection with
the scalpel.

All bleeding was stopped using the Valley Lab electrocautery
device. The elliptical piece of skin and the underlying chest
wall nodule was completely excised in this fashion. After the
specimen was turned over to the pathologist, the operative field

continued...

110

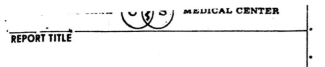
was examined for further bleeding points and all minimal bleeding
was stopped using the Vallen Lab electrocautery device. The
subcutaneous tissue was then closed using interrupted inverted
simple sutures of 4-0 chromic catgut. The skin was then closed
using interrupted vertical mattress sutures of 4-0 nylon.

All counts were correct x2. EBL: Negligible. No drains were
left in place. A dry sterile dressing was applied and the patient
was taken from the OR awake and alert and in good condition.

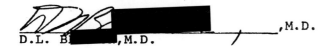 ,M.D.

D.L. B   ,M.D.

DLB:KR/tr
D: 8/24/78
T: 8/25/78

The final needle and sponge counts were correct as per the
Primary Surgical Log.

See also:
8485-76
C-2425-77
C-7776-77
16203-77

HOSP. NO:
ROOM:
AGE
DOCTOR:
RECEIVED:
SPECIMEN:

Patient #4   CA
                                7-20-76
CLINIC
12-06-42
L.M
August 24, 1978

Skin, chest wall

GROSS DESCRIPTION

Labeled "skin, chest wall" and received in Bouin's is an ellipse
of skin measuring 2 cm. in length and 1.0 cm. in width. The
skin is colored yellow from the Bouin's solution. However, in
the center of the ellipse there is an ill defined area roughly
0.8 cm. in diameter that has a somewhat brownish hue. There
are no ulcerations or nodules in this area. The subcutaneous
tissue extends to a depth of 0.6 cm. On serial sectioning the
subcutaneous tissue appears to contain diffuse hemorrhage.

A.   3)
B.   5) All embedded
C.   3)

                                                    JK:rt

DIAGNOSIS: Skin, chest wall (biopsy):
                Adenocarcinoma, consistent with metastatic
                   carcinoma of mammary gland origin
                Granulomas, subcutaneous tissues (no organisms
                   present)
                Cicatrix, skin of chest wall

                                        MF:ms

      T 01 - M 8146
      T 01 - M 4400

      8/28/78   MICHAEL F
                                        , M.D.   , M.D.
      DATE OF REPORT   RESIDENT   PATHOLOGIST
FORM NO. 1794(Rev. 1/78)   DIV. of ANATOMIC PATHOLOGY • LEO K   M.D., DIRECTOR

112

Patient #5

Patient #5 is a 78-year-old woman from Arkansas alive 13 years since diagnosed with metastatic breast carcinoma.

In early spring 1974, Patient #5 noticed a small, painless mass in her left breast, which gradually increased in size over a three-month period. In addition, she experienced chronic fatigue and diminished appetite, associated with a gradual, mild weight loss.

In June 1974, Patient #5 consulted her family doctor who noted a large, 5 cm tumor in the lower outer quadrant of the left breast. Subsequently, on June 20, 1974, she was admitted to Washington Regional Hospital in Fayetteville, Arkansas, where after a biopsy confirmed adenocarcinoma, she underwent a left radical mastectomy.

The final pathology report describes extensive disease invading into the axillary (armpit) region:

> There are lymph nodes throughout the axillary dissection which contain obvious tumor. These measures [sic] up to 2.5cm in greatest dimension. At the site of primary biopsy, there is extensive hemorrhage and additional tissue which suggests further tumor over a fairly large area, measuring up to 3cm in diameter. Some of this tissue is quite necrotic and friable. The breast tissue is not abundant.

In the summary section, the pathologist writes:

> Tissue from radical mastectomy showing extensive additional adenocarcinoma, similar to that seen in biopsy, and metastatic to lymph nodes at all levels of axillary dissection.

A consulting oncologist proposed an aggressive course of radiation to the chest wall, but Patient #5 decided to refuse further conventional treatment. As she told me, as a nurse for 25 years she had seen too many patients with cancer die after chemotherapy and radiation to have much faith in the standard approaches. And Patient #5 already knew of Dr. Kelley from a friend who followed his program; his regimen, she believed, represented her most sensible option.

After her discharge from the hospital on June 27, 1974, Patient #5 quickly deteriorated clinically; her surgical wound began to drain pus, she developed severe

113

anemia associated with fatigue and anorexia, and lost, over a two-week period, 10 pounds. When first seen by Dr. Kelley in mid-July 1974, Patient #5 was very ill.

Patient #5 began her nutritional regimen as soon as she returned home, and in the months that followed gradually recovered. Her incision healed, her anemia resolved, her energy and sense of well-being returned, and within a year she felt better than she had for decades.

Patient #5 continued the full protocol for four years, before tapering to a maintenance program. Today, 13 years since her diagnosis, she remains in excellent health with no sign of cancer. "I owe Dr. Kelley my life," she says simply.

For Patient #5, all signs pointed to a poor outcome. As discussed in the case of Patient #3, for patients with breast cancer the prognosis worsens as the number of positive axillary lymph nodes increases. At the time of diagnosis, Patient #5 had clear evidence of cancerous spread to many lymph nodes at all levels of the axilla, a particularly ominous finding.

For patients with locally metastatic disease, prognosis clearly correlates not only with the number of positive lymph nodes, but also the levels of axillary involvement. Cancerous nodes located higher in the axillary region portend a worse prognosis than disease restricted to lymph nodes lower down or closer to the breast. Hellman describes a study of 182 mastectomy specimens, in which the pathologist found evidence of malignancy in the highest area of the armpit in 15 cases. All 15 of these patients experienced relapse, "indicating," as he writes, "the grave prognosis associated with involvement high in the axilla."[1]

The size of the primary breast mass itself indicated poor-prognosis disease. At surgery, the tumor was judged to be at least 5 cm in diameter and in spite of some disruption during the procedure, the pathologist later identified multiple cancerous sections, each up to 3 cm across. The larger the tumor, the worse the prognosis, particularly when associated with metastases to axillary nodes.

For patients with tumors at least 5 cm in diameter with accompanying nodal involvement, the five-year, disease-free survival ranges from 21% to 35% in the studies reported to date.[2] However, these statistics refer to groups of patients undergoing radiation, chemotherapy, or both in addition to aggressive surgery. The percentages fall off drastically for patients untreated after mastectomy.

In summary, Patient #5 was diagnosed with breast cancer metastatic to multiple nodes at all axillary levels, and after surgery, chose only to follow the Kelley program. It seems reasonable to attribute her long-term disease-free survival, now in excess of 13 years, and her current good health to her nutritional regimen.

REFERENCES

1. DeVita, VT, et al. *Cancer Principles & Practice of Oncology*. Philadelphia; J.B. Lippincott Company, 1982, page 920.

2. DeVita, VT, et al., page 921.

DISCHARGE SUMMARY

ADMITTED: 6-20-74.
DISCHARGED: 6-27-74.

This 66 year old female was admitted on 6-20-74. She had been aware
of a nodule in her left breast for approximately three months, which
had apparently shown some gradual increase in size, but did not have
any other particular symptoms relating to this. She had neglected
consultation in regard to this, as her husband had some antitipated
surgery. However, when first seen by Dr. P▓▓▓▓, and later referred
to me, she was found to have approximately 5 cm. lass in the lower
outer quadrant of the left breast, which had some clinical indications
of a malignant tumor. She then agreed to a biopsy, after her husband
had had his cholecystectomy, and she was therefore admitted at this
time for biopsy and frozen section.

Chemistry 12 Profile was found to be within normal levels. Hb. was
12 grams, with 4,700 WBC, normal differential, and normal urinalysis.
Chest x-ray was normal.

She was taken to surgery on 6-21-74, where biopsy indicated this to
be adenocarcinoma, and a left radical mastectomy was carried out.
Postoperatively, however, she did extremely well, promptly becoming
ambulatory with a minimal amount of pain and discomfort. She became
tolerant of her diet, had no difficulty in voiding, and had return
of her bowel function. After change of her dressing, there did not
appear to be any evidence of accumulation of fluid, though she showed
some ischemic change of the medial flap of the skin. She was allowed
to be dismissed from the hospital on 6-27-74, and will be followed in
the office. Her subsequent pathological tissue report indicated that
she did have evidence of metastatic tumor to regional lymph nodes, and
it is anticipated that she will be given Cobalt therapy following
healing of her wound.

JACK A. W▓▓, M.D.
d. 7-12-74.
t. 7-15-74.
JAW:vrb

DISCHARGE SUMMARY

116

ANL MEDICAL LABORATORY
Fayetteville, Arkansas 72701

TISSUE EXAMINATION

dd: 6-24-74
dt: 6-24-74

WRMC

S-2695-74

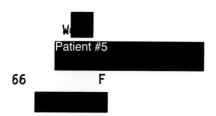

66   F

6-21-74 Mass in left breast.
         Left breast biopsy with FS.
         Carcinoma of left breast - left radical mastectomy.

         A. Biopsy of left breast   B. Left breast

GROSS: A. Specimen consists of a number of small fragments of gray to brownish tissue,
taken completely for microscopic examination. It appears that this tissue has dried out
somewhat following the frozen section and prior to fixation.

FROZEN SECTION DIAGNOSIS: A. Adenocarcinoma of breast.

        B. Specimen consists of tissue from a radical mastectomy. The skin segment mea-
sures 30cm x 12cm. The skin incision for the primary biopsy appears to be in the intra-
nipple area. The skin is somewhat inelastic, but does not appear indurated. The tissue
of the pectorales muscles is not remarkable. There are lymph nodes throughout the axillary dissection which contain obvious tumor. These measures up to 2.5cm in greatest
dimension. At the site of primary biopsy, there is extensive hemorrhage and additional
tissue which suggests further tumor over a fairly large area, measuring up to 3cm in
diameter. Some of this tissue is quite necrotic and friable. The breast tissue is not
abundant. There is abundant fat within the breast.

FINAL MICROSCOPIC DIAGNOSIS: A. Adenocarcinoma of breast.

MICROSCOPIC DIAGNOSIS: B. Tissue from radical mastectomy showing extensive additional
                          adenocarcinoma, similar to that seen in biopsy, and metastatic
                          to lymph nodes ar all levels of axillary dissection.
                          0401-8413, 0871-8146

M. B. N▓▓▓▓▓▓, M. D.

117

Patient #6

Patient #6 is a 78-year-old woman from Colorado with a history of metastatic breast carcinoma, alive 14 years since diagnosis.

Before developing cancer, Patient #6 had undergone a hysterectomy and oophorectomy for benign uterine disease. Otherwise, she had been in good health when in early spring of 1973, she noticed a non-tender mass in her left breast which enlarged over a two month period. Patient #6 consulted her family physician who, suspecting malignant disease, admitted her on May 14, 1973 to Presbyterian Medical Center in Denver for evaluation.

The following day, after biopsy studies confirmed invasive intraductal carcinoma, Patient #6 underwent a left radical mastectomy. Since the tumor appeared to be confined to the breast, at the time of discharge one week later no additional therapy was recommended.

For the next two years, as Patient #6 seemed to do well, her physicians remained optimistic about her prognosis. Furthermore, in December 1974, a follow-up bone scan and X-ray studies were completely clear.

But in mid-1976, three years after her original diagnosis, Patient #6 experienced right rib pain which her doctors initially attributed to a muscle sprain. When over the next several months her symptoms gradually worsened, in May 1977 she was referred for a bone scan and X-rays, both of which showed evidence of metastatic cancer. Her oncologist described the findings in his note:

> One week ago the patient had a repeat bone scan which had previously been negative and is now positive in the ribs and spine. Rib x-rays confirmed metastatic disease. A chest x-ray was negative. Thus, this 68 year old female developed new changes on bone scan and x-rays confirming metastatic bone disease.

In June 1977, Patient #6 began a course of Stilbestrol, a synthetic estrogen used to treat metastatic breast cancer. At the same time, she decided to investigate unconventional cancer therapies, including the Kelley regimen. She later discussed such options with her oncologist, who although skeptical, did not try to discourage her. In a letter to Patient #6 dated July 1, he wrote:

> I received your letter today regarding the Kelly [sic] Institute and nutrition . . .

I have no objections to any nutritional diet, including that proposed by the Kelly [sic] Institute, but I do wish to stress that I do not believe in the theories as proposed, as they are not scientifically founded.

After consulting with Dr. Kelley later that month, Patient #6 began the full nutritional program. She continued hormone therapy as well, and within weeks on this combined regimen, her bone pain improved. Within a year, her symptoms had completely resolved.

Her oncologist, not surprisingly, attributed the progress only to hormone therapy. In an April 1978 letter written to Patient #6's local physician, he discussed her condition but made no mention of Dr. Kelley or his regimen:

[Patient #6] continues to receive Stilbestrol therapy for her breast cancer. She remains clinically stable with no evidence for progression of disease.

But nine months later, in January 1979, Patient #6 decided to discontinue hormone therapy altogether, a decision strongly opposed by her doctors:

As you may know, [Patient #6] has elected to stop all of her hormonal therapy to which she has been responding for the last 1 1/2 years [again he discounted any effect from Dr. Kelley's regimen]. She is very involved in vitamin and nutritional therapy and has elected to see if this helps her as opposed to the recommended hormonal therapy.

At this time she is disease free and in a state of clinical remission.

Patient #6, to her doctors' surprise, continued to thrive. In fact, she did so well her oncologist, despite the obvious evidence, even questioned the original diagnosis of cancer rather than give Dr. Kelley any credit. In another letter, dated July 9, 1979, he wrote:

[Patient #6] has been off all hormonal treatment now for approximately six months with no evidence of any recurrent disease as per a recent bone scan.

As time goes by without therapy [again he dismissed the Kelley program as treatment], I am more concerned that our original diagnosis of bone metastasis was incorrect, but, as you know, she did have confirmatory x-rays of her positive areas on bone scan.

Today, Patient #6 still follows the Kelley program, and at age 78 reports feeling stronger and healthier than at any other time in her life.

Breast cancer, once disseminated, is a deadly disease; both Owens and Haagensen report a 0.0% five-year survival rate for patients with evidence of distant metastases.[1,2]

Although Patient #6 did receive a course of Stilbestrol, this therapy does not cure metastatic breast carcinoma. Only one-third of those treated with the hormone respond, and even in this group the disease inevitably recurs. Hellman reports that a mere 30% of postmenopausal patients with metastatic breast cancer show any benefit with hormonal therapy, with the responses lasting on average 12–14 months.[3]

Patient #6 periodically returns to her oncologist, who claims she is the healthiest cancer patient he has ever known. But Patient #6 herself finds such visits distressing. "It's difficult," she told me, "to sit in his waiting room time after time and watch so many patients be destroyed by chemotherapy."

Despite Patient #6's apparent cure, none of her physicians have expressed any interest in Dr. Kelley or his nutritional programs.

REFERENCES

1. Harvey, AM, et al. *The Principles and Practice of Medicine*, 20th Edition. New York; Appleton-Century-Crofts, 1980, page 629.

2. Haagensen, CD. *Diseases of the Breast*, Revised 2nd Edition. Philadelphia; WB Saunders, 1971, page 623.

3. DeVita, VT, et al. *Cancer Principles & Practice of Oncology*. Philadelphia; J.B. Lippincott Company, 1982, page 947.

TISSUE EXAMINATION

HOSPITAL NO. ▓▓▓ NAME Patient #6 ▓▓▓▓ AGE 64 ROOM NO. ▓▓▓

DATE 5-15-73 DR. J. S▓▓▓

ACCESSION NO.: S-73-2908

PRE-OP. DIAGNOSIS:

CLINICAL HISTORY: Breast mass, left outer quadrant

SURGERY: Left radical mastectomy

SPECIMEN: Left breast

POST OP IMPRESSION:

MACROSCOPIC:

The first submitted specimen, is a 3.5 cm. piece of fat surrounding a 1 cm. firm gray nodule with yellowish streaking. Frozen section diagnosis (F) was Comedo infiltrating carcinoma. The remainder of the tissue is submitted in capsules #1 through #4.

The second submitted specimen, labeled left breast consists of a 190 x 120 x 50 mm. portion of breast with attached pectoralis muscles which display a 35 x 57 mm. ellipse of skin which a central 7 mm. in diameter areola marked by a 9 mm. in diameter raised nipple. In the inner quadrant is a 57 mm. linear scar which is partially closed with silk sutures. The axillary contents are separated from the breast which is frozen. An addendum report of the breast will be submitted at a later date.

The axillary contents are resected as follows:
The level nearest the breast is I. Level furthest of the axilla is level III, The inner level of the areola is II. Four structures felt to be lymph nodes are palpated in level I and submitted in capsule #5. Five structures felt to be lymph nodes are palpated in level II and submitted in capsule #6. Six structures felt to be lymph nodes are palpated in level III and submitted in capsule #6. RPI:mae

MICROSCOPIC:
Examination of slides F-1-A and F-2-A reveal ducts marked by cribriform hyperplasia. These ducts have no myoepithelial layers. They are surrounded by dense fibrosis in which smaller ducts stream out in single file within the fibrous stroma.

Examination of slides #1 through #4 reveal increased intralobular fibrous connective tissue, cystic dilatation of the ducts, with a mild chronic inflammatory infiltrate surrounding these ducts. The lobules are orderly and regular but in two areas it is configured by fibrous connective tissue.

The four lymph node structures in slide #5 reveal sinus histiocytosis. Five structures in slide #6 and slide #7 contain no evidence of tumor tax metastasis. RPI:mae

DIAGNOSIS:
Left radical mastectomy - -
1. Intraductal carcinoma, invasive
2. 14 lymph nodes examined and negative for tumor

E.B. P▓▓▓ Jr., M.D.:mae
Pathologist

PHF 2 48 (Rev 4-45)

To: 434280

PATIENT'S NAME: *(redacted)* Patient #6

HOSPITAL NUMBER: *(redacted)*

ADMISSION DATE: May 14, 1973

DISCHARGE DATE: May 22, 1973

FINAL DIAGNOSIS:

Ca - of breast

COMPLICATIONS:

None -

OPERATIONS:

of Radical mastectomy

DISCHARGE SUMMARY:

This is a 64 year old female with a mass in the upper outer quadrant of the left breast for several months duration. On the day following admission the patient was taken to the Operating Room where breast biopsy and left radical mastectomy was performed. Postoperatively she did well without complications and was discharged home on May 22, 1973, and asked to return to the office in one week for further follow up.

JS/lb

cc: H.K *(redacted)*, M.D.

d: 6-17-73
t: 6-27-73

(SIGNATURE OF ATTENDING PHYSICIAN)

J.S *(redacted)*

122

Asked to see ██████████████████, a 68 year old female, by Dr.
John S█████ for evaluation of the patient's metastatic breast
carcinoma. The patient's internist is Dr. Herbert Ke██████.
The patient's cardiologist is Dr. Robert M████████.

Present Illness: Present illness on May 15, 1973 when the patient
underwent a left radical mastectomy at Presbyterian Medical Center
by Dr. John S█████. At that time all nodes were negative and the
patient was given no therapy including no postoperative therapy
or adjuvant therapy. The patient did well following this until
she has noted some right upper abdominal or rib pain which has
been intermittent over the last two years, but has recently become
progressively severe. One week ago the patient had a repeat bone
scan which had previously been negative and is now positive in
the ribs and spine. Rib x-rays confirmed metastatic disease.
A chest x-ray was negative. Thus, this 68 year old female developed
new changes on bone scan and x-rays confirming metastatic bone
disease.

At the current time, the patient is completely asymptomatic outside
of her right rib pain and is not having any anorexia, weight loss,
fevers or night sweats. The patient is postmenopausal and has
received no hormone medications.

Past Medical History: Past medical history is significant for
floppy mitral valve with associated PAT for which the patient
takes Inderal. Surgically the patient has had a tonsillectomy,
appendectomy, hernia repair, total abdominal hysterectomy and
bilateral salpingoooophorectomy and a right thyroidectomy. The
rest of the past medical and surgical history is unremarkable.

The patient takes Inderal, as above, and is allergic to Codeine,
Morphine derivatives and possibly to female hormones which have
caused severe nausea and vomiting in the past.

Family History: Negative for carcinoma.

Social History: Patient is married and is a retired school teacher.
The patient has had no children for no known specific medical reason.
The patient does not smoke or consume alcohol.

Physical Examination: Height: 5'4". Weight: 116#. Blood pressure:
90/58. Pulse: 80 and regular. Respiration: 16. Temperature: 98.6.
The patient is a very healthy appearing 68 year old female in no
acute distress. Head, ears, eyes, nose and throat: Unremarkable
including a normal funduscopic examination. Neck: Supple without
thyroid enlargement. Lymph nodes: None palpable. Skin: No rashes
lesions or jaundice. Breasts: Left mastectomy scar. Clean: Right
breast without masses or lesions. Lungs: Clear to auscultation and
percussion. Heart: No obvious discernable murmurs, rubs or gallops.
Abdomen: Flat, soft, non-tender without organomegaly or masses.
Pelvic-rectal examination: Not done. Extremities: No edema or
arthritic changes. Neurological examination: Physiologic.

Impression: Metastatic breast disease involving the bones in a postmenopausal female.

123

Plan: Plan to review the patient's hospital records including
x-rays and scans and obtain a liver scan and mammogram. Will also
check a chemistry profile, CBC and CEA.

This patient is a candidate for Stilbestrol therapy if she has
disease limited to bones. Even without estrogen binding protein
this patient is in a good category for estrogen response being
this far post-menopausal with a long disease free interval since
her original mastectomy. Statistically she has a 30% chance of
responding without estrogen binding knowledge.

After the above workup will institute Stilbestrol therapy in hopes
of patient tolerance considering her past history.

KMF/jg   Kyle M. F███, M. D.

HEMATOLOGY-ONCOLOGY ASSOCIATES

███████████████

DENVER, COLORADO 80218

███████████

ROBERT F. E███████, M.D., P.C., F.A.C.P.
PAUL K. H█████████ JR., M.D., F.A.C.P.
MARVIN P. B████████ M.D.
DAVID H. G██████████ M.D.
KYLE M. F████, M.D.

1 July, 1977

Patient #6

███████████████████

Dear ███████████:

I received your letter today regarding the Kelly Institute and
nutrition. I read, of course, your letter and the newsletter that
you sent to me.

I have no objections to any nutritional diet, including that
proposed by the Kelly Institute, but I do wish to stress that I
do not believe in the theories as proposed, as they are not
scientifically founded. I do believe in nutrition possibly
playing a definite role in the cause of cancer and possibly its
therapy. Unfortunately, however, this has not been proven on a
scientific basis.

Thus I have no objections to your obtaining a nutritional consultation
with the Kelly Foundation and believe that it will do no harm, and
possibly good. If Dr. Kelly is right regarding his diet helping
in the therapy of cancer, I am sure it will be for the wrong reasons.

I am returning your check, as I consider this part of my services
in caring for the total aspects of your disease.

If I can be of any further assistance, please do not hesitate
to call.

Sincerely,

Kyle M. F████, M.D.

KMF/p

125

HEMATOLOGY-ONCOLOGY ASSOCIATES

████████████████████

DENVER, COLORADO 80218

████████████

ROBERT F. B██████ M.D., P.C., F.A.C.P.
PAUL K. H██████ JR., M.D., F.A.C.P.
MARVIN P. ██████ M.D.
DAVID H. G██████, M.D.
KYLE M. F██, M.D.

April 10, 1978

John S██████, M. D.
████████████████
Denver, Colorado 80204

Re: Patient #6 ████████████████████

Dear John:

████████████████ continues to receive Stilbestrol therapy for her breast cancer. She remains clinically stable with no evidence for progression of disease. Most of her initial symptoms from the Stilbestrol have now disappeared and she is handling such much better.

Thank you once again for having me see ████████████ It is pleasing to see her doing so well at this time.

Sincerely,

Kyle M. F██, M. D.

KMF/jg
cc: Herbert K████████, M. D.
    Robert M████████, M. D.

126

HEMATOLOGY ONCOLOGY ASSOCIATES

███████████████████

DENVER, COLORADO 80218

███████████

ROBERT F. B███████ M.D., P.C., F.A.C.P.
PAUL K. H███████, JR., M.D., F.A.C.P.
MARVIN P. B███████, M.D.
DAVID H. G███████ M.D.
KYLE M. F███, M.D.

January 15, 1979

John S█████, M. D.
███████████████████
Denver, Colorado 80204

Re: Patient #6 ████████████

Dear John:

As you may know, ████████████████ has elected to stop all of her hormonal therapy to which she has been responding for the last 1½ years. She is very involved in vitamin and nutritional therapy and has elected to see if this helps her as opposed to the recommended hormonal therapy.

At this time she is disease free and in a state of clinical remission. Hopefully she will remain so in the months ahead.

Thank you again for having me see ████████████ I will keep you closely informed of future developments as they occur.

Sincerely,

KMF/jg   Kyle M. F███, M. D.
cc: Herbert B. K█████████, Jr., M. D.
    Robert M█████████, M. D.

127

HEMATOLOGY-ONCOLOGY ASSOCIATES

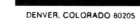

DENVER, COLORADO 80205

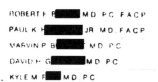

ROBERT F. F█████ M.D. P.C. FACP
PAUL K H█████ JR. M.D. FACP
MARVIN P B█████ M.D. P.C.
DAVID H G█████ M.D. P.C.
KYLE M. F█████ M.D. P.C.

July 9, 1979

John S█████, M. D.
█████████████████████
Denver, Colorado 80204

Re: Patient #6

Dear John:

████████████████ has been off all hormonal treatment now for
approximately six months with no evidence of any recurrent
disease as per a recent bone scan.

As time goes by without therapy, I am more concerned that
our original diagnosis of bone metastasis was incorrect, but,
as you know, she did have confirmatory x-rays of her positive
areas on bone scan. She may just have a long remission off of
therapy, but only time will tell.

Thank you again for having me see ████████████. It is very
pleasing to see her doing so well.

Sincerely,

KMF/jg   Kyle M. F████, M. D.
cc: Herbert B. Ke█████, Jr., M. D.
    Robert M████████, M. D.

128

Patient #7

Patient #7 is a 53-year-old woman alive more than 17 years since first diagnosed with breast carcinoma.

In 1970, Patient #7 first noticed a painless mass in her right breast. After a biopsy confirmed infiltrating carcinoma, she underwent a right radical mastectomy at St. Anthony's Hospital in Florida. Since the disease appeared localized, Patient #7's doctors suggested no adjuvant treatment at that time.

In 1973, after developing a tumor in her remaining breast, Patient #7 proceeded with a left radical mastectomy at St. Anthony's for what proved to be infiltrating carcinoma. At the time, Patient #7 was again assumed to be cured, but over the following year, her health gradually deteriorated. She experienced chronic fatigue, lethargy, and bouts of depression persisting for months at a time. In mid-1974, Patient #7 also developed pain along the length of the vertebral column and into the right shoulder that by late 1974 was so severe at times she was unable to dress herself or walk.

Although Patient #7 consulted her physicians repeatedly, they did not suggest an evaluation to determine the cause of her pain. Finally, at Patient #7's insistence in May 1975 her primary doctor ordered a series of spinal X-rays, which revealed an obvious abnormality in the fifth lumbar segment, described as "indicative of osteolytic metastasis from the breast carcinoma." A bone scan May 14, 1975 documented lesions consistent with metastatic disease in both the skull and right shoulder blade, reported as "focal abnormal uptakes of skull and tip of right scapula [shoulder], possibility of metastatic disease . . . "

On May 27, 1975, Patient #7 was admitted to St. Petersburg General Hospital in Florida for a bilateral oophorectomy (removal of both ovaries), a procedure intended to slow the growth of the tumor and ease her bone pain by reducing estrogen levels. Despite the surgery, Patient #7 was told she most probably would not live out the year, and in desperation, after leaving the hospital on May 31, 1975, Patient #7 decided to investigate alternative cancer therapies. She quickly learned of Dr. Kelley, consulted with him and began the nutritional program in the summer of 1975.

She told me that within six months, the persistent pain and depression completely resolved. According to the patient's statements, a bone scan at the end of 1975 showed some improvement, and a third bone scan, in mid-1976, demonstrated complete regression of the skeletal lesions, though the actual reports of these particular tests were no longer available when requested. Nonetheless, today, 12 years after her last episode of cancer, Patient #7 still follows the Kelley program, and is in excellent health.

As discussed previously, the five-year survival rate for patients with metastatic breast cancer approaches 0.0%, regardless of conventional therapy administered. And oophorectomy, which may lead to symptomatic improvement in this group, does not cure metastatic breast cancer. Hellman reports overall response rates for the procedure, in those women with estrogen-dependent disease, in the range of 30–40%. However, even among these patients, the benefit lasts only nine to 12 months on average, with little survival advantage.[1]

In summary, this patient developed evidence of metastases after successive mastectomies for recurring breast carcinoma. Although she did undergo oophorectomy, Patient #7 continued to deteriorate after the procedure. She received neither chemotherapy nor radiation, and her extensive disease and many symptoms resolved only after she began the Kelley program.

REFERENCE

1. DeVita, VT, et al. *Cancer Principles & Practice of Oncology*. Philadelphia; J.B. Lippincott Company, 1982, page 945.

PROCEDURE: BONE SCAN

REASON FOR EXAMINATION:

	TIME STAMP IN HERE	DATE TO BE DONE

M.

RADIONUCLIDE: AMOUNT: ROUTE OF ADMIN.

REPORT

NMD 715-75   5-14-75

The actual skeleton and skull are imaged after administration of
15 mCi of 99 mTc PP.   There are two or three areas of abnormal uptake
over the skull. There is also increased uptake of the tip of the right
scapula as compared to the left side.

IMPRESSION: FOCAL ABNORMAL UPTAKES OF SKULL AND TIP OF RIGHT SCAPULA.
              POSSIBILITY OF METASTATIC DISEASE SHOULD BE CONSIDERED.
RAE/mlb

Patient #7

Dr. F

age 41

DATE

R. E_____ M.D.

NUCLEAR MEDICINE CONSULTATION

131

DISCHARGE SUMMARY

PATIENT	Patient #7 ████████████		ROOM #	HOSP # ████
ATTENDING PHYSICIAN	Dr. ████	DATE OF ADMISSION 5-27-75		DATE OF DIS. 5-31-75

Physicians utilize order of dictation from suggested outline. Please include name of patient, room, admission and discharge dates.

Brief History of Present Illness

Consultation Findings

Summary of X-rays

Laboratory Summary

Minor Procedures

Operative Procedures and Dates

Course in Hospital

Discharge Medications

Discharge Status

Final Diagnosis

This 41 year old white female was admitted on 5-27-75 with a tentative diagnosis of metastatic CA of the breast.

She had a right mastectomy done in 1970 and had a left radical mastectomy done about 1½ years ago.

She had a chest x-ray done at Dr. ████ on 5-9-75 which showed no evidence of active infiltration of consolidation of either lung field. No pulmonary metastasis. The cardiac silhoutte was normal. Actually the chest x-ray showed little significant change compared to the previous x-ray of 11-4-74.

AP and lateral projection of the lumbosacral spine done on 5-9-75 showed osteoarthritis minimal of the lumbar spine. Also osteolytic defect of body 5th lumbar segment indicative of osteolytic metastasis from the breast carcinoma.

Bone scan done in this hospital on 5-14-75 showed focal abnormal uptakes of skull and tip of right scapula and possibility of metastatic disease.

Patient was taken to surgery on 5-28-75 and had an exploratory laparotomy and bilateral oophorectomy and appendectomy. No metastasis noted in liver or elsewhere.

Pathological exam revealed the ovaries and appendix to be normal.

Following an uneventful post operative course ████████████ is now discharged and I will check her in my office in 10 days.

Prognosis guarded.

DD: 12-16-75
DT: 12-18-75
dr
by M. G████ for

J. Crayton/████ M.D.   M.D.

I
M 6/28/75

ST. PETERSBURG GENERAL HOSPITAL

ADMISSION NO.
53246-5 C

MARITAL ST. DATE OF BIRTH AGE SEX
Marr.   41   F

ADM. DATE   TIME ADM.   TYPE ADM   ROOM-BED
5-27-75   3:00pm   DA   37-2

PERMANENT OR LEGAL ADDRESS
Same as above

RE-ADMISSION   PREV. ADM
YES NO X   No
PRE-ADMISSION   DATE AND ADM. CLERK
YES NO X   5-27-75 CH

PATIENT'S NEAREST RELATIVE (NAME, ADDRESS, PHONE NO.)
Husband: Same address

INSURANCE AND/OR MISCELLANEOUS INFORMATION
Continental National American
Agent: Robert C.
813-966-1356

GUARANTOR OF ACCOUNT
Self

PHONE NO.

ADDRESS
Same as above

ZIP CODE

CODE   ATTENDING PHYSICIAN/SERVICE
Dr. P

REFERRING PHYSICIAN   CONSULTANTS

MEDICARE "B"   MEDICARE NO
YES   NO

CONSULTANTS

HOSPITAL INSURANCE

CODE   ADMISSION DIAGNOSIS
540   Metastatic CA of Breast

SURGE SER

EST. LENGTH OF STAY INITIAL DIET.

POLICY NO.   ACCOUNT STATUS
                         3

CORONERS CASE   RELIGION AND CHURCH AFFILIATION
YES   NO   Cath, Hungarian Christian

GROUP   CERTIFIED

FINAL DIAGNOSIS
(UNDERSCORE CAUSE OF DEATH)   Metastatic carcinoma from breast
to bone

COMPLICATIONS OR
INFECTIONS: none

OPERATIONS/PROCEDURES: 5/28/75 Exploratory laparotomy
Bilateral oophorectomy and appendectomy.

CONDITION ON DISCHARGE
IMPROVED
UNIMPROVED

PATIENT'S CHART

133

CERVICAL CANCER

In 1987, cervical cancer claimed 6,800 lives in the United States.

Pap smears offer a simple and accurate means of detecting this disease, which if diagnosed early can be effectively treated with surgery and radiation. At present, 65% of patients with cervical carcinoma live five years.

Patient #8

Patient #8 is a 74-year-old woman from Canada alive nine years since her diagnosis of metastatic cervical cancer.

In mid-1977, Patient #8 experienced episodic vaginal bleeding that gradually worsened over a six month period. In January 1978, she finally consulted her gynecologist who on examination discovered, and biopsied, a cervical mass. When the tumor proved to be "invasive squamous cell carcinoma of the cervix," in early February 1978 Patient #8 was referred to the W.W. Cross Cancer Institute in Edmonton, Alberta. There, the doctors confirmed the diagnosis and assessed her cancer as early stage, localized (1B) disease.

The physicians at Cross recommended a course of radiation therapy, beginning with radium insertions into the cervical area, to be followed by 3500 rads of external beam radiation to the pelvis. Patient #8, who was already knowledgeable about alternative cancer therapies, suggested to her doctors a nutritional approach. Her physician wrote in his notes:

> Apparently she [Patient #8] is a little worried about radiation therapy treatment but we have tried to explain to her the only orthodox treatments at the present time for her condition are surgical or radiotherapeutic and that in view of the surgical complication rates, it is our policy in this clinic . . . to employ radiation as a routine. . . . I think both she and her daughter are a little doubtful about accepting this and she wonders whether some dietary methods may be helpful. I have informed her that there is no evidence known to me to suggest that diet will influence cancer to any significant degree and that any delay in commencing treatment will almost certainly lead to impaired chances of cure . . .

After Patient #8 returned home to consider her options, her physician continued to press for radiation therapy. In mid-February 1978 he even enlisted family members in his efforts, as detailed in the official records:

> This patient called in to say that she did not want to take our offer of treatment . . . I called her daughter . . . and had a long talk . . . The daughter is to continue to try and change her mother's mind . . .

Because of such pressure, Patient #8 returned to the Cross Institute on February 20, 1978, for her first course of radium insertion therapy. She tolerated the initial treatment without difficulty, but after her second round on March 8, 1978, she experienced constant heartburn, severe abdominal pain, and urinary difficulties, all attributed to the radiation. Despite her symptoms, she began external beam radiotherapy on March 22, 1978, receiving 1150 rads to the anterior and posterior pelvis over a five day period.

Patient #8 was scheduled for additional therapy in early April 1978, but decided, although opposed by her family and physicians, to stop treatment. Her physician wrote in an April 14, 1978 note:

> I had a long talk with her and daughter [sic], the patient is obviously got [sic] an Ostrich Syndrome. She thinks that if she doesn't have any treatment the disease will go away. . . . I have emphasized that her maximum chances of cure and control of her disease are a full treatment now and that we can not add on in the future to the partial treatment she has taken to date.

Patient #8 held her ground, but then quickly began to deteriorate. Later that month she developed severe weakness and fatigue, and when her vaginal bleeding recurred, she returned to the Cross Institute on May 14, 1978.

Though a cervical smear revealed residual malignancy, Patient #8 refused to resume therapy. Instead, after leaving Cross, she consulted Dr. Kelley for the first time, but due to her family's antagonism toward him, Patient #8 did not begin her prescribed protocol.

Throughout the summer, as the patient pursued no treatment, the cancer grew unchecked, and in September 1978, Patient #8 developed a partial urinary tract obstruction brought on by the enlarging pelvic tumors. A renogram confirmed declining function in both kidneys, but Patient #8 still refused all conventional intervention.

In late October 1978, after her vaginal bleeding worsened, Patient #8 was admitted on an emergency basis to Misericordia Hospital. During their evaluation, her doctors noted a large abdominal mass extending into the bladder. Her physician wrote:

> The lower abdomen was tender and it was felt likely that there was some urinary retention. However because of the tumor mass rising up out of the pelvis, it was difficult to assess. Severely anemic, with a hemoglobin of 7.4 (normal 12-16), she required multiple transfusions before finally stabilizing.

137

Patient #8 was seen by a staff oncologist, who, recommending no treatment other than palliative care and pain control, prescribed the Brompton Cocktail, a highly potent pain mixture usually reserved for dying cancer patients.

Family members were told Patient #8 most probably would not live more than several weeks, and at their request, she was discharged from the hospital on November 3, 1978, so she might die at home. On the official summary from that date, the provisional diagnosis reads "CA UTERUS—TERMINAL" with a secondary diagnosis of "METASTATIC SPREAD TO ABDOMINAL CAVITY."

After a difficult night, Patient #8 was readmitted to Misericordia the following day. Her physician again noted the large abdominal tumor, as described in the records: [the] "abdomen showed marked tenderness in the lower abdomen with a hard tumor mass rising up out of the pelvis."

The family planned to place her in a nursing facility for terminal care, but Patient #8 contacted Dr. Kelley, who suggested she start the full program at once. Because of his support, she insisted on returning home during the second week of November 1978, so she might begin her protocol.

Despite the skepticism of her family, Patient #8 quickly improved on her nutritional regimen. Over the following year, her abdominal tumors regressed completely, her kidney function returned to normal, and she was able to discontinue all pain medications without experiencing narcotic withdrawal.

Today, more than nine years after her terminal diagnosis, Patient #8 currently reports good health with no sign of cancer. A recent Pap smear and abdominal ultrasound, she told me, were both negative for malignancy.

Patient #8 regrets only that she didn't refuse all radiation and begin the Kelley program sooner. She feels her course would have been much easier, had she ignored the expert advice of her orthodox physicians and instead followed her instincts.

CLINIC No. ███████

RE: Patient #8 ████████████

EDMONTON ☐   CALGARY ☐   LETHBRIDGE ☐

February 9, 1978

████████ reports to the joint consultative clinic today with a
confirmed diagnosis of invasive squamous cell carcinoma of the cervix.
The story is that she had a menopause at about age 50. She is now
65 years of age. For the past 7 months, she has been having intermittent
bloody discharge. She promptly reported to her doctor and a biopsy
was taken from the cervix. She states that until just before this
biopsy she had not had a Pap smear for several years.

On examination, no enlargement of cervical or supraclavicular nodes.
The abdomen is soft, no masses are felt. The vulva is healthy. The
vagina appears to be healthy. There is an exophytic tumor mass
protruding from the anterior lip of the cervix. There is tumor
involving the posterior lip of the cervix, but is somewhat hidden
by the mass. We do not think that this has encrouched on the vagina,
although possibly on the left lateral fornix is very close and we
will have to defer this impression until we have an opportunity to
examine her under anesthesia. Certainly on rectal and rectovaginal
examination, there is no clinical evidence of spread into the parametrial tissues and on this basis, we would tenatively stage this
as a Stage Ib lesion. Arrangements are being made for her to be
admitted to the W.W.Cross Institute for a preliminary work-up and
for radium insertions followed by a course of external beam therapy.

Dr. L. B. B█████lks

cc: Dr. R. L███

CARD: February 13, 1978 (TBA)

10/2/78

139

CLINIC No. ▉▉▉▉▉▉

RE: Patient #8 ▉▉▉▉▉▉▉▉▉▉▉

EDMONTON ☐   CALGARY ☐   LETHBRIDGE ☐

February 9, 1978

This patient has been referred by Dr. L▉▉ on account of postmenopausal bleeding. A pap smear has been reported as invasive carcinoma and a cervical biopsy shows invasive squamous cell carcinoma. The patient attended the Cancer Clinic today and was seen with Dr. G▉▉▉▉▉▉▉ and Dr. B▉▉▉. On pelvic examination there is an exophytic tumor arising most on the anterior lip but possibly extending onto the posterior lip. There is a slight suspicion as also that it may be into the left lateral fornix in a minimal fashion. Rectal examination confirms the extremely good mobility of the uterus. There were no peripheral pelvic nodules to be felt. Patient also suffers with dyspepsia and excessive flatulence and we note that the flat plate of her abdomen today shows excessive colonic and small bowel gas. This is rather worrying to the patient. She has been on a voluntary diet, has dropped from 250 lbs to her present weight.

Apparently she is a little worried about radiation therapy treatment but we have tried to explain to her the only orthodox treatments at the present time for her condition are surgical or radiotherapeutic and that in view of the surgical complication rates, it is our policy in this clinic along with many other world centres to employ radiation as a routine. The treatment offered to the patient has been two radium insertions and three weeks of external beam parametrial radiation. I think both she and her daughter are a little doubtful about accepting this and she wonders whether some dietary methods may be helpful. I have informed her that there is no evidence known to me to suggest that diet will influence cancer to any significant degree and that any delay in commencing treatment will almost certainly lead to impaired chances of cure. Provisional arrangements have been made to admit the patient on Tuesday, February 14th, 1978 for EUA radium insert the following day. She will also have an IVP, renogram, liver scan, cystoscopy by Dr. B▉▉▉ and Dr. B▉▉▉ will do a sigmoidoscopy at the same time. If the patient ultimately decides against this treatment she will call in and cancel out these arrangements. Note she has had a flat plate of abdomen today which shows gaseous distension and a Barium enema showing no constriction lesions or filling defects. If the patient does not wish to accept this treatment then she will call in and cancel the arrangements. Check card in one week.

cc: Dr. R. S. Y. L▉▉   Dr. G. A. G▉▉▉▉▉/gs

140

PROGRESS NOTES

CLINIC No. ▮▮▮▮▮▮▮

RE:

Patient #8 ▮▮▮▮▮▮▮▮▮▮▮▮▮▮▮▮▮

EDMONTON ☑   CALGARY ☐   LETHBRIDGE ☐

Feb ruary 14, 1978

This patient called in to say that she did not want to take our offer of treatment
for herStage IIB carcinoma of the cervix. I called her daughter, Miss ▮▮▮▮▮
▮▮▮▮, and had a long talk and decided again that the early nature of this
lesion and it has a good chance of a cure and how these are being eroded by
waiting. She is more worried about her gastrointestinal upsets. I explained
that it could be that the cervix cancer is making the gastrointestinal upsets
worse. It is thought a psychological rejection phenomenom and implying that
radiation will have some degree of discomfort, this was on ly temporary
and is not anywhere near as uncomfortable as the cancer would be if left.
The daughter is to continue to try and change her mother's mind and that
the booking which was made for this week should be postponed till next week.

Dr. G.A. G▮▮▮▮▮▮/smg

cc: Dr. R.S. L▮▮
     Dr. L. B▮▮▮

141

CLINIC No. ███████

RE: Patient #8 ████████

EDMONTON ☐   CALGARY ☐   LETHBRIDGE ☐

April 4, 1978

*This patient missed treatments last week ~~during~~ owing to disorderly
action of the heart. I presume that not very much was found
and she has also missed treatment yesterday. I had a long
talk with her and daughter, the patient is obviously got an
Ostrich Syndrome. She thinks that if she doesn't have any
treatment the disease will go away. Her daughter agrees
with this. I have emphasized that her maximum changes of cure
and control of her disease are a full treatment now and that
we can not add on in the future to the ~~powerful~~ partial treatment she
has taken to date. I have agreed with them that there is a
chance amounting to no more than 40% at the utmost that we
have controlled her disease with the treatment she has already
had, that her present supplementary perimetrial irradiation is
to control the probability of lymph node metastases tumor in the
pelvis which I have put at 60% chance of being present at her stage
of disease. I have also, one again, re-emphasized the reactions at
the present time are due to the radium insertions rather than the
8MeV x-rays which she is taking. Inspite of all this I understand
the patient wishes to exert her perogative of refusing further
treatment. Therefore, her treatment for Stage IIA squamous carcinoma
of the cervix has been been by means of 2 radium insertions to
full dosage and partial supplementary 8MeV x-ray treatments from
the 22nd of March to the 31st of March, 1978. Five fractions of
treatment were given over 10 days to a anterior and posterior field
set-up measuring 14x17 cm, central lead shielding to both using
8MeV x-rays at 100 cm SAD. A total dosage of 1150 rads at the
midplane.*

*Appointment = 1 month, gyne follow-up, Monday, pm. In the meantime
she should continue with Pyridium, and a high fluid intake to control
her cystitis which should be settled down in the next 7 to 10 days
and for her mucusy diarrhea I would suggest Anusol HC or Proctosedyl
rectal suppositories, 1 tid. The irradiated skin will probably be
very little trouble at the dosage administered. She will probably
be able to wash and bathe, ad lib in another 1 week.*

Dr. G.A. G████████   /dw

cc: Dr. R.S.L.██
    Dr. L. B:████   FILE COPY

142

ROOM NUMBER	PREVIOUS ADMISSION					27-10-78			
303	PA YES								

PATIENT PHONE			EMERGENCY PHONE			
RES. ███	BUS.		RES.	BUS.		

EMERGENCY NOTIFICATION		ADDRESS	RELATIONSHIP
███	SAME	DAUGHTER	

CONDITION

EMERG. ☒☒ URGENT ☐ ELECT. ☐ OTHER HOSPITAL ☐

PROV.	WELFARE	CHILD	GUARANTOR	ADDRESS
	CITY		SELF SAME	███

W.C.B.	EMPLOYER	OCCUPATION
	RETIRED	

DEPOSIT	SAFEKEEPING	DOCTOR NUMBER	FINANCE USE
NOT RE.Q	YES no ☒☒		10-24-98

TIME	ADM. BY	SERVICE	PROVISIONAL DIAGNOSIS	DISCHARGE DATE
2245	CB		CA UTERUS - TERMINAL	NOV 3 1978

MEDICAL SUMMARY
TO INCLUDE: CLINICAL HISTORY, PHYSICAL EXAMINATION, LABORATORY FINDINGS, X-RAY FINDINGS, TREATMENT, PROGRESS, OPERATIONS, CONSULTANTS.

CLINICAL HISTORY: This 66 year old woman was admitted on Oct 27/78. She came via the Admitting Room. She was known to have carcinoma of the uterus and had had treatment at the W.W.C.C.I. earlier this year. The daughter brought her into the hospital and stated that she had been bleeding for several weeks and felt very weak. There as urinary difficulty (strangury) and there were bowel problems. In view of these difficulties it was decided to admit her for assessment and treatment of her urinary problems.

She was given Morphine and Stemetil in the Emergency Room.

PHYSICAL EXAMINATION: A very anxious and obviously ill 66 year old woman. The patient was fibrillating. BP 162/92 with P 108 and irregularly irregular. Abdomen was bloated. Liver and spleen could not be felt. The lower abdomen was tender and it was felt likely that there was some urinary retention. However because of the tumor mass rising up out of the pelvis, it was difficult to assess.

Initial Assessment was that this patient had Carcinoma of the Cervix with Pelvic Spread.

LABORATORY FINDINGS: Hgb. 7.2 gm. on admission, WBC 31,400, 92% polys, 4% lymphs, 4% monos, 2% bands. BUN 31 mg/dl. Electrolytes essentially normal. Repeat BUN showed it had increased to 45 mg/dl. Urinalysis showed 3+ occult blood, 4+ protein and it was presumed that these findings were indicative of tumor involvement of the bladder. Multi 12 showed marked changes in the biochemistry in that the Albumin was down and BUN was up as indicated and also Creatinine to 2 mg%. There was slight elevation of Alk. Phos.

TREATMENT & PROGRESS: The patient was seen by Dr. F███ in consultation and he noted the marked anemia and the frozen pelvis with carcinoma. He felt that he was unable to examine her adequately rectally because of hemorrhoids and he agreed that she should continue with Foley catheter drainage (continuous) and other supportive measures.

cont'd

DISCHARGE STATUS:
DISCHARGED ALIVE
☐ WITH APPROVAL
☐ AGAINST ADVICE

TRANSFERRED TO
☐ OTHER HOSPITAL
☐ EXT. CARE FACILITY
☐ HOME CARE PROGRAM

DIED (INCLUDING STILLBORN)
☐ AUTOPSY   ☐ IN O.R.   ☐ POST OPERATIVE
☐ NO AUTOPSY   ☐ CORONER'S CASE

PRIMARY DIAGNOSIS: CARCINOMA OF CERVIX

COMPLICATIONS: NONE

SECONDARY DIAGNOSIS: METASTATIC SPREAD TO ABDOMINAL CAVITY
URINARY RETENTION WITH STRANGURY
SEVERE ANEMIA (FOLLOWING HEMORRHAGE)
HEMORRHOIDS
ATRIAL FIBRILLATION
The initial irregularity of the heart settled during her stay in hospital.

INFECTIONS NONE

P.A.S. DONE ☐
I HAVE READ AND APPROVED THE MEDICAL PORTIONS ON
THIS RECORD ON _____ 19___

SIGNATURE OF ATTENDING PHYSICIAN

143

DISCHARGED: Nov 3/78

      Initially he felt that chemotherapy might be considered but subsequently he decided not to. She was also seen by Social Services in consultation and they arranged for VON and homemaker to go into the house.
      The patient was given IV therapy and catheterized. Initially she was given Morphine but subsequently it was decided to start her on Brompton cocktail starting with 30 cc. q3-4h. Subsequently the frequency of this was able to be reduced to q6h. She was also given Stemetil for relief of nausea and Septra. To relieve her bowel problems she was given Surfak. On this regimen she made progress. Pastoral Care was invited to see her. The family obviously responded to the measures which were being taken and she was being discharged home on Nov 3/78 with a prescription for Brompton Cocktail. She had the catheter in when discharged home and arrangements were made for the VON to irrigate the catheter and change when necessary.
<u>CONSULTANT</u>: Dr. C.P. F███, Social Services

D Nov 27/78
T Dec 7/78

cc Dr. A.G. D██████ (2)
    Dr. R. L███
    W.W.C.C.K.   Dr. D██████/mb

_____
DATE   SIGNATURE

144

PATIENT PHONE		EMERGENCY PHONE SA				Patient #8
RES. ████ BUS.		RES.	BUS.			
EMERGENCY NOTIFICATION ████		SA	ADDRESS	RELATIONSHIP		
CONDITION						
EMERG. XXXX URGENT ☐ ELECT. ☐		OTHER HOSPITAL ☐				
PROV. WELFARE CITY	CHILD	GUARANTOR SELF		ADDRESS		
W.C.B.	EMPLOYER RETIRED		OCCUPATION			ABC OR PRIVATE INSURANCE
DEPOSIT 5.00	SAFEKEEPING YES XXX NO	DOCTOR NUMBER	FINANCE USE		MAIDEN NAME — LAST NAME UNDER ████
TIME 2000	ADM. BY EP	SERVICE	PROVISIONAL DIAGNOSIS METASTATIC CA CERVIX		DISCHARGE DATE NOV 11 1978

MEDICAL SUMMARY
TO INCLUDE: CLINICAL HISTORY, PHYSICAL EXAMINATION, LABORATORY FINDINGS, X-RAY FINDINGS, TREATMENT, PROGRESS, OPERATIONS, CONSULTANTS.

NOTE: THIS PATIENT NOT R.C. BUT WOULD LIKE TO HAVE DR. FATHER K████ VISIT WITH HER, WHEN HE RETURNS.

CLINICAL HISTORY: this is a readmission for a patient who had previously been in hospital and is known to have cancer of the cervix with abdominal spread. She had been discharged home with Brompton Cocktail the day prior to admission. She had a Foleys catheter but although arrangements had been made for her to be supervised at home, the family felt they could not cope and she was therefore brought back and readmitted via the emergency room.

PHYSICAL EXAM: she was certainly in better condition then when she had been discharged previously. She was not dehydrated. The catheter appeared to have been blocked by clots. Patient was feeble but in no particular distress at time of admission. H&N clear; heartsounds normal; BP 112/80; lungs clear; abdomen showed marked tenderness in the lower abdomen with a hard tumor mass rising up out of the pelvis. There was some mild edema of the lower legs.

Consultation: she was seen by Dr. W████ because of her urinary problems and he advised that if the foley catheter is not satisfactory, then #22 or #24 2-way catheter should be inserted with the irrigating arm clamped so as to be used as the need arises. He further advised that if the catheter did block with clots, it would have to be changed or irrigated and this could be done at home or in the emergency room. Social service have arranged for nursing and home care services.

LAB DATA: Hg 7.3 gm%; WBC 13,100 with 83 polys, 2% eosin, 10% lymphs, 4% monos, 1% bands; sed rate 141 mm/hr; electrolytes were normal; urinalysis showed 3+ occult blood, protein 4+ with more then 50 rbc/hpf and more then 50 pus cells/hpf. Multi 12 showed albumin to be down and alkaline phosphatase slightly elevated; urine for C&S showed gram positive organisms with colony count greater then 10 to the 5th. Bactrim tabs 2 bid was used during her stay in hospital. She did well and was discharged home on Nov 11th 1978. Consultant: Dr. W████

DISCHARGE STATUS: DISCHARGED ALIVE			Social Services DIED (INCLUDING STILLBORN)		
☐ WITH APPROVAL	☐ OTHER HOSPITAL	☐ HOME CARE PROGRAM	☐ AUTOPSY	☐ IN O.R.	☐ POST OPERATIVE
☐ AGAINST ADVICE	☐ EXT. CARE FACILITY		☐ NO AUTOPSY	☐ CORONER'S CASE	

PRIMARY DIAGNOSIS:	COMPLICATIONS:
CARCINOMA OF THE CERVIX	D – 30 Nov 78
	T – 4 Dec 78
SECONDARY DIAGNOSIS:	INFECTIONS c.c. Dr. D████ (2)
METASTATIC SPREAD TO ABDOMINAL CAVITY URINARY DYSFUNCTION	Dr. R. L████
	Dr. W.W.C.C.I.
	P.A.S. DONE ☐
	I HAVE READ AND APPROVED THE MEDICAL PORTIONS ON
	THIS RECORD ON _____ 19__
	Dr. AG D████/rp
	SIGNATURE OF ATTENDING PHYSICIAN

145

COLON CANCER

In 1987, colon cancer claimed 52,000 lives. Only lung cancer kills more.

Survival figures have improved in recent years, largely because of more effective diagnostic techniques. Today, about 50% of all patients with colon cancer live five years, although the number drops to less than 6% once the disease has metastasized.

Patient #9

Patient #9 is a 74-year-old woman from California alive more than ten years since her diagnosis of colon cancer.

In late 1976, Patient #9 experienced episodes of "stabbing" mid-abdominal pain that worsened over a several month period. When her symptoms persisted, in December 1976, she consulted her family doctor who referred her to a local clinic for tests. After a barium enema revealed a large mass in the region of the midtransverse colon, Patient #9 was admitted to Santa Cruz Hospital on December 15, 1976 for hemicolectomy (removal of half of the large intestine).

At surgery, Patient #9 was found to have a large tumor penetrating through the colon wall, described in the pathology report as a "nearly circumferential centrally ulcerated neoplasm . . . Cut sections through the tumor area disclose infiltration of the entire bowel wall into the subserosa." The malignancy was identified as a moderately differentiated adenocarcinoma, metastatic to the only two lymph nodes examined.

Patient #9 was told her disease most likely would recur and prove terminal, but no additional treatment was recommended at the time. Subsequently, despite the poor prognosis, she seemed to do well for a time. In April 1977, four months after surgery, her blood level of carcinoembryonic antigen (CEA)—a protein antigen that malignant colon cells often produce in large amounts—was reported as 1.1, well within the normal range (less than 2.5). Furthermore, her physical exam was normal, and, though her physicians still assumed the disease would eventually recur, a consulting oncologist again believed treatment unwarranted. He wrote in his records:

> I saw the patient in consultation in the spring of 1977, at which time I reviewed her studies and felt that although there was a substantial risk of recurrence because of the involvement of lymph nodes, that there was no evidence that the addition of chemotherapy would improve her chances for cure.

Only months later, Patient #9 began experiencing sharp pains in her back, chest, and shoulders, associated with the onset of fatigue, depression, and occasional bouts of abdominal discomfort which she described as a "bloated, nauseated feeling."

In July 1977, a barium enema, upper GI series, and proctoscopic examination showed no sign of recurrent disease. A repeat carcinoembryonic antigen level came back at 1.7, slightly elevated from the previous result, but still within the normal range.

Throughout the fall, Patient #9's muscular and abdominal pains, as well as her gastrointestinal symptoms worsened. In November 1977, a third CEA level was reported as 2.8, a slightly abnormal reading indicating, her doctors began to suspect, possible active cancer.

On December 10, 1977, Patient #9 was admitted to Dominican Santa Cruz Hospital for re-evaluation, at which time her various pains were sufficiently severe to require Dilaudid, a very potent synthetic morphine. However, her doctors could find no reason for her declining health, and after an inconclusive investigation, Patient #9 was discharged from the hospital with a supply of pain medication.

Subsequently, over a period of a year, Patient #9 continued to deteriorate, so that by the end of 1978 she had become bedridden. In desperation, she decided to investigate unconventional cancer therapies, quickly learned of Dr. Kelley, consulted with him in January 1979, and started on the full nutritional program. She reported to me that within weeks, she felt herself improving, and within a year, her once disabling musculoskeletal pains, her fatigue, depression, and abdominal discomfort resolved completely. Today, more than ten years since her original diagnosis, Patient #9 at age 74 is in excellent health with no evidence of cancer.

Though Patient #9 is not a definitive case because I cannot provide biopsy or radiographic proof of recurrent disease, for a number of reasons, her chances for prolonged survival were dim. First of all, several characteristics of her initial disease predict a poor prognosis. Ulcerating colon tumors as in this case, and tumors that encircle or nearly encircle the circumference of the large bowel correlate with diminished survival.[1] At the time of surgery the tumor had already infiltrated "well into the perimuscular fat"—another finding associated with a poor outcome.

In addition, the two lymph nodes biopsied were both positive for malignancy. Sugarbaker writes that lymph node involvement represents the single most important variable in terms of prognosis for patients diagnosed with localized colorectal cancer.[2] Copeland et al report a 25% five-year disease-free survival rate in a group of 68 aggressively treated patients with colorectal cancer and two positive nodes.[3]

Patient #9's rising CEA levels during 1978 suggest return of her disease. This tumor marker, as measured by the same laboratory, increased from 1.1 in April 1978 to 2.8 in November.

Patient #9's clinical condition, as documented by the medical records, deteriorated significantly throughout 1978, warranting more than one extensive evaluation. Whether she suffered cancer or not she clearly was very ill. Altogether, the characteristics of her tumor, the positive lymph nodes, the rising CEA levels and Patient #9's weakened state pointed toward a poor outcome.

REFERENCES

1. DeVita, VT, et al. *Cancer Principles & Practice of Oncology*. Philadelphia; J.B. Lippincott Company, 1982, pages 668–669.

2. DeVita, VT, et al., page 672.

3. Copeland, EM, et al. "Prognostic Factors in Carcinoma of the Colon and Rectum." *American Journal of Surgery* 1968; 116:875–880.

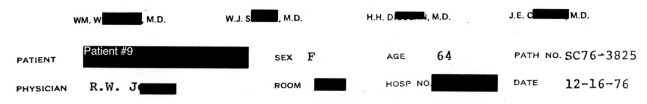

WM. W_____, M.D.   W.J. S_____, M.D.   H.H. D_____, M.D.   J.E. C_____, M.D.

PATIENT Patient #9	**SEX** F	**AGE** 64	**PATH NO.** SC76-3825
PHYSICIAN R.W. J_____	**ROOM**	**HOSP NO.**	**DATE** 12-16-76

GROSS

Specimen consists of a right colectomy specimen. It includes a short 2.0 cm segment of terminal ileum, the cecum, appendix and right colon. The right colon portion of the specimen measures 35 cm in length. Opening the specimen discloses the presence of a nearly circumferential centrally ulcerated neoplasm which is located 8.0 cm from the distal margin or end of resection. Elsewhere the mucosa is grossly unremarkable. The ileocecal valve is normally structured. Cut sections through the tumor area disclose infiltration of the entire bowel wall into the subserosa.

The specimen includes a large 18 x 10 cm portion of omental tissue. Multiple sectioning discloses no gross abnormalities.

Multiple sectioning of the mesentery discloses the presence of only two identifiable lymph nodes, each about 0.4 cm in diameter. WHW

MICROSCOPIC

Sections through the tumor area disclose a moderately differentiated adenocarcinoma that infiltrates well into the perimuscular fat. There is a particularly extensive desmoplastic reaction in the subserosal area. Sections of colon wall distal to the neoplasm disclose no pathological changes. The section of ileum discloses the presence of melanin like pigment within the lamina propria of the mucosa. Sections of the appendix disclose no pathological changes.

Sections of the two grossly identified lymph nodes disclose that both of them are replaced by metastatic tumor with an associated extensive desmoplastic reaction.

DIAGNOSIS: RIGHT HEMICOLECTOMY: MODERATELY DIFFERENTIATED ADENOCARCINOMA OF THE COLON WITH METASTASES TO TWO REGIONAL LYMPH NODES.

PAS 6

MELANOSIS, ILEAL MUCOSA.

colon, adenoca

WILLIAM H. W_____, M.D.
12-20-76   pc

151

☐ HISTORY and PHYSICAL EXAMINATION

☐ OPERATION REPORT

☒ DISCHARGE SUMMARY

☐ CONSULTATION REPORT

DATE: ADMITTED: 12/15/76   DISCHARGED: 12/22/76

The patient was admitted with a lesion in the transverse colon which was a moderately undifferentiated adenocarcinoma. She was taken to the operating room on the day following her admission and bowel prep and a right hemi-colectomy was performed. The abdomen was free of gross metastases and no grossly enlarged lymph nodes were detected. Pathologic report showed two small nodes affected by the tumor and penetration of the tumor into the pericolic fat, with almost complete circumferential involvement of the colon. Her postop course was uneventful and she has made a nice recovery. At the present time, she is eating a soft diet. She is ambulant. The wound is nicely healed. The stitches are removed and she is ready for discharge and outpatient follow up to be carried out at the office in about one week.

ROBERT W. J████, M.D. F.A.C.S.

12/22/76 - 12/22/76 lm

December 9, 1977

Michael A█████████, M.D.
████████████████████
Santa Cruz, California

Re: ⬭ Patient #9 ████████████

Dear Michael:

You will remember having seen ████ on referral by
Dr. R. W. J█████, M.D. She is now one year post op
right hemicolectomy for moderately differentiated
carcinoma of the colon with metastases to two
regional lymph nodes.

She has been quite anxious in recent weeks because
of migratory musculoskeletal aches, without involvement of joints, but being in "back, legs, around
lower thorax", seeming to radiate in this area from
the left scapular area, often described as becoming
worse as the day progresses. There has been no
associated fever or chills. One time she had a
slight cough and claims to have raised some mucus
at times, with a trace of yellow color. No hemoptysis.
She hadn't observed that the cough would aggravate the
discomfort in the left scapular area. She has been
very aware of her bowel function, but none of her
symptoms have suggested serious problems. She does use
bran and Metamucil for bowel function, and occasionally
she states that she uses oil with her salads, and this
seems to benefit the bowel function.

In the Spring, after she returned from Europe, she had
a period of having some loose stools and abdominal
discomfort with associated "bloaty, nauseated" feelings.
At that time, Dr. J████ had three stool specimens checked,
for pathogens or parasites, but those were all normal.
After Bob left for Huston, Texas, I have seen ██████ on
two or three occasions, and, because of persisting
symptoms, I did order a Barium Enema in September.
Dr. M█████ reported it as a normal examination following
right hemicolectomy. An Upper GI Series showed no
evidence of tumor or ulcer. Copies of those reports
are enclosed.

Dr. J████ had also advised that she repeat the liver
chemistries and CEA studies in January, but because o

153

of her recent migratory discomfort and her anxiety,
I ordered these in November and the Panel 13 study
showed alkaline phosphatase, SGOT, LDH, total proteins,
albumen and globulin, and bilirubin values normal.
Urinalysis was normal. CBC was normal, including
a sed rate of 16 mm. CEA report is enclosed, and
was reported as 2.8. Prior values were 1.1 in April
of 1977, and 1.7 in July of 1977, all three by
Solano Labs. When I last examined her on 12/7, I
found no abnormal physical findings. The rectal
mucosa was normal to 20 cm. A swab of the scant
brown mucus in the rectal area was slightly positive
by hemoccult test. She is going to bring other
specimens in after a meat-free diet for occult blood
testing. Her weight has remained stable, (slight gain),
May, 124 pounds; July 126 pounds; August, 127 pounds;
and December 7, 128-3/4 pounds.

She, ~~questioned~~ requested your opinion on her present status and
plans to phone your office and make an appointment.
I told her I would send you this review.

Thank you for your continued interest and support in
Patient #9 problems.

Very truly yours,

Chris J. D█████, M.D.

CJD/cd
enc.

Q.

Patient #10

Patient #10 is a 67-year-old man from Iowa who has survived nearly 12 years since his diagnosis of metastatic colon cancer.

In mid-1974, Patient #10 first experienced persistent fatigue, and severe constipation alternating with episodes of watery diarrhea. Some months later, after noticing bright red blood in his stool, he consulted his family physician who referred him for evaluation at a local clinic. There, a barium enema revealed a large, 5.7 cm mass in the right colon, suspicious for a malignant tumor.

On July 7, 1975, Patient #10 was admitted to Iowa Methodist Medical Center for further evaluation. A liver-spleen scan was positive for a "suspicious defect of the left lobe of the liver," measuring approximately 2.5 centimeters in diameter. Other studies, however, including chest X-rays, showed no additional evidence of metastatic disease.

The following day, Patient #10 underwent exploratory surgery and hemicolectomy (removal of the right half of his large intestine). During the procedure, his surgeon noted unresectable metastases in both lobes of the liver described in the operative note as "two lesions in the liver, one in the right and one in the left lobe of the liver. The right one was larger than the left, measuring about 2 x 2 cm."

Review of the surgical specimen confirmed a huge fulminant grade III adenocarcinoma extending into the adjacent tissues, as described in the formal pathology report:

> The cecal pouch is filled with bulky ulcerated neoplasm which is almost completely circumferential measuring 10 x 6 x 2 cm. Tumor infiltrates directly into the contiguous mesentery [the tissues adjacent to the large intestine].

Patient #10's physicians told him he might live three to six months at most, and believing him to be beyond cure, recommended neither chemotherapy nor radiation. But after leaving the hospital on July 21, 1975, Patient #10 decided to investigate unorthodox approaches to cancer. Later that summer, he learned of Dr. Kelley, consulted with him and began the full nutritional regimen.

Patient #10 continued the full Kelley program for seven years before tapering down to a maintenance program and today, despite the initial dire prognosis, he is in excellent health. Although he has refused further radiographic testing since his original surgery 12 years ago, Patient #10 believes his continued survival is proof enough of his cure.

Colon cancer, when metastatic to the liver, invariably proves rapidly fatal. Pestana and colleagues at the Mayo Clinic report a mean survival of only 9.0 months in 353 patients presenting with liver involvement.[1] In similar studies, Bengmark describes an average survival of only 7.8 months,[2] and Morris a median survival of 11.4 months.[3]

Obviously, Patient #10's progress represents a most unusual outcome for this disease.

REFERENCES

1. Pestana, C, et al. "The Natural History of Carcinoma of the Colon and Rectum." *American Journal of Surgery* 1964; 108:826–829.

2. Bengmark, S and Hafstrom, L. "The Natural History of Primary and Secondary Malignant Tumors of the Liver." *Cancer* 1969; 23:198–202.

3. Morris, MJ, et al. "Hepatic Metastases from Colorectal Carcinoma." *Australia & New Zealand Journal of Surgery* 1977; 47:365–368.

ADMISSION DATE: July 6, 1975   DISCHARGE DATE: July 21, 1975

This 54 year old white male was admitted because of occasional diarrhea and constipation.

PHYSICAL EXAMINATION: Revealed a middle-age white male, cooperative, alert and in no acute distress. The rest of the physical findings was essentially normal.

ADMITTING DIAGNOSIS:
1. POSSIBLE CARCINOMA OF THE COLON.

LABORATORY DATA: Chest x-ray showed fibrotic changes at the left base. There was no evidence of active infiltrate in either lung. IV pyelogram was grossly normal. Liver scan showed suspicious defect of the left lobe of the liver. Spleen was described as normal.

HOSPITAL COURSE: On July 8, 1975 the patient went to surgery with the diagnosis of carcinoma of the right colon with metastases to the liver. Operation done was a right hemicolectomy. The patient tolerated the procedure well and was brought to the recovery room in satisfactory condition. Postoperative course was relatively uneventful and he was discharged asymptomatic on July 21, 1975. Surgical pathology report showed Grade III adenocarcinoma of the right colon with direct infiltration of contiguous mesentery. Five regional lymph nodes were negative for metastases.

FINAL DIAGNOSIS:
1. GRADE III ADENOCARCINOMA OF THE CECUM, WITH DIRECT INFILTRATION OF CONTIGUOUS MESENTERY; HEPATIC METASTASES.

OPERATION: Right colectomy

DOMINADOR G████ M.D.   for WENDELL D████, M.D.

DG:GOS#62
9/24/75

157

NAME: Patient #10　　　　　　　　　　　　　DATE: 7-8-75

SURGEON: Wendell D_____, M. D.　　　ASSISTANTS: Dr. E_____ G_____

ANESTHETIST: K. W_____　　　　　　　SPONGE NURSES: F_____

ANESTHESIA: spinal　　　　　　　　INSTRUMENT NURSES: Ga_____, S_____, Hutchison

PRE-OPERATIVE DIAGNOSIS: Carcinoma of the right colon	OPERATION PROPOSED: Right hemicolectomy
POST OPERATIVE DIAGNOSIS: Carcinoma of the right colon with metastasis to the liver	OPERATION PERFORMED: Right hemicolectomy

Under satisfactory general anesthesia with the patient in the supine position and endotracheal tubing, the abdomen was prepped and draped with sterile towel for this procedure as usual. A smiling incision was performed below the umbilicus, starting at the hip margin and passing down about two inches below the umbilicus and continued up on the other side. After incising the skin, the subcutaneous layer was incised parallel to the skin incision. The fascia was incised. The rectus muscle was clamped and cut between the two clamps and ligated with #0 chromic catgut. All bleeders were ligated with 3-0 chromic catgut. The peritoneum was opened parallel to the skin incision.

After entrance into the abdomen, exploration was performed. There was a big tumor in the ascending colon as far as 6 to 7 cm. to the hepatic flexure. The kidneys were normal. There were two lesions in the liver, one in the right and one in the left lobe of the liver. The right one was larger than the left, measuring about 2 x 2 cm. After exploration, umbilical tape was passed around the colon and was ligated on both proximal and distal part of the lesion. Then by pulling the colon to the left, the attachment to the abdominal wall was excised with the scissor and then was continued to the hepatocolic ligament and downward as far as 6 to 8 cm. proximal to the ileocecal wall. The mesentery of the colon was divided, clamped and ligated with 2-0 silk. Two places, one in the ileum and the other in the mid-colon for anastomosis were made. The mesocolon was ligated and then dissected. The hepato-colic ligament was ligated and then cut between one clamp and then cut between two clamps, and then ligated with 2-0 silk. Then a Kocher was applied in the ileum about 6 cm. proximal to the ileocecal wall and then cut. The Kocher was also applied in mid-colon and then the colon was cut in the mid-colon and the lesion was sent to pathology. After excision of the right colon, we started to do the anastomosis. The anastomosis was carried out between the ileum and the mid-colon in two layers. The first layer was with a running Connell stitch of 3-0 chromic catgut, the second layer with 3-0 silk interrupted stitch. The mesentery was sutured together with running sutures of 3-0 chromic catgut. The abdomen was inspected carefully for any local bleeder. There were several small bleeders which were ligated with 3-0 silk. After this procedure, we started to close the abdomen.

The peritoneum was closed with a running suture of #1 chromic catgut. The fascia was closed with interrupted sutures of 3-0 wire, the subcutaneous layer with a running suture of 3-0 chromic catgut and the skin was sutured with interrupted sutures of 3-0 nylon.

The patient tolerated the procedure well. The sponge count was correct. Blood loss about 200 to 400 cc.

Saeed E_____, M. D. for　　　　　　　　　Wendell D_____, M. D.
SE: v.brown 7-9-75 (10)
1:00 p.m. - 3:00 p.m.

REPORT OF OPERATION

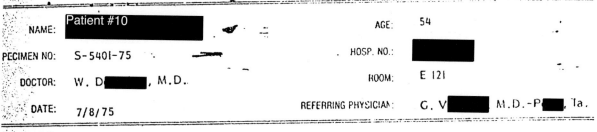

IOWA METHODIST HOSPITAL
DES MOINES, IOWA

NAME: Patient #10

AGE: 54

PECIMEN NO: S-5401-75

HOSP. NO.:

DOCTOR: W. D█████, M.D.

ROOM: E 121

DATE: 7/8/75

REFERRING PHYSICIAN: G. V█████ M.D.-P█████, Ia.

PREVIOUS PATHOLOGY:

FROZEN SECTION DIAGNOSIS:

GROSS DESCRIPTION:
The terminal ileum, cecal pouch, and cecum measure 35 cm. long in the fixed state. The 10 cm. segment of terminal ileum is normal. The appendix is normal. The cecal pouch is filled with bulky ulcerated neoplasm which is almost completely circumferential measuring 10 x 6 x 2 cm. Tumor infiltrates directly into the contiguous mesentery. There is diverticulosis of the ascending colon above the neoplasm. There is sixteen cm. of uninvolved colon distal to the tumor mass.

MICROSCOPIC EXAMINATION:

The terminal ileum is normal. The appendix is normal.

The cecal pouch neoplasm is an ulcerated infiltrating grade III mucinous adenocarcinoma directly extending into the mesentery.

Five regional lymph nodes are negative.

DIAGNOSIS: Grade III adenocarcinoma of the right colon with direct infiltration
of contiguous mesentery.
Five negative regional lymph nodes.
Normal terminal ileum.
Incidental appendix.

SNOP 6

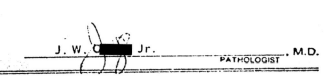

J. W. C█████ Jr. _____, M.D.
PATHOLOGIST

JWC:kdk

159

Patient #11

Patient #11 is a 60-year-old woman from Michigan who has survived over 17 years since diagnosed with carcinoma of the colon.

In 1965, Patient #11 experienced occasional bouts of sharp, stabbing mid-abdominal pain, usually occurring at night and lasting several minutes at most. Initially, attributing these episodes to the residual effects of a recent pregnancy, she did not seek medical advice: however, over a period of three years, the painful bouts increased in severity and frequency. By the end of 1968, she was incapacitated several hours a day, several days out of each week.

Patient #11 consulted a local family physician, who diagnosed her problem as "colitis" brought on by "psychological" stress. He prescribed analgesics which Patient #11 says did little, and within several months, her pain became so severe she had difficulty walking. In addition, she developed chronic constipation, associated with copious amounts of blood in her stool.

In mid-1969, Patient #11 was finally referred for a barium enema, barium swallow, and other tests, which were largely unrevealing. At that point, her doctor modified his diagnosis to include hiatal hernia, resulting from an overly rich diet and, once again, emotional distress. He told her the bloody stools were the result of stress-induced colitis, increased her medication doses, and recommended she not worry so much.

Patient #11 continued deteriorating throughout the first three months of 1970 and finally, on March 9, 1970, in excruciating pain she was admitted to William Beaumont Hospital in Royal Oak, Michigan, with a diagnosis of "possible" bowel obstruction.

A barium enema revealed an area of significant narrowing in the descending colon, consistent with an obstructing large tumor. However, the attending physicians, thinking Patient #11 too unstable for surgery, chose only to perform a series of additional tests during her first week of hospitalization. A pyelogram (a test of kidney function) was unrevealing, but a repeat barium enema on March 16, 1970 again demonstrated a tumor, described as "a 5 cm. long constriction with overhanging borders and with mucosal destruction."

Finally, on March 19, 1970, Patient #11 underwent exploratory surgery and resection of a large 7.0 cm cancerous mass in the descending colon, penetrating through the bowel wall. According to the operative report, the surgeon found no evidence of metastatic disease.

The tumor was classified as an "infiltrating adenocarcinoma of the colon, intermediate differentiation with full thickness involvement of bowel wall but no evidence of regional lymph node metastasis." Though it appeared purely localized, according to what Patient #11 told me, her physicians advised that due to its size, her disease would most likely recur and eventually prove terminal. They discussed with her the therapeutic options but admitted that additional treatment such as chemotherapy would only cause much discomfort without offering significant benefit. Subsequently, after declining further therapy, Patient #11 was discharged from the hospital on March 28, 1970.

Over the following months, Patient #11 recovered slowly from her ordeal, and then did fairly well for a time. Her pain resolved, and although she felt chronically fatigued, she could walk without difficulty and sleep through the night for the first time in years.

Then after a minor traffic accident on December 8, 1971, Patient #11's health rapidly began to deteriorate once again. She experienced persistent abdominal pain as severe as it had been prior to her surgery, associated with constipation and chronic nausea. She became anorectic to the point that over a one-month period, she lost 12 pounds.

During the second week of January 1972, Patient #11 consulted her family physician, who, suspecting recurrent cancer, referred her to a gastroenterologist. At the time Patient #11 underwent, as an outpatient, a complete evaluation including upper and lower GI series, sigmoidoscopy, and colonoscopy. The studies revealed a large, restricting recurrent tumor in the remnant of her descending colon. Although I do not have the records to confirm this, Patient #11 claims her doctor told her the cancer had metastasized widely.

Patient #11's physicians warned that she required immediate surgery to prevent total obstruction of her bowel but when questioned, admitted that her chances of living six months, even with the operation and aggressive chemotherapy, were remote. At that time, Patient #11 decided to refuse all further conventional treatment. She told me:

> I told my doctor I was prepared to die, and would rather die then go
> through the ordeal of another operation. I hadn't even heard of Dr. Kel-

ley yet, but I knew I wasn't going to go through any more suffering at the hands of my physicians.

Shortly afterwards, a good friend spoke to Patient #11 of Dr. Kelley and his program. Though skeptical about the treatment, Patient #11 agreed to a consultation and on January 19, 1971, traveled with her friend to meet Dr. Kelley in Texas, where he practiced at the time.

Patient #11 appears to have been critically ill when she first met with Dr. Kelley: according to what she told me, she felt so weak she could barely walk into Dr. Kelley's office, and her abdomen was visibly distended as she headed for another intestinal obstruction.

Nonetheless, Patient #11 began her nutritional protocol with determination as soon as she returned home, and within days noticed an improvement. Within a week, her bowel obstruction cleared, and her abdominal swelling lessened. From that point, her appetite improved, she gained back her lost weight, and she grew stronger, day by day. Eleven months after beginning her protocol, she reports passing a large globular mass of tissue which she and Dr. Kelley assume was the remnants of her tumor.

Patient #11 followed the full Kelley program for four years, before tapering down to a maintenance regimen which she still follows. At present, 17 years after her original diagnosis, she is in excellent health and apparently free of her cancer. Not surprisingly, she is an enthusiastic supporter of Dr. Kelley.

In summary, in 1970 this patient underwent surgery for a large, invasive tumor of the colon. Less than two years later, she experienced a recurrence, refused conventional treatment, and began the Kelley program. Clearly, this patient's apparent cure and current good health can only be attributed to her nutritional regimen.

william beaumont hospital
royal oak, michigan
549-7000

DEPARTMENT OF RADIOLOGY

PATIENT NAME Patient #11   42   DOCTOR X   X-RAY NO. 30 15 89

DATE 10 March 70 - 11:25 A.M.   ROOM NO. 443   MED. REC. NO.

BARIUM ENEMA

Barium per rectum filled the colon throughout to the cecum and the distal ileum was filled. The sigmoid colon appeared redundant. There appeared a segment of severe narrowing and irregularity in the distal descending colon with rather severe destruction of the rugal pattern and   shelving   effect on its distal portion. This area does not appear distensible. The rest of the large bowel appears intact. The terminal ileum shows no abnormality.

IMPRESSION

Findings in the distal descending colon consistent with malignant neoplasm. I doubt if this represents segmental colitis.

J. F████, M.D./me

_____ M.D.
RADIOLOGIST

RAY REPORT

M 803 REV 7 66

MEDICAL RECORDS

163

william beaumont hospital
royal oak, michigan
549-7000

PATIENT NAME Patient #11   42   DOCTOR   K___ M___   X-RAY NO. 30 15 89

DATE   16 March 70 - 8:40 A.M.   ROOM NO.   443   MED. REC. NO.

BARIUM ENEMA
    There is history of lower sigmoid lesion. Today's film study shows the
rectum and sigmoid loop to be long, large and relatively smooth. In the proximal
sigmoid there is a 5 cm. long constriction with overhanging borders and with
mucosal destruction.

CONCLUSION
    Anular carcinoma, proximal sigmoid.

                                        M. B. S_____, M.D./mc

X RAY REPORT

_____ M.D.
                    RADIOLOGIST

FORM 603 REV. 7-66   MEDICAL RECORDS

164

william beaumont hospital
royal oak, michigan

Dr. M▮▮▮▮▮▮

OPERATIVE RECORD

Preoperative Diagnosis Carcinoma of the descending colon

Date March 19, 1970

Postoperative Diagnosis Same and left ovarian cyst

Time Started 12:30 P.M.

Operation Resection distal descending colon with primary anastomosis.

Time Ended 3:45 P.M.

Room 443

Surgeon Dr. M▮▮▮▮	**Anesthesiologist/Anesthetist** Dr. P▮▮▮
Instrument Nurse P. J▮▮▮▮ - P. S▮▮▮▮	**Assistants** Drs. R▮▮▮ & N▮▮
Anesthetic Epidural	**Sponge Nurse** B. C▮▮▮▮ - E. L▮▮

OPERATION

Findings: A 7.0 cm. irregular mass was present in the distal descending colon. Serosa was puckered but there was no evidence of extramural extension of the tumor. Lymph nodes were not palpable in the mesocolon or along the terminal aorta and iliac vessels. Peritoneal fluid and nodules were not present. The uterus was of normal size, consistency and symmetrical in shape. A 1.5 cm. subserosal fibroid was present on the anterior dome. A 3.5 cm. clear fluid, ovarian cyst was present on the left. The right ovary was normal. The uterus, ovaries and bladder were not fixed within the pelvis. Adnexal areas were unremarkable.

The liver, stomach, gallbladder, spleen, and both kidneys were normal. The small intestine and its mesentery were normal. The appendix, cecum, ascending colon and midportion of the transverse colon were normal. The proximal descending colon, distal sigmoid colon and rectum were normal.

Procedure: The peritoneal cavity was entered through a left paramedian incision. Following exploration the left colon was mobilized. The mesentery was divided in a V shape from the root to the points selected for bowel division. Following excision of this area an end to end two layer anastomosis was performed. The mesenteric rent was closed and hemostasis ascertained. The wound was closed in layers using wires in the anterior rectus sheath. A small penrose drain was placed in the lower pole of the wound.

Blood loss was minimal and transfusion was not given. Sponge count was reported correct following closure of the peritoneum. The patient's condition was stable throughout the procedure.

Form 512

AM/mam

Signature of Operator ▮▮▮▮▮▮

Dr. M▮▮▮▮▮

D: 3-19-70   T: 3-20-70

Name: Patient #11   Age 42 yrs.

Case No.:   Date 3-19-70

Room No.: 443

Dr. M

william beaumont hospital
royal oak, michigan

PATHOLOGICAL REPORT

Specimen: A. Left ovary and tube B. Right ovary   S -   70-2590
C. Portion of bowel

Pre-op Diagnosis: Possible bowel obstruction

Post-op Diagnosis: Bilateral salpingo-oophorectomy, bowel resection

---

A. Left ovary and tube - portion of tube measures 5 x .7 cm. There is an area in the serosa in which there is suture material and a rather solid fibrous-like appearance in the serosa. Rs. re. The ovary is cystic, measures 3 cm. in greatest dimension. The cyst contents are clear and watery and the lining is smooth and glistening both on the inner and outer walls.

B. Right ovary - a portion of fallopian tube 3.5 cm. in greatest dimension with perhaps some thickening of the serosa. Rs. re. The ovary is 3 cm. in greatest dimension and contains one or two atretic follicles. No other unusual gross features. Rs. re.

C. Portion of bowel - a length of colon which in the semi-fixed state is 20 cm. long. There is an area of constriction in the bowel wall near the midportion. This area on the mucosa is occupied by an annular totally circumferential constricting ulcerating and fungating lesion 4.5 cm. long. The entire thickness of the bowel wall is involved. The regional lymph nodes generally do not appear conspicuous. re.

MICROSCOPIC:

A. Examination of the tissue shows the fallopian tube to be histologically unremarkable aside from an occasional nabothian cyst on the surface. The ovary is essentially atrophic and no unusual findings are seen.

B. Section from the fallopian tube again shows no histologic abnormality. Atretic follicles are present in an otherwise unremarkable ovary.

C. Section shows arising from the colonic mucosa infiltrating epithelial neoplasm which is composed of tubular and glandular structures imbedded in a fibrous stroma. Individual tubules are lined by columnar epithelial cells, enlarged nuclei which have lost their basal polarity. Some of the nuclei are very abnormal in appearance. Mitoses are noted. Cytoplasm is moderate to abundant and eosinophilic. The neoplasm appears to infiltrate through the full thickness of the wall. In the stroma there are a few areas of inflammatory cell infiltrate. The regional lymph nodes show some follicular hyperplasia but no neoplasm is seen.

DIAGNOSIS: LEFT FALLOPIAN TUBE AND OVARY WITH SIMPLE CYST
RIGHT FALLOPIAN TUBE AND OVARY
INFILTRATING ADENOCARCINOMA OF THE COLON, INTERMEDIATE DIFFERENTIATED
WITH FULL THICKNESS INVOLVEMENT OF BOWEL WALL BUT NO EVIDENCE OF
REGIONAL LYMPH NODE METASTASIS

R. P. E

FORM 301   REV. 3-59

166

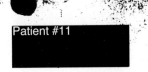

william beaumont hospital
royal oak, michigan

Doctor A. M█████

PROGRESS RECORD

DATE	TIME	DISCHARGE SUMMARY

Admission: 3/9/70
Discharge: 3/28/70

Present illness: This 42 year old female presented with abdominal pain
and was admitted to the hospital with possible bowel obstruction. She
had been seen in the past year and a half by her family physician for
progressive constipation, "colitis", and dyspareunia.

Physical examination was significant for tenderness in the lower abdomen
and induration in the left adnexal area.

Laboratory data: Admission hemoglobin 11.9, WBC 7,100. Urinalysis showed
12—15 WBC. Urine culture showed no growth.

X-rays: Chest normal. Barium enema—annular carcinoma, proximal colon.
Intravenous pyelogram normal. Indentation of upper surface urinary
bladder on the left. Oral cholecystogram normal. Upper GI series and
small bowel series normal.

Electrocardiogram normal.

Consultations: Doctor R. M█████ for evaluation of abdominal symptoms.
Doctor S█████ for evaluation of ? uropathy. Doctor D. Da█████ for
evaluation of several syncope. Doctor T. Ki███ for management of Estrogen
therapy, postoperative oophorectomy.

Operation: 3/18/70 cystoscopy and retrograde pyelogram, normal.
3/19/70, resection, distal decending colon with primary anastomosis and
bilateral oophorectomy for carcinoma confined to the bowel. No evidence of
extramural extension. No abnormality of pelvis. Simple ovarian cyst, left
side.

Microscopic examination: Infiltrating adenocarcinoma of the colon, full
thickness; no evidence of regional lymph node metastasis. Simple cyst,
left ovary. Right ovary normal.

The postoperative course was unremarkable and the patient was discharged
without medication on the ninth postoperative day.

Discharge diagnosis: (1) Adenocarcinoma of the colon, localized.
(2) Ovarian cyst, left.

Complications: None.

Disposition: Doctor K███ for estrogen management. Doctor M█████ for
interval endoscopy and barium enema examination   Doctor M█████ one week.

FORM 510

AM/ljs
D 3/28/70
T 3/30/70

Doctor M█████

167

HODGKIN'S DISEASE

Hodgkin's disease, a moderately rare cancer of the lymphocyte system and associated organs, claimed 1,500 lives in 1987.

Physicians classify this malignancy by a system of four "stages," I-IV. Stage I indicates early, localized disease; stage IV defines advanced, widely disseminated cancer involving many organs of the body. Stages II and III include more intermediate forms. Physicians further categorize Hodgkin's disease by the letters "a" and "b," with the designation "a" referring to patients without associated symptoms, the letter "b" identifying those with symptoms such as fevers, chills, night sweats, and fatigue.

Hodgkin's, if untreated, is usually rapidly fatal. Dr. Vincent DeVita, Director of the National Cancer Institute, describes an old study from 1941 by Croft, completed before the development of modern chemotherapy. In a series of untreated patients diagnosed with Hodgkin's disease, Croft reported a median survival of less than a year, with few living beyond two years, regardless of stage.[1]

The "MOPP" chemotherapy regimen, the most widely recommended drug treatment at present for Hodgkin's, consists of four drugs—nitrogen *m*ustard, Oncovin (vincristine), *p*rocarbazine and *p*rednisone—given once every 28 days for at least six months. Dr. DeVita, who himself helped developed MOPP, advises that "all patients treated with MOPP and other combinations should be given a minimum of six cycles [a dose] or as many cycles needed to achieve a complete remission, plus two additional cycles to consolidate the remission."[2] With protocols such as this, at least 50% of all patients will survive five years.

REFERENCES

1. DeVita, VT, et al. *Cancer Principles & Practice of Oncology*. Philadelphia; J.B. Lippincott Company, 1982, page 1348.

2. DeVita, VT, et al., page 1379.

Patient #12

Patient #12 is a 44-year-old man with a history of widely metastatic Hodgkin's disease, alive five years since his original diagnosis.

In July 1981, Patient #12 noted prominent lymph nodes in his neck that increased in size over a several week period. A biopsy of one of the nodes proved inconclusive, but when the swelling regressed, his doctors believed further diagnostic study unnecessary.

In January 1982, when the lymph nodes in his neck again enlarged, Patient #12 consulted his primary physician who as before was unconcerned. But over the following months, Patient #12 experienced occasional night sweats associated with diminished appetite and a seven-pound weight loss. In June 1982, he noticed sizeable nodes in his left groin, which, when finally biopsied, confirmed nodular sclerosing Hodgkin's disease.

In July 1982, Patient #12 was admitted to St. Francis Hospital in Tulsa, Oklahoma for additional evaluation. On physical exam, his physician detected multiple swollen lymph nodes in the left cervical (neck) region, in the right and left axillae (armpits), and in his right and left inguinal (groin) areas. A CT scan revealed enlarged nodes throughout the chest, the posterior retroperitoneal (abdominal) cavity, and the pelvis. X-ray studies confirmed a mass in the mediastinum (central chest region), suspicious nodules in both lungs, as well as a tumor adjacent to the spinal cord. A bipedal lymphangiogram, a dye study of the lymph node system, showed evidence of cancerous activity along the iliac veins in the pelvis, and finally, a bone marrow biopsy demonstrated myelofibrosis (fibrosis of the marrow), a condition often associated with Hodgkin's.

A consulting oncologist recommended an intensive chemotherapy protocol, the BCUPP regimen, consisting of the drugs Cytoxan, BCNU, Velban, Procarbazine, and prednisone given at monthly intervals for eight months. After agreeing to the treatment, Patient #12 was discharged from the hospital on July 23, 1982, with plans to proceed with therapy as an outpatient.

Between July 27, 1982 and March 15, 1983, Patient #12 received the scheduled eight courses of chemotherapy, which put his disease into remission. However, the improvement did not last very long: a routine chest X-ray on April 12, 1983, less than a month after Patient #12 completed his drug regimen, revealed, as summarized in the radiology report, "a new nodular-like density projected into the right mid lung field."

On April 28, 1983, Patient #12 was admitted to St. Francis for re-evaluation. On exam, many new enlarged nodes were noted in both the axillary and inguinal regions and a repeat bipedal lymphangiogram confirmed persistent cancer along the aorta. "Suspicious" mediastinal nodes were observed on chest X-ray, and a CT scan of the abdomen again documented numerous "enlarged retrocrural lymph nodes."

Patient #12 was discharged, only to be re-admitted to St. Francis on May 30, 1983 for exploratory thoracotomy (chest surgery), though during the procedure, the surgeon could not successfully resect or biopsy the nodules seen on X-ray.

In June, 1983, Patient #12 began a second course of BCUPP chemotherapy, administered on an outpatient basis. After the initial dose of drugs, he developed severe nausea, fatigue, and generalized weakness, and his blood counts fell so low that the protocol had to be delayed on several occasions. Nevertheless, Patient #12 completed the scheduled round of drugs in late October 1983. Although the disease appeared to be under control, he remained anemic, with his hemoglobin falling in the range of 10.5 (normal 14–18).

In late January 1984, Patient #12 began experiencing severe, drenching night sweats, a characteristic sign of advancing Hodgkin's disease, but a CT scan on February 14, 1984 showed no sign of cancer. Though his doctors suspected a recurrence, they decided to hold off restarting chemotherapy at that time.

In March 1984, Patient #12 began investigating unconventional cancer therapies. Although he initially followed no particular regimen, on his own he experimented with a variety of vitamin and mineral supplements. For a time Patient #12 even tried, if only haphazardly, a vegetarian diet as well as coffee enemas under the guidance of a former Kelley patient.

Patient #12 returned to the outpatient oncology clinic at St. Francis in May 1984 at which time significantly enlarged inguinal and axillary nodes were noted, indicating disease progression. His physician broached the subject of chemotherapy, but Patient #12 announced he intended to treat his cancer nutritionally. His doctor wrote in the records:

> He [Patient #12] is also using coffee enemas on a regular basis. He is taking megadose vitamin therapy and was warned about the coffee enemas, about renal stones with vitamin C, about hepatotoxicity of high-dose vitamin A, and about the possibility of hypercalcemia with high-dose vitamin D.

171

At home, as Patient #12 continued his nutritional experiments, his disease continued to progress. During a return visit to St. Francis on July 19, 1984, new large lymph nodes were evident in both the axillary and inguinal regions. His oncologist recommended immediate resumption of chemotherapy, but Patient #12 declined further treatment, even refusing to talk with his doctors. His oncologist wrote:

> [Patient #12] is, according to his girlfriend, quite frightened of rebeginning [sic] chemotherapy. I urged her to get him in contact with me so we could discuss other potential options for treatment.

During the summer and fall of 1984, Patient #12, as he pursued his own nutritional regimen, deteriorated relentlessly. The lymph nodes in his neck, axillae, and groin continued to enlarge, and in September 1984 his left leg suddenly swelled when a large tumor in the inguinal area obstructed lymph flow. Patient #12 also experienced frequent shaking chills, high fevers, ongoing drenching sweats requiring change of sheets at least three or four times a night, and weight loss, at the rate of about two pounds a month.

In October 1984, Patient #12 learned that Dr. Good and I were evaluating "Kelley patients" in our Immunology Clinic at the University of Oklahoma Medical Center. Although he was not then following the Kelley program, Patient #12 came to Oklahoma for an opinion about his condition.

When Dr. Good and I first met Patient #12 on October 9, 1984, he appeared to be in the terminal stages of cancer, emaciated, weighing 171.6 pounds on a large 6′2″ frame. Even aided by a cane, he could barely walk, and his skin appeared diffusely greenish, with the distinctive poison ivy-like rash often associated with advanced Hodgkin's disease covering both arms.

On physical exam, we palpated numerous walnut-sized hard non-tender lymph nodes in the neck, in both axillae, and bilaterally in the groin. The entire left leg, from hip to toes, appeared swollen, cold, and blue from poor blood circulation, and a large tumor mass, measuring 12 cm in diameter, was readily evident in the left inguinal region.

Though both Dr. Good and I advised Patient #12 that without treatment, he most probably would not live another two months, he insisted he would refuse additional chemotherapy regardless of his condition.

After leaving us, Patient #12 flew to Dallas to consult Dr. Kelley, and the following day began the full Kelley regimen. Patient #12 even moved to Dallas, so he might pursue his nutritional protocol under Dr. Kelley's direct supervision.

Patient #12 returned to our clinic for re-evaluation on January 29, 1985, approximately three months after his first visit with us. He arrived in our clinic smiling, walking without a cane, looking not merely improved but healthy, with an added ten pounds on his frame and a normal pink tone to his skin.

The formerly widespread Hodgkin's rash had disappeared, and neither Dr. Good nor I could palpate lymph nodes in any area of his body. The once large tumor in the groin had shrunken to a small, fibrotic mass that felt more like scar tissue than cancer.

Patient #12, in a jubilant mood, claimed he never felt better in his life. He even challenged both Dr. Good and myself to an arm-wrestling match, a suggestion we sensibly declined.

Patient #12's laboratory values from that visit were those of a healthy young man. Even his persistent anemia, initially brought on by the aggressive chemotherapy, had improved.

After his visit with us, Patient #12 returned to Dallas for another two months of treatment under Dr. Kelley's guidance. During this period, I visited with him and Dr. Kelley in Dallas on two occasions, and each time he seemed only stronger and healthier. Finally, in March 1985, Dr. Kelley thought Patient #12 sufficiently stable to return home to Oklahoma.

Patient #12 did well for a time, but then gradually abandoned his nutritional program in favor of more aggressively promoted treatments such as Laetrile. While pursuing such options, he suffered a mild relapse in early 1986. Currently, in the spring of 1987, he is following a modified Kelley protocol and feels strong enough to be back at work full time, competing on the rodeo circuit.

Patient #12's response to the Kelley regimen seemed to us quite remarkable. He was diagnosed with stage IVb Hodgkin's disease that recurred despite two courses of intensive chemotherapy, and when initially evaluated in our clinic he appeared to be only weeks from death. Yet while following the Kelley program, he experienced a complete regression of his disease and although not yet cured, Patient #12 continues to improve.

Saint Francis Hospital
6161 SOUTH YALE AVENUE   TULSA, OKLAHOMA 74177

PATIENT		AGE	SEX	REPORT NO.	ROOM NO.	HOSPITAL NO.
Patient #12		39	M	███	OP	███

SURGEON	ATTENDING PHYSICIAN	DATE RECEIVED—DICTATED
Dr. D. B███		July 12, 1982

PRE-OPERATIVE DIAGNOSIS
Left saphenofemoral lymphadenopathy

POST-OPERATIVE DIAGNOSIS

SPECIMEN
Lymph nodes, left groin

GROSS EXAMINATION:

The specimen is a rounded tan structure which measures 2.5 x 1.5 x 1.7 cm. in greatest dimension. The structure has been fixed in formalin which precludes touch preparation. On cut section the tissue has a pale tan to pink appearance and section is submitted. There are noted some nodules in the mid portion of the specimen which are sectioned and submitted. Also in the same container is a second small rounded structure measuring 2.5 x 1.0 x 0.8 cm. Sections. WPI/rl

MICROSCOPIC EXAMINATION:

Sections of lymph node show diffuse defacement of the architecture of the node which contains rather extensive areas of fibrocollagenous connective tissue. Some of the collagen is forming bands within the lymph node and resulting in lobules of lymphoid tissue formed by the fibrocollagenous bands. These bands of collagen are represented as true collagen since they are noted to polarize. Scattered throughout the lymph node are numerous mono-nuclear lacunar type giant cells with prominent eosinophilic nucleoli. In addition, there are noted scattered typical binucleated Reed-Sternberg giant cells, as well as scattered plasma cells, eosinophils and other histiocytes. The pattern and infiltration of the node is typical of Hodgkin's disease of nodular sclerosing type.

DIAGNOSIS: Left inguinal lymph node: Hodgkin's disease, nodular sclerosing type.

Code 9

08B

WPI/kh
CHART
SFH-402-137-H

WILLIAM P. I███, M.D.
Pathologist
July 13, 1982

174

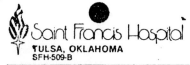
NAME	DATE OF ADMISSION	DATE OF DISCHARGE	HOSPITAL NO.
Patient #12	7/20/82	7/23/82	

FINAL DIAGNOSIS:

    1.   Stage IVA Hodgkins disease -- nodular sclerosing type.

DISPOSITION: The patient is discharged on 7/23/82, to return to the Natalie WArren Bryant Cancer Clinic on 7/26/82, for initiation of out-patient chemotherapy for his Hodgkins disease. His discharge medications include only Motrin 600 mg. 1 PO q. 4-6 h. prn. for pain. Diet and activity are unrestricted.

PROCEDURES THIS HOSPITALIZATION: 7/22/82, repeat lymphangiogram and 7/21/82, bilateral iliac crest bone marrow aspiration and biopsy.

CONSULTATIONS: None.

HISTORY OF PRESENT ILLNESS: The patient is a 39 year old white male who one year previously developed some lymphadenopathy in his neck receiving biopsy done by an osteopathic physician the biopsy being inconclusive because of insufficient specimen size. His lymphadenopathy spontaneously regressed, however 6 months ago they reappeared bilaterally and did not progress and were observed. Four weeks prior to admission he developed 2 left inguinal nodes that were biopsied by Dr. B█ which revealed nodular sclerosing type Hodgkins disease. The patient had no B symptoms although his weight had declined from 195 to 188 lbs. over the last 6-8 months.

Physical examination on admission was largely remarkable for findings of lymphadenopathy with 3-4 mm. nodes in the left neck posteriorly. There was a 2 X 1.5 cm. and a 1.5 X 1.5 cm. right axillary node in the central area. In the left axilla there were central nodes 1.5 X 1.5 cm. and 1.5 X 0.8 cm. These were tiny fibrotic feeling bilateral inguinal nodes. No femoral nodes or epitrochlear or popliteal nodes. Spleen and liver were not palpable. The remainder of the physical examination was unremarkable. His height was 72 inches and weight 188½ lbs.

LABORATORY DATA:

Admission SMAC was unremarkable with the exception of an LDH of 413. Other liver functions were normal. Total bilirubin was 0.4, alkaline phosphatase 111, SGOT 7, uric acid 6.6. Hemoglobin 12.7, hematocrit 37.5, with MCV 84.1, WBC 17.2 with 75 polys, 5 bands, 17 lymphs, 1 mono and only 2 eosinophils. Reticulocyte count 2.9%, platelets 284,000. UA unremarkable. VDRL negative.

Radiologic evaluation included a chest X-ray which revealed a large superior mediastinal mass anteriorly and peripheral pulmonary nodules and paraspinal mass density compatible with Hodgkins disease. CT of the abdomen revealed retro nodes as high as the chest and extending all the way down the

(continued)

DISCHARGE
SUMMARY

175

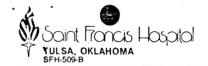
retroperitoneum at least to the bifurcation aorta, and perhaps some pelvic adenopathy as well. X-ray of the left knee was negative for complaints that the patient had in that area. A bipedal lymphangiogram revealed lymphomas involving the right iliac system and nonfilling of nodes in other areas possibly indicating lymphomus involvement.

Bone marrow aspiration was unable to be performed. Biopsy from iliac crest revealed a large amount of fibrosis with many plasma cells and eosinophils. No definite Reed-Sternberg cells were noted however the biopsy was felt to be compatible with Hodgkins disease.

HOSPITAL COURSE:

The patient was admitted and underwent the staging procedures with the findings as noted above. He expressed a desire to be discharged from the hospital and begin his treatment as an outpatient. He will return to the oncology clinic as noted above. He will attempt to be placed on an ECOG protocol No. 1481. He has been given information concerning the procedure and is to look this over this weekend and decide when he returns to the clinic on Monday.

C. S███████ M.D., FOR ALLEN K███████, M.D., ATTENDING

CS:lkc
C: Dr. Donald B███████
    Dr. William S███████

DISCHARGE
SUMMARY

176

HEMATOLOGY-ONCOLOGY ASSOCIATES, INC. PROGRESS NOTE
NATALIE WARREN BRYANT CANCER CENTER, ██████████, Tulsa, OK 74177

DATE	PATIENT'S NAME	R-NUMBER
4-19-83	Patient #12 ██████	

██████ was scheduled for a lymphangiogram on Monday, April 18th and a CT scan of the chest on Tues. the 19th. He will be an in-patient at that time. These were ordered by Dr. S██████.

D. L██████, RN/pd

HEMATOLOGY-ONCOLOGY ASSOCIATES, INC. PROGRESS NOTE
NATALIE WARREN BRYANT CANCER CENTER, ██████████, Tulsa, OK 74177

DATE	PATIENT'S NAME	R-NUMBER
4-28-83	██████████	

DISCHARGE DIAGNOSIS: (1) Hodgkin's disease, nodular sclerosing type, Stage IV-A.

██████ was discharged from the hospital on 4/27/83 after being admitted for diagnostic studies. Bilateral bone marrow aspirates and biopsies were obtained. The results are currently pending. Chest x-ray, PA and lateral, revealed linear streaking in the right upper lobe. CT scan of the chest confirmed this streaking, but it appears to be a benign phenomena, not related to Hodgkin's disease. There was, however, an anterior mediastinal node found 6 to 7 cm above the carina. CT scan of the abdomen revealed some high retroperitoneal adenopathy which is of questionable significance. The lymphangiogram could only be done on the right side and showed no evidence of lymphadenopathy.

██████ will return to see Dr. S██████ on Monday. I feel that he should have a mediastinoscopy for node biopsy to confirm whether this is a complete remission of perhaps simply fibrotic change. Readmission will be scheduled at that time.

Lee N. N██████, M.D./jc

HEMATOLOGY-ONCOLOGY ASSOCIATES, INC. PROGRESS NOTE
NATALIE WARREN BRYANT CANCER CENTER, ██████████, Tulsa, OK 74177

DATE	PATIENT'S NAME	R-NUMBER
5-4-83	██████████	

DIAGNOSIS: (1) Hodgkin's disease, nodular sclerosing type, Stage IV-A.

██████ returns to have his sutures removed from his lymphangiogram. This was done without any difficulty.

Lee N. N██████ M.D./jc

177

DATE	PATIENT'S NAME		R-NUMBER
5/10/84	Patient #12		

████feeling reasonably well. He has been quite active. He is holding his weight. His diet consists principally of a vegetarian diet with two eggs a day, one meat meal per week, other dairy products. He is taking his iron on a t.i.d. basis and has noted some improvement in his hemoglobin and hemato-crit. He is also using coffee enemas on a regular basis. He is taking megadose vitamin therapy and was warned about the coffee enemas, about renal stones with vitamin C, about hepatotoxicity of high-dose vitamin A, and about the possibility of hypercalcemia with high-dose vitamin D. I have encouraged him to bring in his diet supplements and his program for review by our nutri-tionist.

PE: BP 112/88; W 173½.
EENT: Unremarkable.
NECK: No nodes.
LUNGS: Clear.
HEART: Unremarkable.
ABDOMEN: No organomegaly, masses or tenderness.
EXTREMITIES: No joint deformity or edema.
LYMPH NODES;   There are scattered 1-1.5 cm. bilateral axillary nodes

which feel innocent. There is a 1.5 cm. inguinal node on the right. No other nodes are found.

IMPRESSION: (1) No clear-cut evidence of recurrent Hodgkin's disease, though bilateral axillary and right inguinal node are present.

PLAN: (1) WBC 4.5; hemoglobin 10.9; hematocrit 32.8; platelets 207,000; normal diff. (2) Continue to observe and will see again in eight weeks with SMA-20 and CBC. (3) Nutritional consultation as noted above. (4) Continue iron for the present.

                                        G. W. S████████ III, M.D./blk

cc: Donald B████████, M.D.

DATE	PATIENT'S NAME		R-NUMBER
7-5-84	████████		

████did not show for his 10:30 appointment today with Dr. S████████. I attempted to phone him at home, but was unable to reach him.

                                Connie C████, R.N./jc

HEMATOLOGY-ONCOLOGY ASSOCIATES, INC. PROGRESS NOTE
NATALIE WARREN BRYANT CANCER CENTER, ███████████ Tulsa, OK 74136

DATE 7-19-84	PATIENT'S NAME Patient #12 ███████	R-NUMBER

███ returns today for reevaluation. He is feeling perfectly well. He has, however, noted some right-sided axillary lymph nodes which were not present previously.

EXAMINATION:	BP 108/74. Pulse 78. Weight 176 lbs.
EENT:	Unremarkable.
NECK:	No nodes.
LUNGS:	Clear.
HEART:	Unremarkable.
ABDOMEN:	No organomegaly. No masses.
EXTREMITIES:	No joint deformity or edema.
LYMPH NODES:	There is a 1 cm left axillary node. There is a 2 x 1 cm

right axillary node which is very hard. Just below it is another 1 cm node. There is a 2.5 x 2 cm left femoral node, and above it, a 1.5 x 1 cm left inguinal node.

IMPRESSION: (1) Probable recurrent Hodgkin's disease.

PLAN: (1) Needs right axillary node biopsy. He will call me to announce when it can conveniently be done. I have urged haste with completion of the procedure in the next 7 days.

G. W. S████████ III, M.D./jc

cc: Donald B████████, M.D.

HEMATOLOGY-ONCOLOGY ASSOCIATES, INC. PROGRESS NOTE
NATALIE WARREN BRYANT CANCER CENTER, ███████████ Tulsa, OK 74136

DATE 7-23-84	PATIENT'S NAME ███████	R-NUMBER

███ is, according to his girlfriend, quite frightened of rebeginning chemotherapy. I urged her to get him in contact with me so we could discuss other potential options for treatment.

G. W. S████████ III, M.D./jc

179

Patient #13

Patient #13 is a 37-year-old man from Washington State alive nine years since diagnosed with Hodgkin's disease.

In late 1977, Patient #13 experienced persistent mild fatigue and noticed a tender swelling in his neck that rapidly increased in size over a period of several weeks. In January 1978, he consulted his family physician, who, suspecting a low-grade infection, prescribed a course of penicillin therapy. With treatment, the swelling did decrease slightly initially, but then worsened. At that point, Patient #13 began experiencing drenching night sweats as well as sharp pain in the upper part of his chest.

Several weeks later, Patient #13 returned to his physician. A chest X-ray revealed a large upper mediastinal mass, and laboratory studies were significant for an elevated white blood count of 21,000 (upper limit of normal 10,000). Because of these findings, on February 6, 1978 Patient #13 was admitted to Vancouver Memorial Hospital in Vancouver, Washington for evaluation.

During his initial exam, Patient #13 was noted to have extensive lymphadenopathy in the cervical and axillary areas, described in the records as:

> a very large mass present in the left side of the neck with some surround-
> ing smaller masses also present. There were some more discrete masses
> on the right side as well, measuring up to 3 to 4 cms in diameter. There
> is bilateral axillary adenopathy present.

The following day, Patient #13 underwent biopsy of the neck mass, then was discharged from the hospital before the results were ready. Subsequently, the tumor was classified as an aggressive form of Hodgkin's disease, mixed cellularity, well-described in the official pathology report:

> There is no question that nodules are being formed in this lymph node
> but in many areas the picture is more that of mixed cellularity type and
> there are remarkably large collections composed mainly of malignant
> reticulohistiocytic cells with lymphocyte depletion . . . .

With a diagnosis of Hodgkin's confirmed, Patient #13 was readmitted to Vancouver Memorial on February 13, 1978 for additional tests. A chest X-ray showed:

> mediastinal adenopathy which is a little more pronounced on the right.
> There is evidence of . . . .bilateral cervical adenopathy with a hazy den-
> sity caused by the enlarged cervical nodes . . .

And a lymphangiogram, a dye study of the abdominal lymph node system, demonstrated extensive disease, as summarized in the records:

> Abnormal lymphangiogram due to enlarged nodes caused by Hodgkin's disease at L 2, L 3 and probably along the right iliac chain.

On February 13, 1978, Patient #13 underwent a staging laparotomy—exploratory abdominal surgery—and splenectomy (removal of his spleen), often performed in patients with Hodgkin's. Although the organ seemed clear of malignant disease, a periaortic lymph node removed at surgery was infiltrated with cancer. However, a subsequent bone marrow biopsy proved inconclusive.

Patient #13 was told he suffered advanced Hodgkin's disease, officially recorded as Hodgkin's disease, nodular sclerosing type, Stage IIIb. His doctors, advising that aggressive multi-agent chemotherapy offered the only hope for prolonged survival, proposed the standard six-month, six-cycle course of MOPP. Patient #13 agreed to the treatment, which he began in late February 1978 as an outpatient at the Vancouver Clinic.

After the first round of drugs, Patient #13 became extremely weak, fatigued, and anorectic. His symptoms did improve over a two-week period, but during the second cycle of treatment, Patient #13 became acutely ill once again. He subsequently struggled through a third course, but felt so debilitated he decided to discontinue chemotherapy.

His oncologist warned Patient #13 that without finishing the suggested therapy, his disease could prove fatal. When Patient #13 refused to give in, his doctor then suggested a six-week course of radiation to the chest as an alternative. Patient #13 agreed to the plan and in late May 1978 began the proposed regimen. But in mid-July 1978, after receiving a total of 4060 rads to the chest and upper abdomen, Patient #13 reacted so badly to the treatment he refused to continue. At the time, he was not believed to be in remission.

At the urging of a friend, Patient #13 decided to investigate alternative cancer therapies. He learned of Dr. Kelley, met with him in late July 1978, and then began the full nutritional program. Within a month, he noticed improved energy and well-being, and within a year, he told me he felt better than he had for a decade.

Patient #13 followed the full regimen for three years, and today, nine years since his diagnosis, he remains in excellent health. And though MOPP chemotherapy causes sterility in a majority of male patients, while on the Kelley regimen he has fathered two healthy children, currently aged four and six.

Despite his abbreviated courses of both chemotherapy and radiation, I believe Patient #13 is a relatively simple case to evaluate. Although the medical literature does report several cases of patients with advanced Hodgkin's enjoying prolonged survival after incomplete treatment with MOPP, such cases are extremely rare. And while Patient #13 did undergo radiotherapy, all of it was directed to his chest and upper abdomen, not to the extensive disease in the lower abdominal and pelvis.

In summary, Patient #13 was diagnosed with stage IIIb Hodgkin's disease, treated with partial courses of chemotherapy and radiation. When first seen by Dr. Kelley, he was clinically debilitated and not, according to his doctors, in remission; it seems reasonable to attribute this patient's prolonged survival and current good health to his nutritional protocol.

FAMILY HISTORY: Non-contributory. No history of bleeding disorders.

PAST HISTORY: No serious illnesses in the past. Previous operations include appendectomy

No known allergies.

PRESENT ILLNESS: This 26 year old male is admitted to the hospital for biopsy of a cervical node. History reveals that for the past several weeks he has noticed a swelling in his neck, sometimes these have been tender. He was seen by Dr. S███ who felt he had an adenopathy and treated him with Penicillin with some resolution of the neck masses but they did not disappear completely and they shortly began to grow again. While taking the Penicillin he did notice some night sweats each night. Otherwise he has noted no fever or chills. He has felt well and has continued to work during this time. More recently he has noticed some upper anterior chest pain with exertion. Initial laboratory work done on this patient revealed a white count of 21,000. A chest xray done in Dr. S███'s office revealed an upper mediastinal mass with protrusion into the right chest area. He is admitted to the hospital for biopsy of enlarged lymph node.

PHYSICAL EXAMINATION: The patient is a pleasant, young adult male who appears in no acute distress.
Vital signs are normal.
HEENT: Reveals head normocephalic. Pupils equal and reactive. The throat is clear with no lesions. There is a very large mass present in the left side of the neck with some surrounding smaller masses also present. There were some more discrete masses on the right side as well, measuring up to 3 to 4 cms in diameter. There is bilateral axillary adenopathy present.
LUNGS: Clear to percussion and auscultation.
HEART: Regular sinus rhythm without murmurs.
ABDOMEN: Soft. The liver and spleen are not palpable and there are no areas of tenderness.
EXTERNAL GENITALIA & RECTAL: Appear normal. No significant inguinal nodes present.
LOWER EXTREMITIES: Reveal no edema.
SKIN: Reveals multiple pruritic appearing papules, most of which have been scratched off.

IMPRESSION: Probable lymphoma.

Physician's Signature _____ J. D. J████, M.D. /fc

D&T: 2/6/78

Patient #13

J.D. J████, M.D.
STA V-for surgery 2/7/78

vancouver memorial hospital
vancouver, washington
PATIENT HISTORY AND PHYSICAL EXAMINATION
Form ████ (76█-█)

183

GROSS: The specimen is a firm, almost round lymph node about 2 cm. in maximal diameter. Imprints are made and it is submitted as several cross sections, half fixed in formalin and half in Zenker's. Some fat appears to be adherant to surface scarring. C:m

MICROSCOPY: The lymph node is divided into nodule-like aggregates by a sclerotic process which frequently forms dense collagen fibers circumferentially around and in nodules. There are residual, essentially normal lymphoid follicles here and there but, the majority of the lymph node is replaced by granulomatous type infiltrates consisting of reticulohistiocytic cells or "turned-on" lymphocytes, recognizable lymphocytes in various stages of maturity, eosinophils, neutrophils and occasional plasma cells. Mononuclear and multinuclear malignant reticulohistiocytic cells are frequently encountered and classical Reed-Sternberg cells are also identified, especially in the formalin fixed sections and on the Papanicolaou's stained touch preparations. In certain foci, malignant reticulohistiocytic cells constitute 80-90% of the cells and within these areas, it is rather easy to find binucleate mirror image type cells sometimes with large inclusion-like nucleoli. In this respect, these foci resemble the mixed cellularity type of Hodgkin's disease but, there is no question that nodules are being formed. Many of these simulate highly reactive lymphoid follicles except that the centers are malignant in character. Neither large numbers of plasma cells nor proliferation of arborizing blood vessels with thickened walls are found as seen in immunoblastic lymphadenopathy, disease process which resembles Hodgkin's disease morphologically.

DIAGNOSIS:

    CERVICAL LYMPH NODE, RIGHT: HODGKIN'S DISEASE, NODULAR SCLEROSING VARIANT
                        (SEE COMMENT). T-08 M-9673

COMMENT: There is no question that nodules are being formed in this lymph node but in many areas the picture is more that of mixed cellularity type and there are remarkably large collections composed mainly of malignant reticulohistiocytic cells with lymphocyte depletion and I do not understand the meaning of these patterns.

F. R. C_____ M.D. _____   Robert D. J____ M.D. _____

Name:	Patient #13		Date:	2-7-78	Accession #: S-422-78
Age:	27		Specimen(s):		
Sex:	m		(a)	Cervical lymph node, rt	
Case #:			(b)		
Room #:	67-4		(c)		
Doctor(s):	J____		(d)		
			(e)		

Pertinent history and/or diagnosis: Probable lymphoma - neck swelling several weeks - Chest-Xray upper
NS 7070-30   mediastinal mass. M-2783-70

PATHOLOGY REPORT   VANCOUVER MEMORIAL HOSPITAL, VANCOUVER, WASHINGTO

184

RADIOLOGY

TODAY'S DATE	DATE TO BE DONE	WEIGHT	HEIGHT	AGE
2/13/78	2/13/78			

☐ WHEELCHAIR ☐ STRETCHER ☐ PORTABLE

Lymphangiogram
This AM

LYMPHANGIOGRAM

ORDERED BY DR. J_____

TRANSCRIBED BY B∂ W/C

TECH. K

PERTINENT CLINICAL INFORMATION

SPECIAL HANDLING

FORM NO. 7140-24

2-13-77

The lymphangiogram is abnormal, revealing enlarged nodes at the L 2, L 3 level and probably along the right iliac chain.

IMPRESSION: Abnormal lymphangiogram due to enlarged nodes caused by Hodgkin's disease at L 2, L 3 and probably along the right iliac chain.

L/g

L. KRO_____

N. HELGASON, M.D.   J. JUNKER, M.D.

J.D.J_____ MD

119-2   W IV 71

vancouver memorial hospital
vancouver, washington

RADIOLOGY REPORT
CHART COPY

FORM NO. 7140-24 REV. 4/77

185

This 27 year-old man with known Hodgkins disease of a nodular sclerosis type was admitted to the hospital at this time for staging laparotomy. Diagnosis had been confirmed by biopsy of a cervical node approximately a week prior to this admission. Lymphangiogram done the day prior to surgery revealed evidence of multiple nodes in the abdomen which appeared pathologic. At the time of admission his spleen was not enlarged and his liver function was normal.

Following admission he was prepared for surgery and taken to the operating room on 2-14-78 for staging laparotomy. At that time, splenectomy was done, as well as needle biopsy of the liver, and biopsy of periaortic nodes, and a bone marrow biopsy was attempted by Dr. J██████, but was unsuccessful. Also, one of the numerous skin lesions of the patient was excised from his right leg. The procedure was well tolerated and postoperatively he showed good primary wound healing and was tolerating a diet well by the time of discharge and was able to be discharged home on 2-18-78.

Final pathology report revealed the periaortic lymph node to be positive for Hodgkins disease. The liver and spleen were both negative. Skin lesion itself showed no evidence of cutaneous lymphoma.

The patient was to return to the office for removal of sutures and follow up examinations, and institution of therapy.

Hodgkins disease, nodular sclerosis type, Stage III B.

OPERATION: Staging laparotomy with splenectomy, needle biopsy of the liver, biopsy of periaortic nodes, bone marrow biopsy attempted. Excision of skin lesion, right leg.

d3-14 t3-15-78 jj

Patient #13

J.D. J██████, MD.
Discharegd 2-18-78

J.D. J██████, M.D.

vancouver memorial hospital
Vancouver, Washington

DISCHARGE SUMMARY

FORM 8699-212
REV. 12/76

5-23-78: This is a 28 year old white male who has Hodgkin's Disease, Stage III, B.
Original diagnosis was made back in Februauary 1978 when a right cervical lymph
node was biopsied by Dr. J███████ and showed Hodgkin's Disease, Nodular
sclerosing type. Patient then underwent a lymphangiogram, which was positive.
He then underwent a bone marrow biopsy and aspiration, which was negative.
He underwent a laparotomy with splenectomy and liver biopsy. Liver biopsy
was normal. There was no disease found in the spleen. Patient had night
sweats and pruritus, so that his final staging was IIIB.

I discussed his case with Dr. J███████ and at Tumor Board and we decided
a combination of Chemotherapy and radiation therapy would be the best plan
for this patient. He therefore received 3 cycles of Mopp and is nowtaken
into my consideration for total node irradiation therapy.

I first plan to give him Cobalt 60 radiation therapy through a mantle field,
4,000 rads mid-plane tumor dose to the mediastinum and all areas, over a 5 or
6 week period depending on his tolerance. I will start with a dose of 160 rads
daily dose and watch his white blood count and platelet count closely in light
of the fact that he has had 3 courses of Mopp.

Summary: IIIB Hodgkin's Disaese presented in the right neck. The mediasinum
was involved, on chest x-ray. Bone marrow was normal, liver biopsy normal,
spleen was normal, periaortic nodes were positive, both on Lymphangiogram and
aan on biopsy.

Treatment plan Cobalt 60 radiation therapy through a mantle field. Plan 4,000
rads over a 6 week period. Patient will then have a 2 or 3 month rest period
and will be treated through an inverted Y field at that time. Hopefully
patient will receive more cycles of Mop, if he can tolerate the Chemotherapy
after the radtation therapy.   NMH/tf

8-21-78: Patient was in today. His WBC was 6200, differential was fine. He seems
to be doing well, no problems. He will return inSept. 11, 1978 and we will
commence the inverted Y radiation at that time.   NMH/tf

11-3-78: Mantle field on this patient was completed on July 14, 1978 at 4,060 rads.
Patient has refused to complete his Chemotherapy and inverted Y therapy
inspite of multiple warnings by myself that his treatment is incomplete.
It appears that ████ has become convinced that diet therapy is better than
conventional therapy for Hodgkin's Disease. He said that he would go in
and talk to Dr. J███████, but I understand that he has not done this.
I would be happy to complete his radiation therapy if herever shows up.
NMH/tf

187

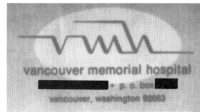

Norman M. H████ M.D.
Radiation Oncology
████████

vancouver memorial hospital
████████ • p. o. box ██
vancouver, washington 98663

RADIATION THERAPY
Hodgkin's Disease

November 6, 1978

J.D. J████████, M.D.
████████████
Vancouver, WA.   98660

Dear Dr. J████:

Patient:	Patient #13 ████████ age 28
Diagnosis:	Hodgkin's Disease - nodular sclerosing, Stage IIIB.
Work-up:	Disease presented in the right neck. Biopsy on February 6, 1978 showed Hodgkin's Disease, nodular sclerosing type. Chest x-ray showed involvement of the mediastinum. Laporotomy revealed the following: Bone marrow biopsy and aspiration normal. Splenectomy - spleen not involved. Liver biopsy normal. Periaortic nodes were positive. Lymphangiogram and I.V.P. showed normal I.V.P., but positive iliac and periaortic nodes.
Treatment modality and dosimetry:	A) A combination of Chemotherapy and radiation therapy: Chemotherapy - Dr. J████████. Patient received 3 cycles of Mopp and this was followed by mantle irradiation therapy as follows:
	B) Mantle field radiation therapy. Collimator size: 24½ x 25 cm. treated at a distance of 140 cm. Mantle field covered from the tip of the mastoids down to the T-12, L-1 junction.

Dosage: 4,060 rads mid-plane tumor dose to the mediastinum. All lymph node bearing areas received at least 4,000 rads by computer dosimetry. Treatment time: May 23, to July 14, 1978.

Inverted Y radiation - patient refused to have inverted Y irradiation therapy and apparently has refused to complete his Chemotherapy, in spite of multiple warnings by myself that his treatment is incomplete.

It appears that ████ has become convinced that diet therapy is better than conventional therapy for Hodgkin's Disease, in spite of multiple warnings by me that he should complete his radiation therapy. He said he would go in and talk it over with you, although I understand he has not done this. I would be happy to complete his radiation therapy if he ever shows up.

Thank you for referring him to me for radiation therapy,

Yours truly,

N.M. H████████, MD.

NMH/tf

188

Patient #14

Patient #14 is a 36-year-old Canadian, alive 15 years since developing Hodgkin's disease.

In January 1971, after noticing a swelling on the left side of his neck, Patient #14 consulted his local physician who, believing the lesion to be a benign cyst, recommended no testing. Over the following year, the swelling fluctuated in size. Finally, when his neck enlarged dramatically in June 1972, Patient #14's physician quickly admitted him to Reddy Memorial Hospital in Toronto. Patient #14 subsequently underwent surgery for removal of the presumed cyst, which proved to be a matted collection of cancerous lymph nodes, fifteen of which were positive for nodular sclerosing Hodgkin's disease.

Patient #14 was then transferred to Princess Margaret Hospital for further evaluation. Serial X-rays of the mediastinum (mid-chest) showed no evidence of malignant disease, but X-rays of the pelvis revealed probable metastatic cancer, as described in the radiology report:

> filling defects with dilated intranodal and peripheral sinusoids in the para-aortic nodes on the left. These changes are typical of early involvement by Hodgkin's Disease.

A bone scan demonstrated abnormalities in the pelvic region consistent with metastases:

> Increased deposition of activity in the left side of the pelvis and the left sacroiliac joint. Appearance suggests the possibiliy [sic] of an abnormality of this site.

A liver-spleen scan indicated an enlarged spleen, and a liver infiltrated with tumor as described in the records:

> appearances on the anterior and right lateral scans are strongly suggestive of the presence of a space occupying lesion located in the anterior right lobe [of the liver]. There is also poor concentration of activity within the left lobe suggesting the presence of an extensive infiltrating lesion. The spleen is moderately enlarged . . .

The patient's oncologist then recommended the standard six-month, six-cycle course of MOPP chemotherapy and after agreeing to the treatment plan, Patient

#14 received his first round as an inpatient on June 30, 1972. He tolerated the chemotherapy without significant side effects, and was discharged from the hospital in early July 1972.

After the second cycle of drugs, Patient #14 developed severe weakness, fatigue and anorexia. He did eventually recover, returning to the hospital for a third round of MOPP in late August 1972. But after falling ill during treatment once again, Patient #14 refused to continue, insisting the chemotherapy be stopped. At the time of discharge several days later, he was told he most probably would not live a year without proceeding with treatment.

Patient #14 then began a long automobile trip through the United States, "to clear my head," as he later told me. In September 1972, while staying with friends in Arizona, he quite by chance learned of Dr. Kelley's work, and obtained a copy of his book *One Answer to Cancer*. Several days later, he was on the road again heading for Dallas and an appointment with Dr. Kelley and within a week Patient #14 began the full regimen.

After several months on the therapy, to his dismay the lymph nodes in his neck and axillary regions suddenly enlarged considerably. Dr. Kelley was unconcerned according to what the patient told me, explaining that lymph nodes often swell before the disease finally regresses, and advising only that Patient #14 continue the nutritional protocol. Subsequently, over a period of several months, the swelling did resolve as Dr. Kelley predicted, and today, 15 years after his diagnosis, he still follows the Kelley program, remains cancer-free and is in excellent health. Although a single course of MOPP can cause sterility, Patient #14 has now fathered three children, all of whom use nutritional regimens designed by Dr. Kelley.

In a telephone conversation with me, the patient's Princess Margaret Hospital oncologist confirmed that in his professional opinion, Patient #14 was not in remission when he stopped conventional treatment.

In summary, Patient #14 was diagnosed with widely metastatic, stage IV Hodgkin's disease, which persisted despite an abbreviated course of MOPP. Subsequently, Patient #14's cancer went into remission, seemingly for good, as he pursued only the Kelley program.

Department of Pathology

SERVICE___Dr. B████_____

TISSUE___Lymph nodes from neck___

Original Diagnosis and
Clinical Data: Hodgkin's Disease,
                     Nodular Sclerosing
                     Type

NAME___[Patient #14]_____

T No.___████_____

AGE___21_____

SLIDE SOURCE___Reddy Memorial H.,
                      Montreal, Quebec

#___1781-72_____

DATE___June 30, 1972___ ACCESSION NO.___R 773-72___

HODGKIN'S DISEASE, NODULAR SCLEROSIS

Totally replacing the node, a series of nodules
partially circumscribed by collagen, are composed of lymphocytes
and histiocytes. Of the latter, the lacunar type dominates.
The capsule is thickened but veins were not involved.

TCB:mr

_____M.D.
PATHOLOGIST

PATIENT'S CHART
75 - 43 - 50 - R70

191

./O.P.	X-RAY NUMBER		DATE	ADDRESS			AGE 21	SEX M.
OPD.	T. 98774		16 June 1972					

	PATIENT'S NAME		CHARGE:		CAT. 3
	Patient #14				

CIAN	Dr. B	EXAMINATION Chest 2. & abdomen 1.

TECHNICIAN	FILMS USED				PROJECTION	KV	MA(S)	TIME	DIST.
	NO.	14" X 17"	NO.	10" X 12"					
	NO.	14" X 14"	NO.	9½" X 9½"					
	NO.	7" X 17"	NO.	8" X 10"					

PLEASE RETURN FILMS and ENVELOPE TO X-RAY DEPT.

THE PRINCESS MARGARET HOSPITAL — [redacted], TORONTO

RADIOLOGICAL REPORT

T. NO.

DATE REPORTED:

June 16, 1972

CHEST PA AND LATERAL

There is a congenital deformity of the lower end of the sternum. The appearances are otherwise within normal limits.

ABDOMEN AND PELVIS

There are filling defects with dilated intranodal and peripheral sinusoids in the para-aortic nodes on the left. These changes are typical of early involvement by Hodgkin's Disease. The right para-aortic nodes, the pelvic nodes on both sides and the inguinal nodes are within normal limits.

PLA   CHAB   HOD-LYM   FIL-DEF   DIL-SIN

DFR/Tt

DR. V.E. V[redacted]   /   DR. D.F. R[redacted]   DR. R. B[redacted]

RADIOISOTOPE SCAN REPORT

THE PRINCESS MARGARET HOSPITAL

DEPT. NO.: 5810.

NAME: Patient #14   T: ▮

ADDRESS: ▮ Montreal, Quebec. AGE: 21.

HOSPITAL: P.M.H.   REFERRING DOCTOR: Dr. A▮ Dr. B▮.

WARD OR FLOOR: O.P.D.   ADDRESS: P.M.H.

TYPE OF SCAN: Liver/Spleen scan.   DATE OF SCAN: 16th June, 1972.

MATERIAL INJECTED: 2 mCi ^{99m}TcS.

DATE OF INJECTION: 16th June, 1972.   INTERVAL: 1/2 an hour.

REPORT:

A liver and spleen scan were carried out 1/2 an hour after the intravenous injection of 2 mCi of technetium-99m sulfide colloid.

The liver is enlarged measuring 23 by 20 cms. At rest however, the lower border does not appear to extend below the right costal margin. There has been considerable technical artifact in spite of this, appearances on the anterior and right lateral scans are strongly suggestive of the presence of a space occupying lesion located in the anterior right lobe. There is also poor concentration of activity within the left lobe suggesting the presence of an extensive infiltrating lesion. The spleen is moderately enlarged measuring 8 by 13 cms on the posterior scan. On the anterior scan it rests well above the left costal margin. The distribution of activity appears to be fairly uniform with no obvious suggestion of a space occupying lesion.

SUMMARY:

Abnormal liver scan; splenomegaly.

G. N. E▮, M.D.

75-92-06

193

Patient	Patient #14	ss

Date	Notes
July 1-72	FINAL NOTE: (Admitted June 30-72, Discharged July 1, 1972) The patient is a 21-year-old male admitted for his first course of M. O. P. P. with a diagnosis of Hodgkins disease, 4a. The patient was reasonably healthy until January 1971 when he had swelling of the left neck. There was no tenderness but the swelling fluctuated in size and his family doctor diagnosed it as a type of cyst. There was no fever, no sweating, no itchiness and apparently no weight loss, though the patient did have a weight loss when he changed to being a vegetarian. It was rather difficult to account for any real weight loss because of his disease. There was no tiredness. On June 5th, 1972 the patient was admitted to hospital in Montreal for cyst removal. However, during the operation 15 lymph glands were removed and the pathological diagnosis was typical nodular sclerosing Hodgkins disease. Thus, he was transferred to P. M. H. for investigation and treatment. A lymphogram was done and showed a defect in the para-aortic nodes on the left side, the chest x-ray was also done but there was no mediastinal or hilar involvement. The abdomen was firm, there was a filling defect of the para-aortic area as well. Liver and spleen scan abnormal. He was diagnosed as Hodgkins disease, 4a, and was admitted for chemotherapy. On functional enquiry of the head and heck he had no headaches, no dizziness, no blurring of vision. No signs of any throat infection. No chest infection or shortness of breath , no cough. G. I. system - No nausea or vomiting, ho history of jaundice, bowel movement always godd. G. U. system - no dysuria, no increase of frequency or nocturia. Extremities - No weakness of any limbs, no tingling or pins and needles sensation. Skin - There was no change at all. No special pigmentation or itchiness. Past Health - The patient had tonsillectomy at the age of 8, he had chest operation because of congenital deformity of the sternal bone, done about 15 years ago. Family History - His grandmother died of ca., specific type unknown, the rest of the family history is negative.

75-44-46-R71

194

PROGRESS NOTES

Patient	Patient #14	ss	T No. ▓▓▓▓

Date	Notes
July 1-72	page 2

PHYSICAL EXAMINATION: He is a healthy looking, young male, of stated age, with long hair.
Head and neck - Eyes- light reflex normal, E. O. M. normal, fundi normal.
Mouth - No sign of any infection, no gum hypertrophy. No sign of any bleeding. Neck - Trachea midline, thyroid not palpable but on the left side there is a scar from recent biopsy just in front of the sternomastoid muscle. Just under the scar there were a palpable cervical chain of lymph nodes, they were non-tender. Each lymph node is about the size of 1 to 2 cm., there was also another suspicious small lymph node on the left supraclavicular area, the size of a pea.
Chest - There is a midline scar from the previous operation, the bony deformity and prominence of the sternum. Otherwise the chest is clear to I. P. P. A., there are also some suspicious axillary lymph nodes on the left side, they are soft but the size cannot really be delineated, the right side was clear.
Abdomen - No tenderness, no ascites. The liver was palpable 8 cm. down the right costal margin at the mid-clavicular line, it is non-tender, smooth in consistency. Spleen not palpable. There are bilateral inguinal lymph nodes palpable on the left more than on the right.
Rectal examination negative.
Cardiovascular system - Pulse rate 64 per minute, regular, b. p. 120/6 0, heart sounds normal, S.1 and S.2 no murmur. Peripheral pulses palpable and equal.
Extremities- No cyanosis, no clubbing, no ankle swelling, no weakness.
Skin generally normal.
Neurological exa m. - Mental status - alert and orientated. Cranial nerves grossly normal. Motor and sensory functions grossly normal and reflexes brisk and bilaterally equal, about ++, plantar reflex downgoing bilaterally.

INVESTIGATIONS: Hgb. 13 grams%, with a white count of 6.8 and 88% polys, platelets 3,400,000. Other biochemistry was also done but the reports are not back yet.

COURSE AND THERAPY: The patient was given Nitrogen Mustard 11.5 mgms. I. V., Vincristine 2 mgms. I. V., Prednisone 40 mgms. per meter square or 80 mgms. per day in divided doses for 14 days and Procarbazine 100 mgms. per meter square or 200 mgms. in divided doses times 14 days.

75-44-46-R71

195

Patient .... Patient #14 .... Address ....

Date	Notes
July 1-72	page 3 with premedication of Valium 10 mgms. I. V. and Stemetil 20 mgms. I. V.. The patient tolerated the procedure well except for slight vomiting about midnight. DISPOSITION: The patient was discharged on July 1st and supposed to be given a return appointment for a bone scan which was arranged for next Thursday, also for direct admission to complete his second half course of M. O. P. P. on Friday. He was also given a prescription for Prednisone 80 mgms. per day for 14 days. and Procarbazine 200 mgms. per day for 14 days. FINAL DIAGNOSIS: Hodgkins disease, 4a. DICTATED: Dr. K. L███ Dr. B. M███ SERVICE: Dr. D. O███ Typed July 4-72 mi
July 7/72	RADIOISOTOPE SCAN . Bone Scan. Summary: Abnormal scan. Dr. G. N. E██ :ca
July 14/72	Haematology report The General Hospital Corporation, St. John's,Nfld.
July 14.72	S.M.A. (see correspondence):map

DEPT. NO.: 5810

NAME: Patient #14   T: ▇▇▇▇

ADDRESS: ▇▇▇▇▇▇▇▇▇▇▇▇▇▇

HOSPITAL: P.M.H.   REFERRING DOCTOR: Dr. P▇

WARD OR FLOOR: O.P.D.   ADDRESS: P.M.H.

TYPE OF SCAN: Bone Scan   DATE OF SCAN: 7.7.1972.

MATERIAL INJECTED: 850 µCi ^{18}F

DATE OF INJECTION: 7.7.1972   INTERVAL: 1 1/2 hours

REPORT:

A bone scan was carried out 1 1/2 hours after the bral administration of 850 µCi of flourin 18. There is uniform distribution of activity throughout the vertebral column and thoracic cage. Increased deposition of activity in the left side of the pelvis and the left sacro-iliac joint. Appearance suggests the possibiliy of an abnormality of this site.

Summary - Abnormal bone scan.

G. N. E▇▇., M.D.

197

Patient #15

Patient #15 is a 37-year-old woman from Ohio with a history of recurrent Hodgkin's disease, alive 23 years since her original diagnosis.

In December 1963, at age 14, Patient #15 developed painless swelling in her right wrist which gradually improved over a three-week period. A month later, in January 1964 after she noted an enlarged, painful lymph node on the left side of her neck, her family physician prescribed a course of antibiotic therapy. When the node subsequently regressed with treatment, no further diagnostic evaluation was believed necessary.

In June 1964, after the neck swelling recurred, a left cervical lymph node biopsy indicated Hodgkin's disease. Patient #15 was then referred to M.D. Anderson Hospital in Houston, where she was first seen in early July 1964. A review of the previous biopsy slides confirmed the diagnosis of Hodgkin's; in addition, chest X-rays revealed enlarged lymph nodes in the left mediastinum (mid-chest) and in the mid-left lung.

Patient #15 then completed a four-week course of cobalt radiation totalling 4000 rads to the neck and 4000 to the chest. At the conclusion of treatment in mid-August 1964, she was thought to be in remission.

Thereafter, Patient #15 did well until early November 1967, when she developed rapidly enlarging masses in the left axilla (armpit) and right clavicle region. After multiple biopsies documented recurrent Hodgkin's disease, Patient #15 returned to M.D. Anderson for treatment. There, she received an additional 4200 rads of cobalt radiation to the neck and chest, with regression of her disease.

After this second episode, Patient #15 appeared to be cancer-free until December 1971 when, while attending college, she noted swelling along the length of her right arm, associated with new onset shortness of breath and severe left rib pain.

In mid-January 1972, Patient #15 returned to M.D. Anderson, where, on physical exam, a 5 cm mass in the left axilla was clearly evident. A chest X-ray showed thickening in the left pleura (the sac enclosing the lung), as well as suspicious lesions in the seventh, eighth and ninth ribs. Biopsies of the axillary mass, the pleura, and the left eighth rib were all positive for recurrent Hodgkin's, nodular sclerosing type, indicating widespread, stage IV disease.

While still hospitalized, Patient #15 began a proposed six-cycle regimen of MOPP chemotherapy. Initially, she tolerated the drugs without serious side effects, but after returning home on January 29, 1972, she experienced constant nausea, frequent vomiting, and anorexia. Over a period of two weeks, she lost a total of 16 pounds.

Reluctantly, Patient #15 returned to M.D. Anderson on February 28, 1972, for her second round of chemotherapy. However, when she became severely ill after the first infusions, against the advice of her physicians—who did not believe her to be in remission—she refused to proceed with treatment.

Though facing a dire situation, Patient #15 then returned home to resume her college studies. At school, a friend who knew about Dr. Kelley gave her a copy of *One Answer to Cancer*. After reading the book, Patient #15 decided to consult with Dr. Kelley, despite objections from her parents who believed him to be a fraud.

Patient #15 subsequently began the Kelley program in the spring of 1972, while still recovering from the side effects of her brief experience with chemotherapy. On the nutritional regimen, over a period of many months her general health improved, her persistent fatigue resolved, and she regained her lost weight.

Patient #15 continued the full Kelley regimen for two years. She subsequently enjoyed excellent health until mid-1986, when she developed a very slow-growing form of thyroid cancer, thought most likely caused by the aggressive radiation treatment administered two decades earlier. Presently, Patient #15 is back on the Kelley program and is in good health.

In summary, Patient #15, beginning at age 14, suffered three bouts of Hodgkin's disease. At M.D. Anderson Hospital, she completed two rounds of intensive radiation and an abbreviated course of chemotherapy, none of which cured her disease. While pursuing only the Kelley regimen, her Hodgkin's disease regressed—apparently for good.

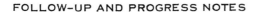
DATE

Jan-29-72   HOSPITAL DISCHARGE SUMMARY:
Admitted to hospital: January 18, 1972
Discharged from hospital: January 29, 1972
Attending physician: J. G█████, M. D.
Patient's age: 22 years.

Chief Complaint and Clinical History of this Hospital Admission:
This 22 year old white female was seen initially at the M. D. Anderson Hospital
in 1964 with a diagnosis of Hodgkin's disease, paragranuloma type involving the
left supraclavicular and mediastinum Stage II-A. She received radiation to
this area at that time and again in 1967 after developing axillary recurrences.
She returned to the clinic in January 1972 with a chief complaint of swelling
in her right arm of recent onset. She gave a history of dyspnea and pain in the
left chest posteriorly. A chest x-ray taken at that time demonstrated what
appeared to be a pleural thickening on the left with evidence of involvement
of the 7th, 8th and possibly 9th ribs posteriorly by destructive process.

Physical Examination:
Examination showed recurrent disease in the right axilla and supraclavicular
areas. There was a 5 cm. mass in the left axilla. It was felt that the patient
had Stage IV Hodgkin's disease involving the pleura, ribs and left axilla and
should be seen in Surgery Clinic for positive proof of probable Stage IV Hodgkin's
disease. This is a young white female in no acute distress. The head, eyes,
ears, nose and throat were within normal limits. The neck was within normal
limits. There were no increased nodes. The chest showed tenderness in the
7th, 8th and 9th ribs posteriorly. There was a questionable pleural fluid present
on the left. The heart was within normal limits. The abdomen was within normal
limits. The extremities were within normal limits. There was a 5 cm. node
palpable in the apex of the left axilla.

Laboratory and X-ray Data:
Hemoglobin 15.6, white blood count 18,050, platelet count 351,000, alkaline
phosphatase 51, BSP 2. Urinalysis was within normal limits. SMA-12/60 was
within normal limits. CBC before discharge showed a hemoglobin of 13.4, white
blood count 10,600, platelet count 445,000 with differential count showing
71 polys, 1 band, 21 lymphs, 5 monos, 1 eosinophil and 1 basophil.

Chest film showed destruction at the posterior aspect of the left 7th and 8th ribs.
Inflammatory versus post-surgical changes in the left lung base. The right arm,
right scapula and dorsal spine were within normal limits. Abdominal lymphangiogram
follow-up showed no definite evidence of retroperitoneal mass. Venogram done
of the right arm was within normal limits. Lateral decubitus chest showed some
evidence of free fluid extending up the left lateral chest wall. The left rib
cage film showed destructive changes in the posterior medial aspects of the left
6th, 7th and 8th ribs.

200

DATE

Hospital Course:
The patient was admitted to the Surgery Service on January 18, 1972 for a
biopsy of the left axillary nodes and left ribs and possible pleural biopsy.
The patient had biopsy of left axillary nodes and partial excisional biopsy
of the 9th rib. A pleural biopsy was done at that time.

The patient tolerated the procedure well. Following the operation, she had a
slight temperature spike, however, this was not felt to be significant at this
time and the patient continued to do well postoperatively.

On January 24, 1972, the patient was transferred to the Hematology Service
for a Stage IV Hodgkin's disease. The pathology report of the pleural biopsy
and the left node axilla showed Hodgkin's disease nodular sclerosing type.
Because of the persistent swelling of the right arm, a venogram was done and
this was negative. ████ therapy was discussed and on January 27, 1972, the
patient was started on MOPP. She received mustargen 0 mg. I.V., Oncovin, 2 mg.
day #3 through 8. Prednisone was also started, 40 mg. p.o. daily for ten days
and then taper. The patient had difficulty approximately seven hours after the
I.V. medication with a bit of nausea and vomiting. However, the following
morning, January 29, 1972, she felt well and was discharged. She was to have a
repeat course of mustargen 2 mg. I.V. and Oncovin, 2 mg. I.V. in one week and
continue the procarbazine and prednisone at home.

Diagnosis for this Hospital Admission:
Hodgkin's disease, nodular sclerosing type, Stage IV.

Operations:
January 19, 1972 - Left axillary node biopsy.
8th rib excisional biopsy, partial.

Condition on Discharge:
Good.

Prognosis:
Guarded.

Recommendations:
1. Mustargen 10 mg. I.V. and Oncovin, 2 mg. I.V. in one week by the family
   physician. A letter was written to the family doctor for instructions on
   this. Continue the procarbazine 150 mg. p.o. daily day #3 through 8.
   Continue prednisone 40 mg. daily for eight days and taper.
2. Return to the Hematology Clinic on February 28, 1972 for evaluation and
   continuation of the MOPP therapy.

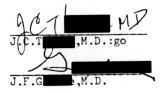

J.C.T████,M.D.:go

J.F.G████e,M.D.

sld: Feb-21-72; t Feb-25-72

THE UNIVERSITY OF TEXAS
M. D. ANDERSON HOSPITAL & TUMOR INSTITUTE
DEPARTMENT OF PATHOLOGY
Surgical Report

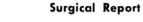

Name: 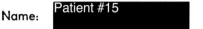 Patient #15   Room: E 301 A   S-   72-0411

Unit No.: _____ Age: 23   Sex: Female   Race: White
Physician: Dr. M█████████   Service: Chest   Date: 1-19-72

Clinical Diagnosis:

Diagnosis and report
by: B. M█████, M.D.

DIAGNOSIS:
(A) Pleural biopsy:
          Hodgkin's disease with nodular sclerosis
(B) Portion of 8th rib:
          Submitted for decalcification
(C) Node left axilla:
          Hodgkin's disease with nodular sclerosis

533-8891
535-8891

BM:kk:pb
S+2
1-21-72
1-21-72

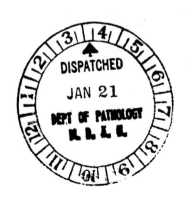

202

S-72-0411

GROSS DESCRIPTION:

(A) Pleural biopsy - consists of a fragment of gray, soft tissue, 1 x 0.5 x 0.2 cm. This tissue is somewhat tan and indurated.

(B) Portion of 8th rib - consists of a curved fragment of rib measuring 5 x 1.2 x 0.8 cm. Multiple sections are submitted following fixation and decalcification.

(C) Node left axilla - consists of a large fragment of fibroadipose tissue containing a large lymph node. The overall dimensions of the specimen are 2.9 x 2 x 1.5 cm. The specimen has been previously opened revealing a tan parenchyma of the lymph node. The surface is marked by poorly defined depressed septa.

DATE

Feb-28-72 HEMATOLOGY CLINIC:
This patient is a 23 year old white female whi has been followed in the
Hematology Clinic for Stage IV Hodgkin's disease. She was started on January
27, 1972 on the first course of MOPP therapy. She returns today for evaluation
and continuation of the MOPP therapy.

The patient states that after her Mustard and Oncovin were given on day #7 by
the family physician, she was very nauseated and vomited for approximately three
days. She is also having some side effects from the drugs in that she is noting
acne with the Prednisone and hair loss over the last three weeks. She has obtained a wig in preparation for more hair loss.

Physical examination today reveals no nodes palpable at this time. The right
arm is still swollen, the same size as when the patient was in the hospital. The
lungs are clear bilaterally. The surgical incision in the left ninth rib area
is well healed. Heart is within normal limits. The abdomen shows no increase
in the size of the liver or spleen. There are no masses. Extremities are within
normal limits.

Disposition:
1) Continue MOPP therapy today with Mustargen, 10 mg. IV; Oncovin, 2 mg.IV; Procarbazine, 50 mg. tomorrow, 100 mg. the following day and 150 mg. days #4
   through 9. Prednisone is also being started at 40 mg. daily for ten days and
   then rapid taper.
2) In one week, the patient will have an injection of Mustargen, 10 mg. IV and
   Oncovin, IV if her CBC and platelet counts are normal.
3) The patient is to return to the clinic in one month.
4) CBC today has not been obtained fully yet and will hold off on the chemotherapy until the total CBC is back; thus far, the hemoglobin is 13.4 and
   white blood count is 5,150. The platelet count has not been done yet.

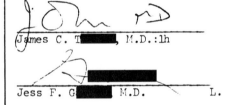

James C. T█████, M.D.:lh

Jess F. G████ M.D. █████ L.

Apr-7-72 HEMATOLOGY CLINIC
Patient #15 █████ has not kept her appointments and this is important since she has been
on MOPP chemotherapy. I need to write her family doctor to find the reason for
her not returning. It may be that distances are involved or that she will not take
any more MOPP chemotherapy.

Jess F. G█████, M.D.:rb   G

10-3-75 Telecon Dr. Stant, A███████ —
Patient is living and well and is
teaching school in Ohio. Her address
(next page)

204

LEUKEMIA

Hematologists currently recognize four major types of leukemia, and many sub-types. Overall, the various leukemias killed 17,800 Americans in 1987.

In this section, I present three cases, one each of acute lymphocytic leukemia, acute granulocytic (myelocytic) leukemia, and chronic granulocytic leukemia.

With aggressive chemotherapy, approximately 30% of all leukemic patients live five years.

Patient #16

Patient #16 is a 50-year-old man from Texas who has survived nearly 13 years since his diagnosis of acute lymphocytic leukemia (ALL).

In June 1974, Patient #16 developed noticeable pallor associated with the onset of chronic fatigue, diminished appetite, and a gradual 15-pound weight loss. During the following months, he noticed multiple petechiae, or small hemorrhages, on his legs that would come and go, though he did not at that time seek medical advice.

In September 1974, after experiencing a bout of severe abdominal pain, Patient #16 consulted his family doctor and was admitted to High Plains Baptist Hospital for evaluation. There, on physical exam, his physician noted an enlarged liver and spleen, and blood studies revealed severe anemia, with a hematocrit of 26 (normal 40-50). In addition, his white count was significantly elevated at 40,100 (normal less than 12,000), with 39% "blasts"—a primitive white cell often associated with active leukemia. A bone marrow biopsy then confirmed acute lymphatic (lymphocytic) leukemia.

A staff oncologist recommended an intensive chemotherapy protocol, the COAP regimen, consisting of the drugs Cytoxan, Oncovin, Cytosar and prednisone. Although told his chances for prolonged survival were dim, Patient #16 agreed to the treatment, which he began in September 1974.

After a second cycle of COAP in early November 1974, a repeat bone marrow biopsy indicated residual leukemic infiltrate. Disappointed with the results despite the intensive chemotherapy, Patient #16 decided to investigate unconventional cancer approaches, and in late November 1974 began the full Kelley program. He also continued chemotherapy, and with this combined approach his leukemia quickly went into remission.

Patient #16 received a total of ten cycles of COAP chemotherapy over a two-year period, all the while continuing the Kelley program. After finishing with drug treatment, he then complied with his nutritional regimen for another two years until 1979, when he quit primarily because of financial considerations. He told me he would have continued with the therapy, had his insurance company been willing to reimburse the cost of the supplements. Nevertheless, he remained cancer-free and in excellent health for 12 years, until early 1987, when he experienced a second bout of leukemia. Once again, Patient #16 has chosen to combine chemotherapy with the Kelley program and currently appears to be improving.

Even when aggressively treated, only 15-20% of adults with acute lymphocytic leukemia live five years. Prolonged survival, as rare as it is, has only been associated with use of the drugs daunorubicin and L-asparaginase, neither of which Patient #16 received.[1] Without these agents, five-year survival approaches 0%, and I have found no evidence in the literature that any patient treated with the COAP protocol—that used in Patient #16's case—lived ten years after diagnosis.

Wiernik, writing in *Cancer Principles & Practice of Oncology*, reports, for patients diagnosed with ALL who do respond to COAP, remissions lasting on average only 15–21 months, with a median survival only marginally longer than two years.[1]

Multi-drug regimens such as COAP are now known to *cause* secondary leukemias in a significant number of patients, most often occurring years after the original treatment. Possibly, Patient #16's current problem may be a new, drug-induced cancer rather than a recurrence of his original illness.

In summary, Patient #16 was diagnosed with acute lymphocytic leukemia, treated with—in addition to the Kelley program—an outdated chemotherapy protocol that only rarely induces long-term survival. Even with his recent recurrence, this patient's 12 year cancer-free remission represents, therefore, a most unusual outcome.

REFERENCE

1. DeVita, VT, et al. *Cancer Principles & Practice of Oncology*. Philadelphia; J.B. Lippincott Company, 1982, page 1420.

The following to be included in discharge summary as indicated: 1. Admitting diagnosis; 2. Pertinent results of laboratory, x-ray, and clinical findings; 3. Treatment; 4. Course while in the hospital; 5. Final diagnosis; 6. Prognosis.

Admission Date: 9/23/74
Discharge Date: 10/13/74

PATIENT PROFILE: Patient #16 is a 38 year old male, admitted to the hospital for evaluation of weakness, 15 pound weight loss over the past 3 months, right upper quadrant pain and an abnormal CBC.

FINAL DIAGNOSIS: 1.) Acute lymphocytic leukemia.

OBJECTIVE FINDINGS: This 38 y/o farmer was in good health until approximately 3 to 4 months prior to admission when he became pale and noted a general decrease in his strength. His appetite has been fair, but there has been a 15 pound weight loss over the past 4 months. He also complains of some dizziness while standing over the past several weeks. He is the father of a 17 year old girl with histiocytic lymphoma, diagnosed earlier this year. His right upper quadrant pain had been bothering the patient for approximately one week prior to admission, especially with taking deep breaths or after eating a large meal.

OBJECTIVE FINDINGS: Height 6'1", weight 173. Vital signs, include a 98 temp, pulse of 100, respiratory rate of 20 and BP 140/70.

PERTINENT PHYSICAL FINDINGS: He has a rather pale appearance.

SKIN: Reveals petechial lesions, especially on the legs, some are fresh, some are old. There is no palpable adenopathy except for a few small nontender nodes in the inguinal region, on both sides.

ABDOMEN: Reveals a liver edge, 7 cm. below the right costal margin and full inspiration. Spleen is also palpable 1 to 2 cm. below the left costal margin.

NEUROLOGICALLY: He appears intact, there is no evidence of any paralysis or sensory deprivation.

PERTINENT LABORATORY AND X-RAY FINDINGS: Admission CBC includes a white count of 40,100; hemoglobin 8.3; hematocrit 26; platelet count 137,000; 38 blast forms; 3 stabs, 4 segs, 54 lymphs and 1 mono. Urinalysis is normal. SMA-12 on 9/24/74, reveals an LDH of 295; uric acid of 9.2, inorganic phosphorous 5, cholesterol of 130, there is a normal pattern to the serum protein electrophoresis, mono spot was negative, heterophile no titer. Latex RA was negative. Leukocyte, alkalin phosphatase was 254, on 10/24/74.

Discharge CBC on October 13, hemoglobin 7.5; hematocrit 25; WBC chamber count 1210; platelet count 199,000; differential 1 blast, 2 eosinophils, 6 stabs, 5 segs, 86 lymphs. Chest x-ray on September 24, was within normal limits. Bone marrow biopsy, September 24, reveals diffuse dense leukemic infiltrate suggestive of acute lymphocytic leukemia.

HOSPITAL COURSE: The patient had a rather uncomplicated hospital course. COAP chemotherapy begun on September 26, finished on September 30th. He remained

HOSPITAL NO.	NAME	ROOM NO.	ATTENDING PHYSICIAN
			C. S M.D./ L. M. H M.D.

DISCHARGE
SUMMARY

FORM 613 REV. 2-69

The following to be included in discharge summary as indicated: 1. Admitting diagnosis; 2. Pertinent results of laboratory, x-ray, and clinical findings; 3. Treatment; 4. Course while in the hospital; 5. Final diagnosis; 6. Prognosis.

Admission Date:
Discharge Date:

afebrile throughout his hospital course and was discharged on October, 13, on Combid spansules, 1 po, q, 8h; prn and Alopurinol 300 mg. every day. He was instructed to return to the office of Dr. T█████ and Dr. H█████ on Wednesday, October, 16, for an appointment.

CS/db
D. 10/12/74
T. 10/14/74
line 2

HOSPITAL NO.	NAME	ROOM NO.	ATTENDING PHYSICIAN
Patient #16			C. S█████, M.D./ L. M. H█████, M.D.

DISCHARGE SUMMARY

FORM 613 REV. 2-69

209

HIGH PLAINS BAPTIST HOSPITAL

AMARILLO MEDICAL CENTER, Amarillo, Texas 79106

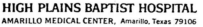

DATE: 9/24/74	TISSUE EXAMINATION	TISSUE: #	H-84-74

Specimen & How Obtained:

· Bone marrow

Patient's Name: Patient #16

Room No.: 517 1

Age: 38 y

Sex: male

Hospital No.:

Doctor: H

CLINICAL HISTORY: (Provisional diagnosis, duration of Lesion, etc.)

(Gross)

Smears of the marrow reveals the marrow to be highly cellular with no
fat cells recognized. There are scattered megakarocytes still seen.
The predominent cell is immature appearing mononuclear cell which is
suggestive of lymphocyte and these are seen to have very little pale
blue slightly vacuolated cytoplasm and nuclei that have rather uniform
chromatin though there is clumping of the chromatin. A few mature
appearing lymphocytes are seen which have course clumping of the chromatin
but approximately 50 % of the atypical cells are immature with rather
large but very finely dispersed chromatin in the nucleus and few of the
cells show rather indistinct single to two nuclei. Scattered among these
cells can be seen a few myelocytic cells and occasional erythrocytic
cell as well as an occasional plasma cell but the atypical lymphocytic
cells make up approximately 95 % of the cells present. An occasional
lymphocyte has notched nucleus but the majority of the nuclei are rounded
with pale immature chromatin networks.

DIAGNOSIS:
Highly cellular marrow with acute lymphatic leukemia.

FORM 35 REVISED 11-72
SURGEON

RALPH J. Z   M. D., F.A.C.P.
J. R. D   M. D., F.A.C.P.

PATHOLOGIST

TISSUE EXAMINATION

210

ANATOMICAL and CLINICAL PATHOLOGY

P. O. BOX ██████   PHONE ██████
AMARILLO, TEXAS 79106

RALPH J. Z██████, M.D.

Patient's Name:	Patient #16 ██████	Specimen No.	T-356-74
Age:	Sex: Male	Date Received:	11/5/74
Physician:	R. T██	Date Completed:	11/6/74

Specimen: Bone marrow biopsy

Clinical Diagnosis:

GROSS:

The specimen consists of a plug of light tan to gray, rather soft tissue measuring 1.8 x 0.5 x 0.5 cm. All will be embedded.

MICRO: Sections of the bone marrow reveals spicules of the bone to be rather narrow but viable. The marrow tissue is hypocellular with more than half of the marrow filled with fat. Within the marrow, where cells can be seen, adequate numbers of megakaryocytes are present; however, the myelocytic series appears to be depleted and there are patchy areas of infiltrate of brown cells which appear to be the size of the lymphcytes with scant cytoplasm and round, rather large, nuclei which have a homogenous dark basophilic staining. An occasional cell shows a nucleolus. There are a few recognizable clusters of erythroid cells. An occasional eosinophil is seen. An occasional neutrophil is present. A few plasma cells are present, also. There is some edema of the fatty tissue. Deposits of brown pigment can be seen in the stroma.

DIAGNOSIS: Hypocellular bone marrow with focal infiltrates of atypical mononuclear cells consistent with leukemic infiltrate.

COMMENT: Though the megakaryocytes appear to be adequate and some erythrocytic cells are present, the myelocytic cells appear to be really depleted. The atypical cells suggest lymphocytic cells.

be

R J. Z██████, M. D.

PATHOLOGIST

FORM 387 (R-1-72)

211

Patient #17

Patient #17 survived for seven years after his diagnosis of acute myelocytic leukemia (AML) in 1977, before succumbing in September 1984 at age 68 from causes unrelated to cancer.

Prior to developing leukemia, Patient #17 had a long history of chronic osteomyelitis (bone infection) in his right calf, first occurring at age 17 after a severe injury to his leg. His past medical history was also pertinent for longstanding peripheral vascular disease, atherosclerosis and angina pectoris. In 1971, after surviving a severe myocardial infarction (heart attack), he underwent coronary artery bypass surgery—and almost died on the operating table. After a very difficult recovery, he developed congestive heart failure associated with atrial fibrillation (a chronically irregular heart rhythm), liver function abnormalities, chronic fluid retention and respiratory problems. In early 1972, Patient #17 began an intensive drug regimen for his cardiac disease that included digoxin, diuretics, and quinidine, an anti-arrhythmic agent.

For a time, in the mid-1970s, Patient #17 managed to lead a fairly active life despite his many health problems, running a busy law practice and on vacations, traveling extensively. However, in January 1977, he developed a flu-like illness associated with anemia and leukopenia (a low white blood count). His physician attributed his symptoms and blood abnormalities to the quinidine, but Patient #17 did not improve after discontinuing the drug in February 1977.

Patient #17 was then referred to the hematology service at the Ochsner Clinic in New Orleans in May 1977, at which time he was found to be severely anemic, with a hematocrit of 32.3 (normal 40-50). His white count measured a low 2,400 (normal 4,200—10,000), with only 5% "polys," usually the predominant white cell. After an extensive evaluation, the Ochsner physicians, diagnosing an "early malignant process" but not active cancer, elected to observe his progress rather than begin treatment. Subsequently, in April 1977, after developing a scrotal abscess, Patient #17 was admitted to the Ochsner Clinic for antibiotic therapy and another hematological evaluation. A bone marrow biopsy at that time clearly revealed acute myelocytic leukemia.

His doctors recommended a chemotherapy protocol consisting of the drugs thioguanine and cytosine arabinoside, though they informed Patient #17 his chances of surviving a year, even with treatment, were not good. He was also warned that his other health problems might make therapy particularly risky.

With no perceivable alternatives, Patient #17 agreed to his doctor's plan. Subsequently, he was discharged from the hospital, then re-admitted to Ochsner in September 1977 for his first cycle of chemotherapy. During treatment, Patient #17 lapsed into acute congestive heart failure and almost died, though he eventually stabilized sufficiently to return home for several weeks, before re-entering the hospital in early October 1977 for a second round of therapy.

After another difficult course, Patient #17 was released from Ochsner in early October 1977, but several days later, when routine testing revealed significantly depressed blood counts, Patient #17 was admitted to a local hospital for blood and platelet transfusions. A bone marrow biopsy confirmed persistent leukemia: "it was felt that he is not in remission at this time," his physician wrote in his notes.

Patient #17 failed to enter remission even after a third course of treatment administered in late October 1977. At that point, the attending oncologist at Ochsner prescribed additional doses of oral thioguanine and cytosine arabinoside, to be taken every day indefinitely. But several weeks later, Patient #17 became so ill on the treatment he simply threw the medication away.

As Patient #17 worsened clinically, his wife began, on her own, investigating alternative approaches to cancer including the Kelley method. In early December 1977, Patient #17, although skeptical about the treatment, agreed to consult Dr. Kelley. Only days later, the patient and his wife ventured through the high Cascades in the middle of a blizzard to meet Dr. Kelley, then living in Winthrop.

When we spoke about that visit, Patient #17's wife admitted to me that she and her husband were not initially impressed. "We expected a medical institution," she explained to me, "with doctors in white coats scurrying around—not a man in a flannel shirt sitting in a one room office in the middle of nowhere." Despite their misgivings, Patient #17 felt sufficiently encouraged after his consultation to begin the program—and refuse further chemotherapy.

On his nutritional protocol, Patient #17 experienced a gradual but steady improvement in his overall health. In July 1978, he developed recurrent fevers, but a repeat bone marrow biopsy showed no evidence of leukemia. When last seen at the Ochsner Clinic in August 1978—six months after beginning the Kelley program—Patient #17 was again found to be cancer-free.

Thereafter, his cardiac status, his liver and respiratory function improved considerably, to the point he eventually discontinued the cardiac medications—digoxin, diuretics, and antiarrhythmics—previously required for six years. Patient #17 told me that after 12 months on the Kelley program, he enjoyed a sense of well-being he hadn't known for decades.

Patient #17 remained in good health until the summer of 1983 when, after re-injuring his right leg, the long-festering osteomyelitis worsened. Because of scarring and poor circulation to the lower leg, the infection did not improve with antibiotics. Nevertheless, Patient #17 did fairly well until September 1984, when he became acutely septic and died. However, according to his wife, an autopsy revealed he was free of leukemia at the time of his death.

The survival statistics for acute myelocytic leukemia remain abysmal, with the literature reporting an average lifespan for untreated patients diagnosed with the disease of only three months.[1] Even with aggressive therapy, only 10–15% of patients—at most—live five years, with survival rates declining considerably with increasing age.

In adults with AML, prolonged survival, as rare as it is in any case, has been documented only with chemotherapy regimens that incorporate the drug dauno-rubicin, never given Patient #17.[2] In a group of leukemic patients followed since 1967, the five-year survival rate for patients receiving only cytosine arabinoside and thioguanine approaches 0%.[2]

After searching through the medical literature, I could find no evidence for an adult patient surviving five years on the drug regimen administered Patient #17. I decided to write an authority in the field of acute leukemias, Dr. Peter Wiernik, currently head of the Department of Oncology at the Albert Einstein College of Medicine, to ask if he knew of any such patients. Dr. Wiernik kindly responded:

> I do not know of any five year or longer survivors of acute granulocytic [myelocytic] leukemia treated only with cytosine arabinoside and 6-thio-guanine . . .

It seems only reasonable, therefore, to attribute Patient #17's long-term survival to the Kelley program.

As a footnote to this case, I asked Dr. Kelley why Patient #17's nutritional program had not protected him, finally, from the osteomyelitis. Dr. Kelley responded by saying that the extensive scar formation most likely prevented sufficient nutrients from reaching the wound to allow for adequate healing.

REFERENCES

1. Petersdorf, RG, et al. *Harrrison's Principles of Internal Medicine,* 10th Edition. New York; McGraw-Hill Book Company, 1983, page 807.

2. DeVita, VT, et al. *Cancer Principles & Practice of Oncology.* Philadelphia; J.B. Lippincott Company, 1982, page 1422.

Patient #17   CLINIC ▮▮▮▮▮

ADMITTED: 8/31/77   DISCHARGED: 9/6/77

This 61 year old white male was in his usual state of health
postoperatively AC bypass five years ago when he developed a
flu-like syndrome in January of 1977. At that time, he was
found to be leukopenic and neutropenic. This was, at the time,
attributed to Quinidine sensitivity. He was referred to Ochsner
Foundation where evaluation for collagen-vascular disease was
negative, and he was found to have positive leuko-agglutinins.
Two weeks ago, the patient developed a scrotal abscess with
purulent drainage from a skin fistula in the scrota. Culture
grew Pseudomonas and the patient was started on oral Geocillin
with some improvement. Patient was seen in the clinic on 8/29/77,
at which time he had a white blood count of 2000, differential
of 18% PMN's, 40% lymphs and 32% monocytes. Bone marrow was
performed which was felt to show acute myelocytic leukemia.
Patient was also felt to have an increased number of atypical
lymphocytes on the bone marrow. Serum protein electrophoresis
showed a polyclonal increase in gamma globulin. The patient
was admitted and begun on intravenous Ticarcillin and Gentamicine.
Skin tests were applied for TB, mumps, Varidase, Trichomephyton
and Candida. His Trichomephyton and Candida skin tests were
strongly positive but TB skin test was negative. It was suggested
that the patient begin chemotherapy for his myelocytic leukemia.
He preferred, however, to have several days of pass before
instituting treatment.

LABORATORY ON ADMISSION: Hemoglobin 7.1, hematocrit 22.8, white
                          blood count 3000, 2% metamyelocytes,
2% myelocytes, 2% eosinophils, 34% lymphocytes and 60% monocytes.
Platelet count 146,000, MCV 98, MCHC 32.2, sedimentation rate 95.
Creatinine 0.9. Urine was normal under analysis. Creatinine
clearance was 99 cc./min. RPR was negative. Stools were negative
for ova, cysts, parasites and blood. Gentamicine level was 1.2 mcg./ml.,
4.8 mcg./ml. peak. Chest x-ray showed transverse diameter of the
heart was 17.8 with some increased markings in both lower lung
fields.

DISCHARGE
DIAGNOSIS: 1) Acute myelocytic leukemia.
                    2) Pseudomonas scrotal abscess.
                    3) History of cardiovascular disease.
                    4) SPO AC bypass.

DISCHARGE RECOMMENDATIONS: The patient will continue to have
                            intramuscular Gentamicine administered
at home and to take oral Geocillin, 2 tabs p.o. q. 6 hrs. He was
advised to return to the clinic in 1 week for chemotherapy. He was
also advised to return for any fever, chills, or bleeding.

                        Wayne G▮▮▮▮▮, MD
                        fcl

216

ALTON OCHSNER MEDICAL FOUNDATION

WILLIAM G. HELIS MEMORIAL LABORATORIES

NEW ORLEANS, LOUISIANA 70121

Date_____

Room No._____Clinic_____

Name_____ Patient #17 _____

████████████ H

Patient's Age ___61 Years___ Sex ___Male___

Specimen _____ Marrow, right posterior iliac spine.

Preoperative diagnosis _____ Leukemia; lymphoma?

CBC: 8/29/77, Hgb 8.7, Hct 26.0, RBC 2.73, WBC 2,000, Retic 29% Platelets 166,000, Seg 18, Lymph 40, Mono 42, Aniso 2+, Poly 2+, MCV 94.

Comments: Rouleaux formation.

Postoperative diagnosis _____ Lymphocytic infiltrate.

Submitted by Dr. _W. A████████/Same_

PATHOLOGY REPORT

Date ___9/1/77___ Path. No. _S-77-9550_

GROSS: The specimen consists of two irregular shaped pieces of dark brown blood coagulum, which measures 1 cm in greatest dimension. In addition there is a light brown bony spicule which measures 1.5 cm in greatest dimension. Submitted in toto.

Soheir N████, M.D.
bf

MICROSCOPIC: Peripheral smear: Platelets are present in every oil power field. The red cells are generally normocytic and normochromic with mild anisocytosis and mild poikilocytosis. There is relative neutropenia on the peripheral smear. Rouleaux formation is prominent.

Bone marrow aspiration: The aspiration smear is very cellular. The M-E ratio is estimated at around 4 or 5:1. There is relatively smooth maturation sequence in the red cell series. There is a marked shift to the left in the granulocytic series. Numerous myelocytes and promyelocytes are present. The number of blasts very from field to field, but in some areas they are remarkably abundant. I believe that this represents an acute leukemia. Since there is partially arrested maturation along the granulocytic line, I would favor that diagnosis. This could also possibly represent an acute myelomonocytic leukemia.

Bone marrow clot section: There are several particles of marrow present. The cell:fat ratio is approximately 2:1. Megakaryocytes are present and appear to be very slightly reduced in number. There is no evidence of metastatic tumor, granuloma, or lymphomatous infiltrate.

Bone marrow biopsy specimen: The marrow biopsy specimen consists of spicules of cancellous bone and marrow. The marrow is essentially identical to that described in the clot section above.

DIAGNOSIS: Bone marrow aspiration and biopsy, right posterior iliac spine: acute leukemia (please note description above).

Form 5178-A-Rev. 2-76

G. W. W████, M.D.   6

217

Patient #17 ███████████   CLINIC ██████

ADMITTED: 10/24/77   DISCHARGED: 10/30/77

CHIEF COMPLAINT: Admitted for chemotherapy.

█████████████ is a 61 year old white male with a history of acute
myelogenous leukemia, diagnosed eight weeks prior to admission,
recently discharged on 10/13/77 after being treated with Cytosar,
200 mg. q. 12 hrs. for five days, and Thioguanine, 200 mg. p.o.
q. 12 hrs. for five days. Since discharge, the patient states
that he has been feeling very well with no indication of fever,
chills, bleeding, bruising, or evidence of infection. Approximately
one week prior to admission, he received two units of full blood
in Alexandria for decreasing hemoglobin and hematocrit, and five
days prior to admission, received six units of platelets from his
brother for a platelet count that had decreased to 24,000. Patient
had several petechiae at that time which cleared since that time.
The patient had a bone marrow examination five days prior to
admission which was interpreted as having an increased percentage
of blasts again, and it was felt that he is not in remission at
this time and admitted for chemotherapy.

PHYSICAL EXAMINATION: Examination of his head and neck was
unremarkable. The blood pressure was 114/80,
lungs were clear to auscultation and percussion. Cardiac examination
revealed a grade II/VI systolic murmur at the base without radiation.
Abdominal examination was unremarkable with the liver palpated 3 cm.
below the right costal margin. There were a few petechiae on the
anterior of his left lower leg. The remainder of the physical
examination was unremarkable.

LABORATORY FINDINGS: On admission, the patient's white count was
1.5 thousand, hematocrit 26.5, hemoglobin 8.8,
platelet count 114,000. On discharge, his white blood count was
1.2 thousand with a hematocrit of 28.8, hemoglobin 9.7, there were
20% polys, 65% lymphocytes, and 10% monocytes. During the
hospitalization, other blood tests included a glucose of 100, BUN 8,
creatinine 1.0, calcium 8.2, phosphorus 3.3, sodium 134, potassium
3.9, CO_2 32, chloride 96, uric acid 4.4, cholesterol 106, triglycerides
63, total protein 6.8, albumin 3.0, total bilirubin 0.6, SGOT 20, SGPT
24, LDH 128, alkaline phosphatase 64. Urinalysis was within normal
limits. Stool was negative for ova and parasites and blood.

SUMMARY OF HOSPITALIZATION: The patient was given a second course of
chemotherapy consisting of Cytosar, 200 mg.
over a 12 hour period for 5 days (that is, 400 mg. of Cytosar daily
running continuously 5 days), and Thioguanine, 200 mg. p.o. q. 12 hrs.
for 5 days. During the hospitalization, the patient remained afebrile
and ambulatory. He received his usual medications consisting of
Digoxin, .25 mg. p.o. q.d., Quinidex, 1 p.o. q.i.d., and Dyazide,
1 p.o. q.d. He was discharged on 10/30/77 with no complaints, to be

218

followed by his local physician, and to return to Ochsner
Hematology Clinic for follow up of acute myelogenous leukemia.

DISCHARGE
DIAGNOSIS:

1) Acute myelogenous leukemia, status post
   chemotherapy (just completed second course).

RECOMMENDATIONS
ON DISCHARGE:

1) The patient will continue his maintenance
   medications as listed above.
2) Digoxin, .25 mg. p.o. q.d.
3) Quinidex, 1 p.o. q.i.d.
4) He will be followed by his home town physician
   for his blood count and platelet count.
5) He will return to Ochsner Hematology Clinic
   for follow up of his acute myelogenous leukemia.

George P. C█████, MD
fcl

Dictated: 10/31/77
TRANSCRIBED AS DICTATED: 11/4/77

219

ALTON OCHSNER MEDICAL FOUNDATION

WILLIAM G. HELIS MEMORIAL LABORATORIES

█████████████████████

NEW ORLEANS, LOUISIANA 70121

Patient's Age_____ Sex ___Male_____

Specimen_____ Outside slides BM 141-77 (8) (5 broken). Marrow.

Preoperative diagnosis_____ AML in partial remission.

Slides from: Pathology Department, Rapides General Hospital, Alexandria, La.

Postoperative diagnosis_____

Submitted by Dr._____ W. An████████

PATHOLOGY REPORT

Date____ 11/1/77 ____Path. No.___ S77-12000_____

MICROSCOPIC: There is a modest decrease in the cellularity of this
marrow. There is a moderate relative increase of erythroid elements.
There is distinct megaloblastic changes involving all stages, but espcially
apparent in the more mature stages. All stages of myeloid series are present
as there is good maturation. There is, however, a modest relative increase
in the number of myeloblasts and promyelocytes indicating that the leukemia
is probably not in complete remission. Since this is not a hypocellular
marrow with marked depression of marrow elements, it is less likely that
the relative increase in blasts is the result of a regenerative marrow.
Infrequent megakaryocytes are present.

INTERPRETATION: Bone marrow: acute myelogenous leukemia in partial remission.

Edwin N. B████████, M. D.
Pathologist   js   6

Slides returned.

220

PATHOLOGICAL EXAMINATION OF SURGICAL SPECIMEN

Name Patient #17   Room #   OP   Case #

Date of   Marital
Operation   7-26-78   Age   Sex   Race   Status

Specimen   Bone Marrow

Clinical History in Brief:

Post-Operative Diagnosis:

                             M. M███████   M. D. Surgeon

PATHOLOGICAL REPORT

                                 Date   7-27-78

PERIPHERAL BLOOD SMEAR:

The red blood cells are normochromic, normocytic. The
leukocytes appear slightly decreased. The platelets are
adequate.

BONE MARROW:

The bone marrow appears essentially normocellular. There
is a mild megaloblastoid dyspoiesis probably secondary to
drug therapy. The M:E ratio appears essentially normal.
There appears to be a slight increase of immature forms but
in the face of the therapy there is questionable
significance. Mitoses are common. Megakaryocytes are
present. Iron stores are adequate.

IMPRESSION:

Acute myelocytic leukemia in remission.

Examined by: _____ M. D., Pathologist

RGH Form 9-4

Patient #18

Patient #18 is a 55-year-old woman from Illinois, alive more than 12 years since diagnosed with chronic granulocytic leukemia.

In mid-1974, Patient #18 experienced fatigue and depression which gradually worsened over a several month period. During that time, her appetite diminished, her weight began to drop, and she developed intermittent bouts of severe pain in her right thumb and middle finger. Patient #18 consulted her local physician, who during a routine evaluation discovered an elevated white blood count. After a bone marrow biopsy revealed chronic granulocytic leukemia, Patient #18 was referred to the hematology unit at the Mayo Clinic in Minnesota in December 1974.

At Mayo, laboratory tests were significant for a white count of 89,000 (normal 4,200–10,000) as well as an elevated platelet count of 686,000 (normal 150,000–450,000), findings consistent with leukemia. Review of the bone marrow biopsy slides confirmed chronic granulocytic leukemia with evidence of the Philadelphia chromosome, a genetic marker usually present with this particular cancer.

The Mayo doctors then recommended a course of the drug busulphan, long the treatment of choice for chronic granulocytic leukemia. However, they warned that even with treatment, the long-term prognosis was poor. The attending oncologist wrote:

> I have discussed in some detail with the patient and her husband the nature of this disease pointing out that at the present time we have very satisfactory treatment to control this disease, but do not ordinarily 'cure it.'

After returning home in December 1974, Patient #18 began chemotherapy under the supervision of a local oncologist. Within months, the leukemia went into remission as predicted, but since her disease was considered ultimately incurable despite the response, Patient #18 began exploring other options.

She first learned of Dr. Kelley toward the end of 1975, after completing ten months of her drug protocol. Several weeks later, Patient #18 began the program under the direction of a local chiropractor trained by Dr. Kelley, at the same time discontinuing chemotherapy.

Patient #18 subsequently followed the full nutritional regimen for more than seven years, before slacking off in 1983. During this time, she enjoyed excellent health and appeared cancer-free. In fact, Patient #18 stopped the program only because she felt confident her disease was cured.

In January 1984, her local hematologist, during a routine check, noted an elevated white blood count in the range of 20,000. A subsequent bone marrow biopsy on January 31, 1984, performed only six months after Patient #18 had discontinued the Kelley therapy, confirmed a "mild" recurrence. Her physicians suggested maintenance therapy with low-dose hydroxyurea, one of the least toxic chemotherapeutic drugs currently available. Patient #18 agreed to the regimen, but at the same time resumed the Kelley program.

Today, three years after her relapse, and 12 years since her original diagnosis, Patient #18 continues on both hydroxyurea and a nutritional regimen. At present, she appears to be in remission, with her most recent white blood counts falling in the normal range.

Even with aggressive chemotherapy, only rarely do patients with chronic granulocytic leukemia survive ten years. The *Merck Manual* describes the dismal prognosis for patients diagnosed with this disease:

> The course is invariably progressive and ultimately fatal. Average survival time is 3 to 4 yr from clinical onset; about 20% of patients survive longer than 5 yr; 2% longer than 10 yr. During most of the disease, treatment may maintain the patient in almost normal health and activity but does not appear to prolong survival time appreciably.[1]

In summary, Patient #18, diagnosed with chronic granulocytic leukemia, initially entered remission while pursuing an abbreviated, ten-month course of the drug busulphan. After that time, she followed only the Kelley program and for a period of eight years remained cancer-free. In 1984, she suffered a relapse after straying from her nutritional regimen, but her disease again went into remission after she resumed both her nutritional protocol and chemotherapy.

REFERENCE

1. Berkow, R, et al. *The Merck Manual*, 13th Edition. Rahway, New Jersey; Merck, Sharp and Dohme Research Laboratories, 1977, page 331.

December 16, 1974

3-108-362

John R. F█████ M.D.
████████████████████
Rockford, Illinois   61108

Dear Doctor F██████

Patient #18 ████████████████████ of Rockford, Illinois has recently been at the
Mayo Clinic for evaluation and has requested that we write you concerning our
findings. As I believe you know, during the course of a workup for an atypical
Raynaud's phenomenan in Rockford, she was noted to have leukocytosis. She comes
here for confirmation of the diagnosis of chronic granulocytic leukemia. Of interest
is the fact that in July of 1973 she apparently had some type of hematologic
change on routine blood counts since a sternal bone marrow aspiration was done,
and as far as she knows, was regarded as normal at that time. We have asked the
laboratory to send for these slides so that we may review them but as yet they
have not been received. At the time of our examination here on December 11 of this
year, she really felt quite well, except for anxiety and tension regarding the
recently established diagnosis of leukemia. She specifically denied sweats, fever,
anorexia and abdominal pain.

On physical examination her height was 66½" and her weight 119 pounds. The blood
pressure measured 125/80. There were shotty lymph nodes palpable in the axilla
and groins bilaterally, but I did not believe that these were clinically significant.
The spleen was not palpably enlarged nor was the liver. The uterus was enlarged
about twice normal size, and slightly irregular and had the feel of a fibroid
uterus. The palmar surface of the right thumb and right index finger had a
dusky cyanosis, and the rest of the general physical examination was unremarkable.

The hemoglobin was 13.3 gm.%, the erythrocytes 4.50 million, and the leukocytes
89,000 with the following differential: segmented neutrophils 55.5, band
neutrophils 6, lymphocytes 6.5, monocytes 3, eosinophils 3, basophils 7,
metamyelocytes 4.5 and myelocytes 14.5. The platelet count was increased
at 686,000 with the upper range of normal in our laboratory being 370,000.
The erythrocyte sedimentation rate measured 3 mm. in the first hour by the
Westergren method. The serum protein electrophoretic pattern was normal with
a gamma globulin fraction of 1.15 gm.%. The leukocyte alkaline phosphatase score
was markedly reduced to 1, with the range of normal in our laboratory being 30-70.
The serologic test for syphilis was nonreactive, and the serum total thyroxine was
within normal limits measuring 8.1 mcg.%. The cold agglutinin titer was normal
measuring less than 1/4, and the test for serum cryoglobulins was negative.

224

The serum sodium, potassium, calcium, phosphorus, glucose, alkaline phosphatase, G.O. transaminase, bilirubin, and uric acid levels were normal. The serum creatinine measured 1.0 mg.% with the upper range of normal for females in our laboratory being 0.9. Urinalysis was normal. X-ray of the chest was normal. A film of the urinary tract with tomograms over the kidneys to demonstrate the spleen showed no evidence of splenomegaly. Bone marrow aspiration from the iliac crest showed markedly hypercellular smears with an erythroid-granulocytic ratio of 1:20. The marrow was quite consistent with the diagnosis of chronic granulocytic leukemia.

She appears to have classical early chronic granulocytic leukemia, as is manifested by the hypercellular bone marrow, the markedly reduced leukocyte alkaline phosphatase score, the markedly elevated leukocyte count and the 7% basophils in the peripheral blood smear. We did do cytogenetic studies on the bone marrow aspiration, and this showed the presence of the so-called Philadelphia chromosome, which again confirms unequivocally the diagnosis of chronic granulocytic leukemia. The reason for her atypical Raynaud's phenomenon in the right thumb and index finger is not clear, and I personally have not seen this previously in patients with chronic granulocytic leukemia.

I have discussed in some detail with the patient and her husband the nature of this disease pointing out that at the present time we have very satisfactory treatment to control this disease, but do not ordinarily "cure it." I feel she should not receive any treatment whatever at the present time but that weekly or bi-weekly leukocyte counts should be done over the next several weeks so that we can get some idea of the rapidity of rise of the white blood cell count, and thus have some idea as to the tempo of her disease. When the time for treatment does come (at the time her leukocyte count is doubled to a value of about 160,000 or when she begins to develop significant splenomegaly or systemic symptoms, then I would suggest the use of Myleran in low dosage. I did discuss with her some of the newer experimental work involving early splenectomy and then intensive antimetabolite therapy including the use of cytosine arabinoside in an attempt to wipe out the leukemic "clone" in the hope that one might permanently cure the leukemia rather than simply control it, as is usually accomplished with Myleran therapy. I would be very happy to cooperate with you in any way that I can in her future management and would appreciate a copy of her leukocyte counts after 10 or 12 of them have been accumulated over the next several months. I am sending under separate cover a bone marrow smear for your review.

Sincerely yours,

J.M.K█████, M.D.

JMK:jl

Bone Marrow Report

Re: ████████████

Aspiration and biopsy performed 1-31-84.

Read 2-2-84

Pre-biopsy diagnosis: Chronic myelogenous (granulocytic) leukemia
in relapse. A posterior iliac spine bone marrow aspiration and
biopsy was performed with ease under local Xylocaine anesthesia
with a Jamshidi needle.

NARRATIVE REPORT:

Microscopic evaluation revealed the specimen to be significantly hypercellular with increased numbers of myelocytes and metamyelocytes as well
as increased numbers of bands and segmented neutrophils. A modest increase
in blast is also noted. Granulopoiesis is generally markedly increased
in comparison to erythropoiesis. Megakaryocytes are present in adequate
numbers.

The marrow pattern is consistent with chronic myelogenous (granulocytic)
leukemia.

DIAGNOSIS:

1. Chronic granulocytic (chronic myelogenous) leukemia in relapse.

NOTE:

The biopsy specimen has been sent to the pathology laboratory at
SwedishAmerican Hospital for interpretation and confirmation of
the above diagnosis is expected.

Donald F. H█████, M.D./lkc

LIVER (METASTATIC TO LIVER)

Gastrointestinal malignancies, such as colon and pancreatic cancer, and tumors of the breast commonly metastasize to the liver. In such cases, survival is usually measured in months.

Patient #19

Patient #19 died in September 1980 at age 69 after surviving six years with carcinoma to the liver, metastatic from an unknown primary.

In mid-1973, Patient #19 noted, while leaning over, a painless mass on the right side of her abdomen. Since she otherwise felt well, she did not initially consult her family physician.

Throughout 1973 and 1974, the mass gradually enlarged, eventually becoming tender to touch. During this period, Patient #19 also experienced persistent fatigue, associated with anorexia and a moderate, gradual weight loss. Finally, on October 12, 1974, when her symptoms noticeably worsened, Patient #19 consulted her doctor, who admitted her to Lancaster General Hospital in Lancaster, Pennsylvania for evaluation.

A barium enema revealed an abdominal tumor, described in the radiology report:

> There is a very large abdominal mass present in the midabdomen and in
> the left upper quadrant which causes an extrinsic pressure defect upon
> the colon and depresses the transverse and splenic area of the colon.

An ultrasound study documented:

> a large intrahepatic mass localized predominantly in the left lobe of the
> liver. This measures at least 12 cm. across . . . In addition, there are some
> areas of internal echoes in the right lobe of the liver . . .

Patient #19 then went for exploratory surgery, during which metastatic cancer was seen throughout her liver. Although biopsied, the tumors were too extensive for resection, as tersely reported in the hospital records:

> She [Patient #19] was explored . . . and a liver full of metastatic disease
> was discovered.

The malignancy was classified as an "undifferentiated malignant neoplasm" believed to represent metastases from some other site, not primary liver cancer, though the tissue or origin could not be determined.

After surgery, Patient #19's doctors, though informing her she suffered terminal disease, proposed a round of chemotherapy they hoped might prolong her life, if only for a few months. After considering her options, while still hospitalized she completed a five-day course of the drug 5-fluorouracil.

Patient #19 was discharged from the hospital on October 25, 1974 in a very unstable condition, with plans to continue chemotherapy as an outpatient. But once home, she and her husband decided to investigate alternative approaches to cancer. Patient #19 learned of Dr. Kelley in November 1974, consulted with him and began the nutritional program, thereafter declining further conventional treatment.

Patient #19 responded very quickly to her regimen with improved energy and appetite, and within months, her husband reported to me the large abdominal masses regressed completely. Subsequently, Patient #19 followed the Kelley regimen for five years until 1980, when she discontinued her prescribed diet and supplements because she believed herself cured. Although she never again became overtly ill, Patient #19 passed away peacefully in her sleep in September 1980, six years after her diagnosis of terminal disease.

Experts consider cancer metastatic to the liver deadly, particularly when originating from an unknown primary. "Liver metastases are considered by most doctors to be incurable," writes Foster, who reports that despite intensive research efforts over a 20-year period, neither systemic nor intra-arterial chemotherapy, alone or coupled with radiation, offers much benefit. He describes a 60% one-year survival for patients with solitary, untreated metastases from colon and rectal carcinoma, a 5.7% one-year survival when both lobes of the liver contain widespread disease—as in this case—and a mean survival in this latter group of only 3.1 months.[1]

Patient #19 did receive a very brief, five-day course of 5-fluorouracil chemotherapy, but this drug has never been shown to extend life in patients such as Patient #19. As Foster writes:

> For solid carcinomas of GI [gastrointestinal] origin, most would agree that the systemic use of 5-fluorouracil for hepatic metastases will usually be followed by an objective response of 3 months or more duration in about 15% [of patients], but that such therapy will not prolong survival.[2]

Patient #19, in summary, presented initially with inoperable, metastatic cancer involving both lobes of her liver. With such disease, by the standards of conventional oncology, her chances of living one year were in the range of 5% yet she survived for six years in good health after her original diagnosis. Furthermore, Dr. Kelley believes that had Patient #19 continued her nutritional program, she might still be alive today.

REFERENCES

1. DeVita, VT, et al. *Cancer Principles & Practice of Oncology*. Philadelphia; J.B. Lippincott, 1982, page 1553.

2. DeVita, VT, et al., page 1557.

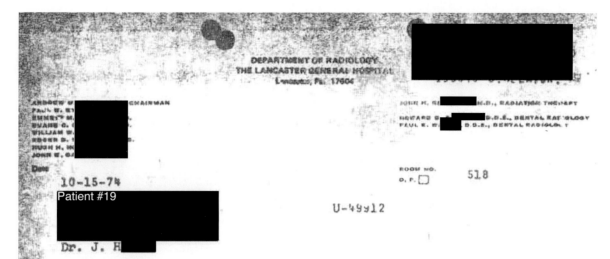

DEPARTMENT OF RADIOLOGY
THE LANCASTER GENERAL HOSPITAL
Lancaster, Pa. 17604

ANDREW W.   CHAIRMAN
PAUL W. E
BURNETT M.
EVANS G.
WILLIAM W.
ROGER D.
HUGH H. H
JOHN E. G

JOHN H.   M.D., RADIATION THERAPY
HOWARD   D.D.S., DENTAL RADIOLOGY
PAUL E.   D.D.S., DENTAL RADIOLOGY

Date   10-15-74

Patient #19

ROOM NO.   518
O. P. ☐

U-49912

Dr. J. H

BARIUM ENEMA:

The contrast flowed from the rectum to the cecum with reflux into
the terminal ileum. There is a very large abdominal mass present
in the midabdomen and in the left upper quadrant which causes an
extrinsic pressure defect upon the colon and depresses the
transverse and splenic area of the colon. There is also some
diverticulosis present within the area. There are also some changes
of diverticulitis in the sigmoid colon but there are no other
abnormalities.

IMPRESSION:

Huge abdominal mass causing extrinsic pressure defect upon the
colon. No evidence of a colonic neoplasm.

Diverticulosis.

Wm. W. Y   M.D.

sme

231

DEPARTMENT OF RADIOLOGY
THE LANCASTER GENERAL HOSPITAL
Lancaster, Pa. 17604

ROOM NO.
O. P. ☐   518

10-16-74   U-50309

Patient #19

Dr. J. He███

ABDOMINAL SONOGRAM:

An abdominal sonogram on 10-16-74 with specific reference to the
liver reveals what appears to be a large intrahepatic mass localized
predominately in the left lobe of the liver. This measures at least
12 cm. across and appears to be displacing liver tissue around it.
It appears solid/nature.
                    in

In addition, there are some areas of internal echoes in the right
lobe of the liver which are also suspicious of some smaller masses
in this area.

IMPRESSION:

A large intrahepatic mass is seen involving the left lobe of the
liver. Some questionable changes are seen in the right lobe of the
liver.

This patient will not be charged for this exam.

                                John W. G████, M. D.

cl

232

LANCASTER GENERAL HOSPITAL

DISCHARGE SUMMARY

Patient #19

█████████ was admitted October 12 and discharged October 25. Her history was of having a mass increasing in size in her upper abdomen. Finally it was determined that she had known of this mass for a long while. Prior to admission, it had become extremely tender so that if she rolled or lend against the area she would have pain. On first examination, I suspected that she had a ruptured aneurysm because of the extreme tenderness of the area. Later as the tenderness subsided it was possible to delinate the mass as part of the liver.

She was studied preoperatively, barium enema, liver scan, cardiogram, blood work. She was explored by Dr. W████ and a liver full of metastatic disease was discovered. The biopsy was taken and it was read as section containing liver with undifferentiated malignant neoplasm.

She recovered from her surgery. She was given 5 Fluorouracil, five injections of 1,000 milligrams each. She will be followed as an out patient. Chemotherapy will be maintained, then Prednisone and ████ maybe added if no response to the Fluorouracil.

OUr diagnosis is metastatic carcinoma involving the liver, primary site undetermined.

Dictated: 10-25-74

Transcribed: 10-25-74 dme

John D. H█████ Jr., M. D.

233

SURGICAL PATHOLOG

,998

| Patient #19 | SURGEON Dr. Robert W | DATE 10/18/74 | ROOM NO. 518 |
| | AGE 64 | DURATION OF SYMPTOMS | |

OPERATION
EXPLORATORY LAP. AND BIOPSY LIVER.

ORGANS SENT FOR EXAMINATION
Biopsy of liver.

HISTORY
Weight loss.

PHYSICAL FINDINGS
Large mass epigastrium.

FINDINGS AT OPERATION
Metastatic carcinoma of liver.

DIAGNOSIS
Metastic Carcinoma of liver.

PREVIOUS SURGERY

Dr. Robert W

GROSS DESCRIPTION

One cm. fragment of gray soft tissue.   2 NS

GRF:ljb

Gerald R. F   M.D.
Pathologist

HISTOLOGICAL EXAMINATION

DIAGNOSIS:

Section contains liver with undifferentiated malignant neoplasm.

Gerald R. F   , M. D.

jh

LUNG CANCER

Lung cancer, the leading cancer killer in the United States, claimed 136,000 lives in 1987. Tumors of the lung resist most therapy, and only 13% of all patients diagnosed with the disease, considering the various subtypes together, live five years.

Patient #20

Patient #20 was 59 years old when in November 1986 she died from complications resulting from bronchoscopy. At the time she had survived nearly 12 years after being diagnosed with metastatic, recurrent lung carcinoma.

Prior to developing cancer, Patient #20 had smoked at least two packs of cigarettes a day for 25 years. As a result of her habit, for decades she was afflicted with chronic sinusitis, associated with a dry, hacking "smoker's cough." In 1955, she experienced a bout of pneumonia so severe her doctors prescribed a course of radiation to clear her lungs. Unfortunately, the treatment destroyed a significant portion of her thyroid gland, so that Patient #20 subsequently required daily hormone supplementation.

Patient #20 said after the radiation, she never felt completely well, living for years with chronic fatigue, mood swings and a constant "worn out" feeling. Then in 1971, her husband developed colon cancer, initially thought cured by surgery. Despite the "good" prognosis, Patient #20 worried constantly about her spouse's health, and experienced frequent bouts of depression alternating with anxiety. Her physician, attributing these various problems to "menopause," prescribed a variety of tranquilizers as well as a synthetic estrogen preparation during the early 1970s.

In 1974, after her husband's colon cancer recurred, Patient #20 began investigating alternative cancer therapies for his use. She even bought Dr. Kelley's book, *One Answer to Cancer,* in a local health food store, but her husband refused to pursue such an unconventional treatment.

Throughout 1974, Patient #20's own health deteriorated. She frequently coughed up purulent, blood-tinged sputum, and experienced a chronic low grade fever. In January 1975, when an X-ray revealed a possible "abscess" or cyst in the region of the left lower lung field, she completed a two-week course of antibiotics for a presumed infection. Although Patient #20 improved slightly, her cough eventually worsened. Finally, after she became bedridden, on February 28, 1975, Patient #20 was admitted to St. Joseph's Hospital in Kirkwood, Missouri, for evaluation.

At St. Joseph's, an X-ray again revealed the lung lesion previously noted, which the radiologist this time around believed to be more consistent with malignancy than with infection. After a laminography evaluation, a more sophisticated X-ray study, the diagnosis of cancer seemed more certain: the official report describes the finding as a "mass lesion at the left lower lobe region . . . A neoplastic process should receive first consideration again." Further tests, including liver and brain scans, showed no sign of metastatic disease, and bronchoscopy (examination of the airways with a flexible tube) was inconclusive.

On March 6, 1975, Patient #20 underwent exploratory chest surgery, during which she was found to have a large tumor, reported in the operative note as "a large firm mass infiltrating the greater portion of the left lower lobe . . . " After a frozen section biopsy confirmed malignancy, the attending surgeon proceeded with resection of the lower left lung.

The lesion, measuring 9.5 cm in diameter, was classified as a bronchogenic adenocarcinoma, one of the more aggressive forms of lung cancer, with three regional lymph nodes positive for metastatic disease. Because of the nodal involvement, her doctors recommended additional surgery, so on March 17, 1975, only 11 days after her first operation, Patient #20 underwent a left pneumonectomy (removal of the entire left lung).

Subsequently, a consulting oncologist recommended a course of intensive chemotherapy, to be administered on an outpatient basis. But after her discharge from the hospital in late March 1975, Patient #20 returned home to find a very sick husband, himself about to begin both chemotherapy and radiation. Only days later, after beginning treatment, he became extremely ill—and never again left his bed.

As she watched her husband deteriorate, Patient #20 decided to refuse all further conventional treatment herself and instead follow the "Kelley program" as outlined in *One Answer to Cancer*, the book she had purchased for her husband. Although she did not contact Dr. Kelley at this time, Patient #20 adhered faithfully to the directions as provided. Within a week, she had given up cigarettes, alcohol, "junk food," and her tranquilizers. She found a source for the various recommended nutritional supplements and enzymes, taught herself how to administer the coffee enemas, and began her own "cancer diet." To her own surprise, she noticed an almost daily improvement in her health.

Meanwhile, her husband, who had been rapidly worsening, suffered a major convulsion, was hospitalized, and died.

Despite her many stresses, Patient #20 continued the "Kelley program" using only *One Answer to Cancer* as a guide, ultimately following the full nutritional regimen for two years before tapering off because she felt herself cured.

237

Thereafter, Patient #20 became careless, even discontinuing her thyroid medication, and gradually reverting to a "junk food" diet. Throughout the first half of 1978, she experienced constant fatigue, depression, and general ill health. When her symptoms worsened in September 1978 she finally returned to her family physician, whom she hadn't seen for years.

Several days later, Patient #20 was admitted to Missouri Baptist Hospital for a thorough re-evaluation. Though severely hypothyroid, after extensive testing she appeared to be cancer-free. Subsequently, although Patient #20 resumed her thyroid medication, her symptoms did not improve; her fatigue persisted, and over the following year, she experienced vague, persistent aches and pains throughout her body.

In October 1979, Patient #20 consulted her physician once again. This time, a chest X-ray performed at Missouri Baptist revealed a 1 cm nodule in the right mid-lung, as well as a possible second nodule in the region of the right fifth rib. Both lesions were believed to be consistent with recurrent cancer, as described in the official radiology report: "The possibility of metastatic nodules to the right lung deserves consideration . . . "

Patient #20's doctors elected to observe her progress for a month before re-evaluating the situation. Then in early December 1979 a tomogram study of the right lung—a procedure involving a series of X-rays—showed "two lesions in the right lung most in keeping with metastatic disease." Although bronchoscopy was recommended, Patient #20 initially decided to refuse further testing. But in March 1980, she agreed to a follow-up chest X-ray at Missouri Baptist which clearly indicated that the nodules had enlarged, as described in the official report: "two nodules right mid lung field which have increased in size compared to October, 1979—these are compatible with metastases."

At that point, Patient #20 resumed her nutritional program under the guidance of a former Kelley patient whom he had trained as a counselor to administer his therapy. On the treatment, Patient #20's multiple health problems improved and the lung masses gradually regressed. Thereafter, Patient #20 remained in excellent health until November 1986, when, after developing influenza complicated by pneumonia, she was admitted to a local hospital for bronchoscopy. During the procedure, Patient #20 began to hemorrhage profusely after her physician punctured one of the pulmonary arteries, and within an hour she had bled to death. At the time she had survived nearly 12 years since her original diagnosis, and seven years from her recurrence in early 1980.

The statistics for bronchogenic carcinoma of the lung are dismal. Minna et al describe a 12% five-year survival rate for all patients with the disease,[1] including those aggressively treated with surgery, radiation and chemotherapy; after her recurrence, Patient #20 chose to follow only the Kelley regimen.

When I last spoke with Patient #20 in the fall of 1986, she was, at age 59, actively making plans for what she called her "second" life. She had gone back to graduate school, and was writing a book about her experiences with the Kelley program. Her only regret was that her husband put too much faith in his conventional doctors. "If he hadn't believed in them so much," she told me, "he might still be alive today."

REFERENCE

1. DeVita, VT, et al. *Cancer Principles & Practice of Oncology*. Philadelphia; J.B. Lippincott Company, 1982, page 403.

Patient #20		AGE 47	RADIOLOGY NUMBER 02-05-64
3-1-75	ROOM NUMBER 1115	ATTENDING PHYSICIAN	

NGS:

CHEST

Examination of the chest with laminographic technique again
reveals thepreviously described mass lesion at the left lower
lobe region. This is a solid mass lesion without the calcification or a cavity formation. The left main stem bronchus is outlined and appeared intact. A neoplastic process should receive
first consideration again.

HDS:las   3-2-75   H. DOGAN S_____, M.D.

_____   _____ M.D.
D-4 REV.10-74   CHART COPY   RADIOLOGIST

240

DICTATED: 3-26-75
CHART: 176597

ST. JOSEPH HOSPITAL

OPERATIVE REPORT

Date   3-6-75

Name   Patient #20   Room No.   1115
                                                              2102

Preoperative Diagnosis Suspect carcinoma left lower lobe

Postoperative Diagnosis Adenocarcinoma left lower lobe

Surgeon   Dr. V███   Anesthetist   Dr. C███████   Anesthetic   General

Assistants   Dr. L███
             Dr. P███

Name Of Operation

                 Left lower lobectomy

Operation Began   12:45 p.m.   Closed   3:00 p.m.

Findings and Procedure

The patient was given general endotracheal anesthesia, placed in the left lateral position,
left hemi-thorax prepared and draped by Betadine technique. Posterior-lateral thoracotomy
and subperiosteal resection of the 6th rib was performed using cautery for hemostasis.
Exploration revealed several hundred cc's of clear yellow fluid in the pleural cavity.
This was aspirated. There was a large, firm mass infiltrating the greater portion of
the left lower lobe basil segments region. The very adjacent regional nodes were enlarged,
but soft and pliable. The upper lobe and hilum appeared relatively free of disease.
A single node in the anterior hilum at the upper lobe level was resected and reported as
not involved. Exploratory dissection was carried out in the inferior pulmonary ligament
area. Ligament divided and inferior vein dissected and ligated with 2-silk prior to
any further manipulation. A biopsy of the mass was then made and a report of adenocarcinoma
returned. It was felt that lobectomy would be an adequate procedure, therefore, the pulmonary
artery to the lower lobe was completely dissected, ligated above the origin of the superior
segment artery with one silk, suture ligated with 0-silk and divided. The inferior pulmonary
ligament was now firmly ligated with 2-silk, suture ligated with 0-silk and divided. The
inferior pulmonary ligament was completely dissected about the bronchus, the bronchus totally
dissected to the origin of the left upper lobe bronchus. No gross evidence of tumor could
be found. Additional small nodes and inferior pulmonary ligament and beneath the pulmonary
artery were submitted separately. The bronchus was stabilized at its origin and closed
with the auto suture stapler technique. The lobe was then resected. The wound thoroughly
irrigated with normal saline solution. Closed drains were placed in the second interspace
in the midclavicular line and in the 10th interspace in the posterior axillary line. The
incision was closed with 0-silk intercostal muscle and 1-chromic to each layer of the
thoracic muscle with 3-0 Dexon in subcutaneous fascia and 4-0 Ethilon to the skin. Simple
dressing applied. Procedure well-tolerated.

Immediate Postoperative Condition
Transcribed: 3-27-75
JCV/asd

Signature Of Surgeon _____

                                    James C. V███, M.D.

Form 118

241

SURGICAL PATHOLOGY REPORT

Name: Patient #20   Date: 3-6-75   Adm. No.

Doctor: Dr. V█   Room   Age

Specimen Labeled:
       A.   needle biopsy of lung tumor
       B.   hilar lymph nodes
       C.   lower lobe of left lung
       D.   lymph nodes
       E.   rib, left side

GROSS EXAMINATION:

Special A. Specimen consists of two pieces of needle biopsy tumor tissue, 1 cm each. Frozen section diagnosis: mucinous adenocarcinoma.

Specimen B. Specimen consists of two anthracotic lymph nodes 0.8 and 1.2 cm. Frozen section diagnosis: negative for tumor.

Specimen C. Specimen consists of lower lobe of left lung, average size, with a large mucinous tumor replacing the anterior medial basal segment and extending to the pleura but not through the pleura. The tumor measures 9.5 cm in diameter, and a bronchus from which it appears to be arising is identified and sectioned for microscopic examination. There are no satellite tumor nodules. The small anthracotic hilar nodes are grossly negative for metastatic tumor. One hilar node somewhat suspicious of tumor is negative on frozen section.

Specimen D. Specimen consists of two anthracotic lymph nodes, 1 and 1.5 cm.

Specimen E is a rib 19 x 1 cm, grossly unremarkable.

MICROSCOPIC EXAMINATION:

Sections demonstrate large mucinous bronchogenic adenocarcinoma arising in anterior medial basal segment of the left lower lobe. The tumor is a typical mucinous adenocarcinoma. There are no metastases demonstrated in the hilar lymph nodes, but two of the nodes submitted with the left lower lobe contain metastatic carcinoma and one of the nodes submitted as just lymph nodes (specimen D) also contains metastatic bronchogenic mucinous adenocarcinoma. The lymph nodes submitted for frozen section are negative for metastatic tumor.

DIAGNOSIS: Lung, left lower lobe needle biopsy and lobectomy
            :   bronchogenic adenocarcinoma, mucinous type, 9.5 cm extending
               to but not through pleura.
            :   metastatic mucinous bronchogenic adenocarcinoma to broncho-
               pulmonary lymph nodes of left lower lobe (two out of seven).
            :   metastatic bronchogenic mucinous adenocarcinoma in one of four
               separately submitted lymph nodes.
            :   hilar lymph nodes negative for metastatic tumor.

(continued)   SURGICAL PATHOLOGY REPORT   St. Joseph Hospital
                                                               Kirkwood, Missouri

242

Path. No.   75-1165   No. 82 A

SURGICAL PATHOLOGY REPORT

Name   Patient #20   Date   3-6-75   Adm. No.

Doctor   Dr. Vest   Room   1115   Age   47

Specimen Labeled: A.   needle biopsy of lung tumor
                          B.   hilar lymph nodes
                          C.   lower lobe of left lung
                          D.   lymph nodes
                          E.   rib, left side

GROSS EXAMINATION:

DIAGNOSIS: (continued)

          Bone, left thoracic rib, thoracotomy
          : no pathologic findings.

William H. S█████████, M. D. 3-7-75

CODE ☒ Y
      ☐ N

243

DEPARTMENT OF RADIOLOGY
CONSULTATION REPORT

10/15 03:12 PM 0068

TYPD 10/15/79   3:09 PM   DISCH

PAGE	1
X-RAY NO.	915510
EXAM DATE	10/15/79
ORDER NO.	0001

Patient #20   F   OUT-PT

PATIENT NO.	PATIENT NAME	BIRTH DATE	SEX	ROOM - BED
W█████, HARVEY JR.	321			

ATTENDING DOCTOR	CODE	REFERRING DOCTOR	CODE

PROC: 1020 CHEST, PA & LATERAL

SUMMARY: POST-OP LEFT THORACOTOMY AND PNEUMONECTOMY. SHIFT OF THE MEDIA-
STINAL STRUCTURES TO THE LEFT. INTERVAL DEVELOPMENT SINCE 9-12-78 OF A 1 CM
NODULE RIGHT MID LUNG WITH QUESTIONABLE SECOND NODULE OVERLYING PROXIMAL

END OF THE 5TH RIB. POSSIBILITY OF METASTATIC NODULES DESERVES CONSIDERATION.
LAMINAGRAMS OF THE RIGHT LUNG WOULD BE OF FURTHER VALUE.

    PA AND LEFT LATERAL VIEWS OF THE CHEST WERE OBTAINED AND COMPARED TO
PREVIOUS EXAM OF 9-12-78. POST-OPERATIVE LEFT THORACOTOMY CHANGES AND LEFT
PNEUMONECTOMY CAN BE SEEN. THE MEDIASTINAL STRUCTURES AER SHIFTED FROM
RIGHT TO LEFT. SMALL, APPROXIMATELY 1 CM NODULE, IS NOW SUGGESTED IN THE
MID PORTION OF THE RIGHT LUNG. A QUESTIONABLE SECOND NODULAR DENSITY MAY BE
PRESENT OVERLYING THE COSTAL AND OF THE 5TH ON THE RIGHT. THE POSSIBILITY
OF METASTATIC NODULES TO THE RIGHT LUNG DESERVES CONSIDERATION AND WHOLE
LUNG LAMINAGRAMS OF THE RIGHT LUNG ARE RECOMMENDED FOR FURTHER STUDY. NO
OTHER CHANGES ARE SEEN OF THE RIGHT LUNG. PLEURAL FLUID IS NOT IDENTIFIED.
BONY STRUCTURES ARE UNREMARKABLE EXCEPT FOR THE THORACOTOMY CHANGES ON THE
LEFT.

10-15-79LY

L█████ J.H. M.D.

244

RADIOLOGY CONSULTATION REQUEST
NUCLEAR MEDICINE REQUEST

PATIENT IDENTIFICATION AREA

Patient #20

PATIENT TRANSPORT		PATIENT AVAILABLE	
WALK	STRETCHER	ANYTIME	AFTER NO ROUTINE LAB
WHEEL CHAIR	BEDSIDE	AFTER 9 A.M. ROUT. LAB WK	OTHER

Dr. D   12/7/79

DATE OF REQUEST   DATE EXAM TO BE DONE   REQUISITION PREPARED BY

P. C

RADIOLOGY CONSULTATION REQUEST

ORGANS	AREAS	VERTEBRAE	BONES Rt Lt	JOINTS Rt Lt
☐ IVP	☐ Chest Pa Lat R☐ L☐	☐ Cervical	Humerus ☐☐	Shoulder ☐☐
☐ Gall Bladder	☐ Abdomen Upr Decub☐	☐ Thoracic	Forearm ☐☐	Elbow ☐☐
☐ Esophagus Ba Swallow	☐ Pelvis	☐ Lumbo Sacral	Hand ☐☐	Wrist ☐☐
☐ Upper G.I.	☐ Skull	BONES Rt Lt	Femur ☐☐	Hip ☐☐
☐ Sm. Bowel	☐ Sinuses	Ribs ☐☐	Leg ☐☐	Knee ☐☐
☐ Colon Ba Enema	☐ Facial Bones	Clavicle ☐☐	Foot ☐☐	Ankle ☐☐

OTHER EXAM. **Tomogram right lung**

OTHER EXAM.

REMARKS:

NUCLEAR MEDICINE REQUEST

NUCLEAR MEDICINE		THERMOSCAN
Brain Scan C.F. / Histo	Renal	Breast
Brain Scan	Bone — Total Body	Abdomen
C.F. Study	Xenon	Extremities
Liver	Pancreas	Total Body
Liver / Spleen	Placenta	OTHER
Lung	OTHER	PHONE
Thyroid		
Thyroid / Uptake		

Isotope	Time	Delay	Initials

PREVIOUS X-RAY   YES ☐ NO ☐   IS PATIENT PREGNANT   YES ☐ NO ☐   UNKNOWN ☐

CONTRAINDICATIONS? GLUCAGON ☐   ANTICHOLINERGICS ☐   OTHER ☐ _____

X-RAY _17538_   EXAM COMPLETED _____ AM-PM   DATE COMPLETED _____

CLINICAL HISTORY (SYMPTOMS, LAB DATA, DX TO BE R/I OR R/O) ____ Ca of lung

TOMOGRAPHY:

Tomograms of the chest were taken, to evaluate the possibility of a lesion in
the right lung. Preliminary film does show what appears to be a density in the
right lower mid-lung. In retrospect, this is not seen on examination of
12-4-79, probably because it is underlying a rib.

Multiple tomographic cuts were taken of the right lung, and do demonstrate the
presence of two lesions suggested beneath the anterior interspace between the
2nd and 3rd ribs. These lesions appear to be adjacent to the minor fissure.
They are compatible with metastatic disease.

IMPRESSION:

Demonstration of two lesions in the right ~~lung~~ most in keeping with metastatic
disease.

12-10-79 BFB/lo   Barry F. B_____, MD

12-779 chest tomograms

FORM 10958-11/78

MISSOURI BAPTIST HOSPITAL

ST. LOUIS, MISSOURI 63131

DEPARTMENT OF RADIOLOGY
CONSULTATION REPORT

TYPD   3/10/80   3:11 PM   DISCH

Patient #20

PAGE	1
X-RAY NO.	04229
EXAM DATE	3/10/80
ORDER NO.	0001

PATIENT NO.	PATIENT NAME	BIRTH DATE	SEX	ROOM	BED
			F	OUT-PT	
W▮▮▮, HARVEY JR.	321				

ATTENDING DOCTOR	CODE	REFERRING DOCTOR	CODE

PROC: 1020 CHEST, PA & LATERAL

SUMMARY: STATUS POST-LEFT THORACOTOMY AND LEFT PNEUMONECTOMY. TWO NODULES
RIGHT MID LUNG FIELD WHICH HAVE INCREASED IN SIZE COMPARED TO OCTOBER, 1979 -
THESE ARE COMPATIBLE WITH METASTASES.

PA AND LEFT LATERAL VIEWS OF THE CHEST SHOW EVIDENCE FOR A PREVIOUS LEFT
THORACOTOMY (LEFT PNEUMONECTOMY). LEFT HEMITHORAX IS OPACIFIED AND THE
MEDIASTINAL STRUCTURES ARE SHIFTED TO THE LEFT. THERE ARE AGAIN NOTED TWO
NODULES IN THE RIGHT MID LUNG FIELD. BOTH OF THESE HAVE INCREASED IN SIZE
COMPARED TO 10-15-79. THE NODULE MEDIAL TO THE ANTERIOR ASPECT OF THE RIGHT
THIRD RIB MEASURES APPROXIMATELY 1.5 CM IN DIAMETER AND A NODULE IN THE RIGHT
4TH ANTERIOR INTERSPACE MEASURING APPROXIMATELY 1 CM IN DIAMETER. THESE ARE
COMPATIBLE WITH METASTASES. NO EVIDENCE OF RIGHT PLEURAL EFFUSION.

3-10-80 JR

H▮▮▮▮▮ w▮▮▮ M.D.

246

Patient #21

Patient #21, a 52-year-old man from Ohio, has survived 13 years since his diagnosis of metastatic squamous cell carcinoma of the lung.

In early 1974, Patient #21, with a long history of heavy smoking, developed a persistent, dry hacking cough. He consulted his family doctor, who, diagnosing an infection, prescribed a course of antibiotic therapy. Despite the treatment, the symptoms only worsened, and in March 1974, Patient #21 returned to his physician. After a chest X-ray revealed a 3 cm mass in the upper lobe of the right lung, Patient #21 was admitted to Akron City Hospital on April 7, 1974 for exploratory chest surgery. During the procedure, he was found to have a large inoperable tumor in the right lung that had metastasized to many lymph nodes, findings described in the operative note:

> A tumor approximately 4 cm. in greatest diameter was found in the periphery of the posterior segment of the right upper lobe [of the lung]. In the area below the azygos vein were multiple nodes which extended posteriorly up along the vena cava and acquired a maximum diameter of about 3.5 cm . . . Because of the massive involvement of the mediastinum curative resection obviously was not feasible.

A biopsy of the tumor confirmed "Poorly differentiated carcinoma consistent with squamous cell type . . . " In addition, a lymph node removed at surgery was positive for metastatic disease.

Patient #21's doctors then recommended a course of cobalt radiation treatment, though they informed him that even with such therapy, his chances of surviving one year were dim. Nonetheless, he agreed to the treatment, which he began while still hospitalized. In the discharge summary, the attending physician wrote: " . . . the patient, due to the metastatic nature of this carcinoma does have a poor prognosis."

Patient #21 completed the suggested regimen of 5000 rads to the lungs as an outpatient, but when the tumors continued to grow despite radiation, his doctors proposed a course of intensive chemotherapy. Since his disease appeared to be incurable, Patient #21 refused all further conventional treatment, instead choosing to investigate unconventional cancer therapies. He soon learned of Dr. Kelley, consulted with him and began the full program in late spring of 1974.

Subsequently, over a several month period his persistent respiratory symptoms resolved, and within a year Patient #21 says he felt better than he had for a decade. Today, 13 years after his diagnosis, Patient #21 still follows his nutritional protocol and remains in excellent health with no sign of his once metastatic disease.

For squamous cell carcinoma of the lung, one of the most deadly of cancers, the literature reports a five-year survival rate for patients with stage III disease, regardless of treatment, of less than 5%.[1] Stanley describes a median survival of only 24-27 weeks in 32 symptomatic patients such as Patient #21 with unresectable tumors despite aggressive standard treatment.[2]

In summary, Patient #21 was diagnosed with inoperable, metastatic lung cancer which did not respond to a course of cobalt therapy. It therefore seems appropriate to attribute this patient's long-term survival to the Kelley program.

REFERENCES

1. DeVita, VT, et al. *Cancer Principles & Practice of Oncology*. Philadelphia; J.B. Lippincott Company, 1982, page 409.

2. Stanley, KE. "Prognostic Factors for Survival in Patients with Inoperable Lung Cancer." *Journal of the National Cancer Institute* 1980; 65:25–32.

Name

Age 39

Preoperative Diagnosis

Tumor of the right lung

Postoperative Diagnosis

Eperdermoid carcinoma of lung,
right

Operation   33.1   92.2

360-11 Excision of lesion of lung,
right: 350-40 Bronchoscopy

Began 11:45 AM   Closed   2:45 PM

Sponge Count: Before 10-4x4 10-DLG After

Admission No.

Date   4-8-74

Surgeon   Dr.W.

Assistants   Dr. P   B

Anesthetist   Dr.T

Instrument Nurse   J. F   J.B

Preoperative Drugs

Anesthetic

Nurse J.S   , J. F

Findings: Gross (Describe all pathological findings and all organs explored, normal and abnormal.)

Referral: Dr.Charles M

There was a clinical history of one month and a half cough with radiographic
evidence of radiopaque 3 cm. in diameter mass in the region of the right upper
lobe in the posterior segment.

On bronchoscopy there was no remarkable abnormality and no specimen.

On right thoracotomy a tumor approximately 4 cm. in greatest diameter was
found in the periphery of the posterior segment of the right upper lobe. In the area
below the azygos vein were multiple nodes which extended posteriorly up along the
vena cava and acquired a maximum diameter of about 3.5 cm. These were really not in

Operative Procedure:

the anterior mediastinum as much as they were laterally and posteriorly located.
On frozen section the tissue was positive for epidermoid carcinoma. There was no
other significant intra-thoracic abnormality.

Because of the massive involvement of the mediastinum curative resection
obviously was not feasible.

OPERATIVE PROCEDURE:

The above was carried out under general anesthesia. Following bronchoscopy,
through a right posterolateral 6th rib bed incision the thora was opened and a
portion of the hilum removed. _Closure was then effected in layers using silk to the
intercostal bundle, two layers of thoracic wall muscles and skin with one tube
for drainage purposes.

Immediate Postoperative Condition: Hemorrhage, Shock, Etc.

WF; mh;
Typed 4-17-74
Dict- 4-8-74

Signature of Surgeon _____

OPERATIVE RECORD
AKRON CITY HOSPITAL

TISSUE EXAMINATION

ICU.

NAME _____ AGE 39 NO. ▓▓▓ DR. W. P▓▓ WARD 5 3 W

GROSS EXAMINATION

Lab. No. 74-3851

Date 4-8-74

I. "Lung tissue"---to lab by Dr. K▓▓
Frozen Section: Two pieces of grayish-pink soft tissue. One measures
1 by 0.8 by 0.1 cm. The other one 0.8 by 0.6 by 0.3 cm. (2 ns)

II. "Rib"
A piece of rib plus two fragments from the same, 16 by 1.5 cm. (ss no micro)

TA/js

MICROSCOPIC EXAMINATION

I. FROZEN SECTION DIAGNOSIS: Carcinoma (probably epidermoid). SK

Controlling Frozen Section: Two separate sections, one is fibrous tissue
fragment totally replaced by discrete to confluent nests of poorly
differentiated carcinoma more compatible with squamous cell type rather
than adenocarcinoma. Chronic inflammation, fibrosis and moderate
artefacts. No pulmonary alveoli or any specific structures are present
to identify the exact anatomic location of this fragment. The second
fragment is a section of lymphnode with metastatic focus of poorly
differentiated carcinoma which histologically resembles the neoplasm in
the other fragment. Fibrosis, focal anthracosis and moderate artefacts.

II. No sections made.

DIAGNOSIS -6

Poorly differentiated carcinoma consistent with squamous cell type totally
replacing one biopsy fragment from hilum of right lung.
Metastatic poorly differentiated squamous cell carcinoma in lymphnode.
Segment of rib.

L. R▓▓ M. D.

Form F-201

AKRON CITY HOSPITAL

250

PATIENT NAME

DISCHARGE DATE

UNIT NUMBER

Patient #21

Dr. W. F█████

4-17-74

REASON FOR ADMISSION: This 39-year-old white male was in his usual state of good health until approximately 1-1/2 months prior to admission, when being treated for an upper respiratory tract infection that failed to resolve. X-ray at this time revealed a tumor mass of the lung. The patient denied any history of shortness of breath, wheezing or hemoptysis.

SIGNIFICANT FINDINGS: On physical examination the chest was clear to auscultation and percussion. The abdominal examination was within normal limits. Admission CBC revealed the patient to have a hemoglobin of 14 with hematocrit of 41.5 with a WBC of 18,500 with 57% neutrophils, 5% bands, 29 lymphocytes, 6 monocytes and 3 eosinophils. Admission urinalysis, SMA-12 and EKG were within normal limits. Admission chest X-ray revealed a mediastinal mass on the right, involving the right hilum.

TREATMENT RECEIVED: On 4-8-74, patient was taken to surgery at which time a right thoracotomy and mediastinal node biopsy were performed. Pathologic examination of the specimen revealed poorly differentiated squamous cell carcinoma. Due to the mediastinal involvement, resection was impossible, and the patient was started on cobalt therapy and this will be continued as an outpatient.

FINAL DIAGNOSIS: METASTATIC SQUAMOUS CELL CARCINOMA OF THE LUNG.

CONDITION ON DISCHARGE: Satisfactory, but the patient, due to the metastatic nature of this carcinoma does have a poor prognosis.

PLANS FOR FUTURE CARE: Patient will be seen in three weeks by Dr. F█████ and will continue cobalt therapy as an outpatient.

R. B█████, M. D.
RB: bg
dictated - 4-17-74
transcribed - 4-23-74

DISCHARGE SUMMARY
Akron City Hospital
F-487 Rev. 1-74

HOUSE PHYSICIAN

ATTENDING PHYSICIAN

251

LYMPHOMA

Pathologists divide the lymphomas into at least eight major types, distinguished by very specific molecular and genetic characteristics. Altogether, the various lymphomas claimed 15,400 lives in 1987. Approximately 50% of all patients diagnosed with the disease survive five years, although great variation in prognosis exists depending on the subtype.

In the following section, I present cases of diffuse histiocytic lymphoma, diffuse mixed histiocytic and lymphocytic lymphoma, diffuse poorly differentiated lymphocytic lymphoma, and nodular poorly differentiated lymphocytic lymphoma.

Patient #22

Patient #22 died in November 1986 at the age of 63 from renal failure and other complications of cancer, after surviving nearly seven years with a diagnosis of widely metastatic diffuse histiocytic lymphoma.

Toward the end of 1979, Patient #22 first experienced gradually worsening fatigue, associated with a persistent sensation of fullness in his chest, distressing enough to interfere with sleep. Despite his symptoms, Patient #22 did not seek medical attention until spring of 1980, when his abdomen suddenly enlarged. At that time, his physician noted a large palpable mass in the upper left abdomen on physical exam. A subsequent ultrasound study revealed, as described in the radiology report, "a large bulky mass within the left side of the abdomen, measuring on the order of 13 to 14 cm's [sic] in diameter . . . "

Patient #22 was then admitted to Sacred Heart Medical Center in Spokane on April 13, 1980 for further evaluation. The following day, during exploratory surgery he was found to have a huge retroperitoneal (posterior abdominal) tumor, which, although biopsied, was too large for resection.

The tumor was initially classified as an undifferentiated "high grade malignancy." The biopsy slides were then sent for further assessment to the University of Washington, where the pathologist diagnosed diffuse histiocytic lymphoma, summarized in the records as "Retroperitoneal mass: malignant lymphoma, histiocytic type (Rappaport) associated with extensive sclerosis."

At this point, the patient's oncologist at Sacred Heart then recommended intensive chemotherapy with the CHOP regimen, consisting of the drugs cyclophosphamide, Adriamycin, vincristine, procarbazine and prednisone, to be administered on a monthly basis. Patient #22 agreed to the treatment, which he began on May 2, 1980.

Patient #22 tolerated the first round of chemotherapy without significant side effects, but after returning home May 5, 1980, he decided to investigate unconventional approaches to cancer, including the Kelley program. In June 1980, when he was not thought to be in remission, he began the Kelley regimen, thereafter refusing further conventional treatment.

Within weeks, as he followed his nutritional regimen, Patient #22 noted an improvement in his general health. When next seen by his physician in August 1980, an ultrasound study revealed the tumor had stabilized.

254

Patient #22 continued his nutritional protocol and continued doing well. An ultrasound performed December 14, 1981, as the patient followed only the Kelley program, showed noticeable shrinkage of the abdominal mass. And when evaluated some eight months later, on August 30, 1982, a third ultrasound documented further regression of the tumor, as described in the radiology report:

> The mass is again well visualized but has diminished in size since the previous examination. On today's examination, it measures 61 mm. [millimeters] in its maximum width, 39 mm. in depth, and 72 mm. in length. This compares with previous measurements of 77 mm. in width, 51 mm. in depth, and 102 mm. in length.

Patient #22 followed the Kelley program for approximately four years, until July 1984, when he discontinued his protocol, thinking himself cured. Subsequently, over a period of several months he developed recurrent fatigue associated with a gradual weight loss. With his health deteriorating, Patient #22 resumed the prescribed supplements, but on his own decided to incorporate two other alternative therapies into his regimen and adopt a strict vegetarian diet—a serious mistake by Dr. Kelley's standards, since he emphasizes lymphoma patients invariably worsen unless they consume red meat frequently, usually daily. To complicate matters, during 1985, according to Dr. Kelley, the quality of available supplements, particularly the pancreatic enzymes, deteriorated.

Thereafter, Patient #22 suffered a gradual decline due to recurrent lymphoma, eventually succumbing to his disease in November 1986, more than six and a half years after his initial diagnosis.

Although Patient #22 did ultimately fall victim to his cancer, his prolonged survival is most unusual. Experts consider diffuse histiocytic lymphoma a very aggressive cancer that requires intensive chemotherapy, radiation, or both, for prolonged survival. DeVita describes DHL as "biologically aggressive," a malignancy that if untreated nearly always kills within two years.[1]

With aggressive chemotherapy, between 25–45% of patients with advanced diffuse histiocytic lymphoma will survive five years.[2] Oncologists recommend that for optimal benefit, the drug regimens be administered for a minimum of 6–12 months, or at least until the patient achieves a complete remission. Patient #22 completed only one cycle of chemotherapy before discontinuing the treatment to search out alternative approaches when he was clearly not yet in remission. Furthermore, his cancer regressed, as documented by sequential ultrasound studies, only after he began the Kelley program.

Dr. Kelley believes that the vegetarian diet used by this patient severely compromised his chance for recovery. Had Patient #22 continued his prescribed diet, Dr. Kelley feels he might still be alive today.

REFERENCES

1. DeVita, VT, et al. *Cancer Principles & Practice of Oncology*. Philadelphia; J.B. Lippincott, 1982, page 1387.

2. Harvey, AM, et al. *The Principles and Practice of Medicine*, 20th Edition. New York; Appleton-Century-Crofts, 1980, pages 565-566.

SACRED HEART MEDICAL CENTER
DEPARTMENT OF RADIOLOGY

NAME	Patient #22			AGE	X-RAY NO.

ADDRESS	59 Years		

PHYSICIAN	A. Logan			DATE

ABDOMINAL ULTRASOUND

Gray scale scanning was carried out in multiple projections
showing a large bulky mass within the left side of the abdomen,
measuring on the order of 13 to 14 cm's in diameter, containing
numerous internal echo's consistent with a solid lesion.
The mass lies anterior to the left kidney and spleen, but
cannot be separated with certainty from the left lobe of
the liver. Differential diagnostic possibilities would
include a large tumor of mesenchymal origin such as a
leiomyosarcoma or fibrosarcoma, possibly a lymphoma, (although
there are no obvious abnormal changes in the peri-aortic region)
of possibly a hepatoma arrising from the left lobe of the liver.
It would appear to lie somewhat far anteriorly to be arrising
within the tail of the pancreas. Right lobe of the liver
appars normal.

DIAGNOSIS: LARGE BULKY SOLID MASS WITHIN LEFT MID AND UPPER ABDOMEN
AS NOTED ABOVE. A TUMOR OF MESENCHYMAL ORIGIN, HEPATOMA OR
LYMPHOMA WOULD BE CONSIDERED POSSIBLE ETIOLOGIES.

Edmund I. _____ M.D.

RADIOLOGIST

PHYSICIANS COPY

X-RAY REPORT FORM 06-2379

257

Age ___58__ Sex ___M__ Race_____

Operation

Specimen(s)

Attending Surgeon:
Service:

Referring Hospital: Sacred Heart Medical Center

	A.M.	P.M.
Date Specimen Removed	____	____
Date Received in Lab.	____	4/22/80
Date Reported	____	5/7/80

Clinical Data

ANATOMIC FINDINGS

GROSS:
Received are seven slides and subsequently two blocks and a fragment of tissue fixed in formalin (less than 1 cm. in greatest dimension), all labeled S-80-3089; and the corresponding pathology report.

MICROSCOPIC:
Sections are from tissue covered on one surface by a flattened layer of serosal cells, the remainder being small groups of large malignant cells with a high mitotic rate supported by and divided into compartments by thin layers of collagen. The malignant cells have multilobulated nuclei, many with prominent nucleoli, and scanty poorly defined cytoplasm. In many areas the center of these compartments contains a finely granular amorphous pale eosinophilic deposit which is weakly P.A.S. positive and negative for amyloid on a Crystal Violet stain included. A reticulin stain confirms the sclerosing pattern present on H&E, but does not show reticulin around each individual cell.

ULTRASTRUCTURAL REPORT: (by Dr. J. B████)
Ultrastructural preservation is excellent. The most conspicuous cell type includes a malignant lymphoid cell ranging up to 16 to 17 microns in cross sectional diameter. It features a prominently hyperlobated nuclear contour, marginated chromatin and prominent nucleoli. Cell organelles are relatively simple and consist of mono- and polyribosomes, small aggregates of mitochondria, and occasionally prominent perinuclear Golgi complexes. The latter is not associated with observable numbers of lysosomes. The peripheral cell membrane is relatively straight to areas of undulation without evidence of cell membrane specialization in the form of cell junctions. The malignant lymphoid cell is oftentimes intimately admixed and often outnumbered by reactive mesenchymal cells featuring elongate nuclei, marginated chromatin, and cytoplasmic organelles concerned with the elaboration of extracellular collagen. This includes prominently dilated segments of rough endoplasmic reticulum containing a granular proteinaceous product. In addition, there are conspicuous bundles of myofilaments along their cell membrane associated with dense body formation. The myofibroblasts are intimately associated with bundles of type I collagen. Infrequent mononuclear inflammatory cells are also noted. A conspicuous change accounting for the pinkish extracellular material noted by light microscopy is the accumulation of cellular debris in the extracellular space. This includes

Page___1___ of __2___ pages

_____ M.D.
Pathologist

bas 5/8/80

UNIVERSITY OF WASHINGTON HOSPITALS
HARBORVIEW MEDICAL CENTER
UNIVERSITY HOSPITAL
SEATTLE, WASHINGTON
PATHOLOGY REPORT

UH 0503   REV. OCT 79   1-79-2700

PATHOLOGY NO.:

multiple small vesicles admixed with residual cell organelles. One can find a transition from degenerating cells exhibiting nuclear pyknosis, progressive dilatation of their cytocavitary system to eventuating into an aggregate of cellular debris. It's not possible to determine whether it's predominantly the mesenchymal myofibroblasts or malignant lymphoid cells are is in the process of cell degeneration creating this peculiar extracellular material.

DIAGNOSIS:
Retroperitoneal mass: Malignant lymphoma, histiocytic type, (Rappaport) associated with extensive sclerosis.

COMMENT: (by Dr. J. B█████)
This lesion is distinctive for a number of reasons. [1,2] The pattern of scarring simulates the sclerosing lymphoma described initially by Rappaport. [1,2] The ultrastructural findings generally parallel those observed by Katayama, et al [3] and include a population of malignant lymphoid cells and reactive mesenchymal myofibroblasts; the latter cell type is likely responsible for the elaboration of the extracellular collagen. The prominent nuclear hyperlobations and perinuclear Golgi complexes of the lymphoid cells raise the possibility of a "T cell lymphoma" however cell markers would be required to confirm this suspicion.

REFERENCES:
1. Rosas-Uribe A, Rappaport H: Malignant lymphoma, histiocytic type with sclerosis. Cancer 29:946-953, 1972.
2. Bennett MH: Sclerosis in nonHodgkin's lymphoma. British Journal of Cancer (supplement II) 44-52, 1975.
3. Katayama, et al: Histocytic lymphoma with sclerosis arising from a nodular lymphoma with special stromal reaction. Cancer 40:2203, 1977.

COMMENT by Dr. Marshall E. K█████
The remarkable degree of nuclear pleomorphism hyperlobation seen in this case is very infrequent in lymphomas other than Hodgkin's disease. I find no diagnostic Reed-Sternberg cells to make the latter diagnosis. Mulberry-like nuclear segmentation has been described in T-cell lymphomas (Am J Clin Path 72:540, 1979) and we have seen this also in rare non-T cell lymphomas, probably of follicular center cell origin, but surface marker data relating the origin of the neoplastic cells in this case are not available. Interestingly one of our previous cases with hypersegmented nuclei presented as a mediastinal mass, was associated with extensive fibrosis and amorphous cellular debris compartmentalizing the tumor cells and giving the impression of a metastatic undifferentiated tumor as in the present case. By electron microscopy, however, Dr. B████ found no intercellular junctions and a likely lymphoid origin in both cases. Although sclerosis has been found to be associated with a more favorable prognosis in the usual non-Hodgkin's lymphoma (Br. J. Cancer 31, Supp. II:44, 1975), the degree of pleomorphism and frequent mitoses seen in the present case suggests a more aggressive course in my view.

Marshall E. K█████ M.D.

M. █████ M.B., Ch.B.   M.D.
                                                             Pathologist

Page __2__ of 2 ____ pages
bas 5/8/80

NT   AT
UNIVERSITY HOSPITAL
UNIVERSITY OF WASHINGTON
SEATTLE, WASHINGTON 98195

PATHOLOGY REPORT

UH 0603   REV JUL 78   1-78-1605   (Continued)

Patient's No.:   Patient #22
Patient's Name:

Pathology No.:

259

Dr. Kenneth K█████
Standardized Record Form Developed By Northeastern Washington Hospital Council

Admission Date: 5-2-80

Discharge Date: 5-5-80

16386 (handwritten)

ADMISSION DIAGNOSIS:
1) Retroperitoneal lymphoma. In for chemotherapy.

DISCHARGE DIAGNOSIS:
1) Retroperitoneal lymphoma.

SUMMARY: This 50-year-old male was admitted to Sacred Heart Medical Center (SHMC) for chemotherapy for abdominal lymphoma. This mass was discovered by his physician approximately a month prior to admission. Laparotomy was performed by Dr. Z█████, and biopsies confirmed the nature of the tumor.

Physical examination showed normal vital signs in a healthy appearing 59-year-old white male. Physical exam was only remarkable for the obvious firm, slightly movable, 8x12cm mass in his abdomen, to the left of midline and superior to the umbilicus.

LABORATORY DATA and PROCEDURES: SMA-12 - LDH elevated at 325 (207 - upper limits of normal), alk phos 149 (88 - upper limits of normal). Hemoglobin and hematocrit were 11.8 and 37.4, respectively, with normal indices. Urinalysis was normal. Platelet count 265,000. Electrolytes were within normal limits. Creatinine 1.2, sed rate 18. There were no X rays obtained.

HOSPITAL COURSE: The patient was begun on CHOPP therapy on Saturday morning, 5-3-80. Cytoxan, adriamycin, vincristine, procarbozine were begun, and the patient tolerated administration of therapy extremely well, with only mild nausea for a complaint. Zyloprim was begun on 5-2-80, and this will be continued.

DISPOSITION: The patient is discharged to home, where he will continue medications orally. Followup to be arranged by Dr. Ken K█████.

Discharge medications include: Compazine - 10mg q 6 hours, prn. Procarbozine - 50mg, one b.i.d. Senokot tabs, one b.i.d. Allopurinol - 300mg, one daily. Prednisone - 20mg, two t.i.d. for six days.

JWL/lt
5-5-80d
5-9-80t
cc: Dr. Kenneth Kraemer

Jeffrey W. L████, M.D.
R-2, Internal Medicine
HOSPITAL: SACRED HEART MEDICAL CENTER

Dr. Kenneth K█████

DISCHARGE SUMMARY

GOOD BUSINESS FORMS CO. SPOKANE   (23501)

260

3-31-80   Dr. L█████   age 58
        IVP. The preliminary film of the
abdomen shows a vague fullness in the left
upper quadrant but a definite well-defined mass
is not identified. Following the injection of
contrast media, tomograms were obtained and
show both renal outlines to be intact. The
calices, pelves and ureters show no abnormality. The urinary bladder outline is generally normal, although the base of the bladder
is indented by an enlarged prostate gland.
Following voiding there was fair emptying of
the bladder with a small to moderate post-
voiding residual.
        DIAGNOSIS: Prostatic enlargement
with some post-voiding residual. Vague fullness of the mid and left upper abdomen suggesting a mass.
        CHEST.   PA and lateral views of the
chest show heart, mediastinal and hilar structures to be normal.   There is slight widening
of the left paraspinous line at the level of
the diaphragm. This is somewhat more prominent
than on previous examinations, and while this
may be of no significance, the findings would
at least raise the possibility of some
paraaortic lymphadenopathy in this region.
The lung fields are clear and there is no
pleural fluid.
        DIAGNOSIS: Slight widening of
the left paraspinous line at the level of the
diaphragm, raising the possibility of some
paraaortic lymphadenopathy.   These findings
are equivocal. Chest otherwise negative.
br   Michael L. B█████ M.D.

1-2-81   Dr. L█████   age
        PA AND LEFT LATERAL OF THE CHEST.
The cardiovascular structures appear normal.
The lungs are well expanded and clear. Again
is noted some fullness in the paraspinal region on the left and this is unchanged since
the exam nine months ago.
        THREE VIEWS OF THE RIGHT SHOULDER
show roughening of the cortex of the greater
tuberosity and some subcortical cystic change
compatible with osteoarthritis. There is
spurring of the inferior lip of the glenoid
fossa. No soft tissue calcifications are
noted.
        IMPRESSION: Osteoarthritic change
of the right shoulder. No active pulmonary
disease with no change in the appearance of
the chest since the exam nine months ago.
jb   P. A. B█████ M. D.

12-14-81   Dr. L█████   age 59
        ABDOMINAL ULTRASOUND. Ultrasound
evaluation of the abdomen was performed with
emphasis on a previously demonstrated mass
in the left mid and upper abdominal region.
Today's examination demonstrates a solid, but
relatively echofree mass which measures 7.3 cm.
x 10.2 cm. in its greatest dimensions. It is
situated just medial to the left kidney and
lies between the mid and lower pole of the
left kidney and the abdominal aorta. A small
portion of the mass extends over the aorta
and elevates the superior mesenteric artery.
Note is made of slight prominence of the calyces and pelvis in the left kidney and I suspect that there is at least a lowgrade associated hydronephrosis with the mass. The
right kidney is normal. Scanning through the
liver shows no abnormalities. Ultrasonograph-
ically, the appearance of the mass is most
consistent with either a retroperitoneal sar-
coma or a lymphomatous process. Our examination is compared with the previous examinations from Sacred Heart and comparison is very
difficult as the mass is considerably better
visualized on our examination with well defined margins. Nevertheless, it would appear
that the mass has generally reduced in size.
Future comparison, however, should be quite
accurate because the mass is well demonstrated
on our examination.
        DIAGNOSIS: Lobulated, 7 cm. x 10 cm.
mass in the left retroperitoneal area between
the left kidney and the aorta as discussed.
jb   Michael L. E█████, M. D.

8-30-82   Dr. L█████   age 60
        ABDOMINAL ULTRASOUND. Ultrasound
evaluation of the previously noted retroperitoneal mass was performed and is compared with the previous examination. The
mass is again well visualized but has diminished in size since the previous examination. On today's examination, it measures
61 mm. in its maximum width, 39 mm. in depth,
and 72 mm. in length. This compares with
previous measurements of 77 mm. in width,
51 mm. in depth, and 102 mm. in length. The
mass is solid but relatively sonolucent
compatible with a mass of lymph nodes.
jb   Michael L. E█████, M. D.

Patient #23

Patient #23 is a 67-year-old woman from Minnesota alive more than ten years since her diagnosis of diffuse mixed histiocytic and lymphocytic lymphoma.

In 1957, Patient #23 was diagnosed with breast carcinoma, treated initially with a right radical mastectomy. Although the cancer had metastasized to multiple axillary lymph nodes, after a course of radiation therapy she was assumed to be cured.

Patient #23 subsequently did well until January 1976, when she experienced chronic fatigue associated with frequent colds, sore throats, and an episode of shingles. Then in the spring of 1976, she noted several large, painless lymph nodes in her neck. She consulted her family physician who believed a full evaluation was unnecessary, but when Patient #23 failed to improve over a period of six months, she was referred to the Mayo Clinic in Rochester, Minnesota, in October 1976.

At Mayo, a cervical lymph node biopsy confirmed, as described in the pathology report, "Malignant lymphoma, Diffuse (Partially nodular) Mixed lymphocytic histiocytic type."

X-rays of the chest and a bone survey showed no sign of metastatic disease. However, a bipedal lymphangiogram revealed suspicious-looking nodes in the region of the lumbar spine, and a bone marrow biopsy was positive for metastatic lymphoma.

Overall, the findings indicated advanced cancer, as described in the official Mayo summary: "On the basis of the lymphangiogram and the histologic pattern of the lymphoma, we felt that [Patient #23] most likely had disseminated disease."

The Mayo physicians painted a grim picture, telling Patient #23 her cancer would most likely ultimately prove terminal. Nonetheless, initially they recommended no therapy, wishing to hold off treatment until her disease worsened, but when her tumors grew more rapidly than expected, in January 1977 she returned to Mayo for palliative radiation.

The records describe in detail the precise extent of the treatment:

> She has completed a course of radiation therapy to the left supraclavicular, left axillary and mediastinal region because of the local progression of her malignant lymphoma in the left supraclavicular region.

Her doctors then suggested a course of intensive chemotherapy, which Patient #23 refused, instead choosing to investigate unconventional cancer therapies. Within weeks, she learned of Dr. Kelley, visited him, and in late January 1977 began the full nutritional regimen.

Over a five month period, as she followed the Kelley program, Patient #23's symptoms improved, with her lymphoma apparently going into remission. At a follow-up visit to Mayo in May 1979, she was believed, as reported in her doctor's summary, to be "free of disease." Today, more than ten years after her diagnosis, Patient #23 is in good health with no sign of her once metastatic malignancy.

Diffuse mixed histiocytic lymphocytic lymphoma is a deadly cancer with a dismal prognosis. Even with intensive treatment, the majority of patients do not survive five years; DeVita describes the diffuse mixed lymphomas as "clinically aggressive," with long term survival possible only after treatment with intensive multi-agent chemotherapy.[1]

Patient #23 did complete a short course of localized radiation therapy, administered to slow the growth of her large neck tumors, but the suspicious area of the vertebral column evident on the lymphangiogram was untreated. Since she never received chemotherapy, I think it reasonable to attribute this patient's continued good health and apparent cure to the Kelley program.

REFERENCE

1. DeVita, VT, et al. *Cancer Principles & Practice of Oncology*. Philadelphia; J.B. Lippincott Company, 1982, page 1372.

SURGICAL RECORD
MAYO CLINIC — ROCHESTER, MINNESOTA

No. ███████   Age 56   Sex F   Section Monc   Date 1976

Name Patient #23 ████████   Address NORTHFIELD, MN.

Name of Dr. Bernard S████   Dr's. Address Northfield, Mn.

Not Referred   Accompanied Patient   Sends Letter to................   Referred Only   Wishes to be notified date of operation

Operation advised by, Medical Consultant................   Surgical Consultant................ N.O█

Preoperative Diagnosis LEFT SUPRACLAVICULAR MASS, STATUS POSTOPERATIVE RIGHT
RADICAL MASTECTOMY FOR CARCINOMA.

Operation Indicated BIOPSY MASS

4-104B   Meth. NO   Recorder FCT
Date opr. 10-6-76(1)   Opr. Room X-1   Su N.O███ 060) 1st D. M████   2nd M████ -MS

SURGICAL SERVICE OF DR. MC█

Oper.
Diag.:   Mass, left supraclavicular area (postoperative right radical
            mastectomy for carcinoma elsewhere).

            Removal of left supraclavicular lymph nodes for diagnosis.

Oper.:

Drainage

Add. cond. to index:
Detail: Skin antiseptic: betadine

Under local anesthesia, an incision was made in the left supraclavicular
area and carried down to the strap muscles. These were retracted laterally
thereby exposing two enlarged lymph nodes. These were completely excised and
sent for histologic identification. The preliminary diagnosis was lymphoma.
The incision was closed in two layers first by approximating platysma
with 4-0 plain catgut and the skin with 3-0 subcuticular dexon.   *closure
10/6/76 Delayed Path report. Left supraclavicular lymph node. C21063-76,
C21064-76. Malignant lymphoma, Diffuse(Partially nodular) Mixed lymphocytic
histiocytic type.(LHW).

264

October 13, 1976

3-231-507

Bernard S█████, M.D.
█████████████████████████
Northfield, MN 55057

Dear Doctor S█████:

██Patient #23████████████████████ was recently evaluated in the Lymphoma
Clinic. She had originally been evaluated by Dr. Stephen C█████████
in the Department of Oncology. Enlarged left supraclavicular lymph
nodes were noted. Biopsy of the left supraclavicular lymph nodes
on October 6, 1976, revealed malignant lymphoma, diffuse (partially
nodular) mixed lymphocytic-histiocytic type. When seen in the Lymphoma
Clinic, there was no sign of residual mass in the left supraclavicular
region and no other sign of active lymphoma on physical examination.

    Chest x-ray was negative. Metastatic bone survey showed no
definite sign of malignancy. Excretory urogram was normal. Bipedal
lymphangiogram revealed suspicious lymph nodes in the region of the
L-2 interspace. Chemistry profile was entirely satisfactory. White
blood count was 5500; hemoglobin, 13.6; platelets, 314,000. Bone
marrow aspiration revealed several focal aggregates of lymphocytes,
suggesting marrow involvement by lymphoma. Bone marrow biopsy, however,
was interpreted as showing no definite evidence of malignant lymphoma.

    On the basis of the lymphangiogram and the histologic pattern
of the lymphoma, we felt that █████████████ most likely had disseminated
disease. Because she is asymptomatic and has no sign of impending
complications from her lymphoma, we have not advised initiation of
specific therapy at this time.

    We have arranged for a complete re-evaluation in approximately
six weeks. We do intend to initiate treatment at the first sign of
symptomatic progression of her disease.

    Please let us know if we could be of assistance with her case
prior to her scheduled return.

                              Sincerely,

                              M. J. O'█████ M.D.

MJO:jmh

265

January 17, 1977

3-231-507

Bernard S███████ M.D.
█████████████████████
Northfield, MN 55057

Dear Doctor S█████:

Patient #23 █████████████████ was dismissed from the Mayo Clinic on January 14, 1977. She has completed a course of radiation therapy to the left supra- clavicular, left axillary and mediastinal region because of the local pro- gression of her malignant lymphoma in the left supraclavicular region. She has developed some mild dysphagia and cutaneous inflammation related to the radiation treatments. These do not appear to be serious problems and I ex- pect them to resolve without specific therapy.

Physical examination revealed no evidence of progression of lymphoma in other sites. I plan to see her again in two months for a repeat evaluation, I will be glad to keep you informed as to significant changes in her clinical status.

Sincerely,

Michael J. O'████████ M.D.

MJO:clm

266

May 10, 1979

3-231-507

Bernard S█████ M.D.
███████████████████ Street
Northfield, MN 55057

Dear Doctor S█████:

It was my pleasure to see ██████Patient #23███████ in Lymphoma Clinic during Dr. Michael J. O'█████'s absence. As you are aware, she has previously received radiation therapy treatments after documentation of progressive diffuse mixed lymphocytic histiocytic malignant lymphoma. Her treatments were in late 1976 and she has been clinically free of disease since that time. She returns to the Mayo Clinic now essentially asymptomatic with no particular complaints except recently noting some increased mucus with tiny flecks of blood in her stools. She specifically denies fevers, sweats or weight loss.

On physical examination, there is no evidence of progressive lymphoma. I find no suspicious lymphadenopathy or any enlargement of the abdominal viscera. Her chest x-ray is normal. Her hematology and chemistry screening tests are all within normal limits.

The finding of increased mucus and blood in the stool needs to be followed up. She does use irritative enemas as a part of a treatment course to which he subscribes and I suspect her bowel complaints are from these treatments, however, I have strongly advised her to continue with the work-up and have a barium enema at home as I understand that she is scheduled for this. Otherwise, I would continue following her clinically. We have not set a date for return appointment, however, she will contact us in approximately six months. If problems arise before this, I have urged her to contact us sooner.

I was happy to see ███████████ and hope that she remains free of her disease. We appreciate the opportunity of working with you.

Sincerely,

William C. N█████, M.D.
Assistant to
M. J. O'██████ M.D.

WCN:ct
cc: J. G. B██████ M.D.

267

Patient #24

Patient #24 is a 64-year-old man from North Dakota alive nine years since his diagnosis of diffuse poorly differentiated lymphocytic lymphoma.

In late 1977, Patient #24 first experienced persistent fatigue associated with decreased appetite and a mild weight loss. In December of that year, he developed pneumonia, which quickly resolved with antibiotic treatment. However, several weeks later he noticed enlarged lymph nodes in his right and anterior neck region. When the swelling did not regress, on January 30, 1978 Patient #24 was admitted to St. Luke's Hospital in Fargo, North Dakota, for evaluation.

On physical exam, he was noted to have multiple non-tender swollen lymph nodes in the right cervical (neck) area, in both axillae (armpits), and in the groin. In addition, his spleen and liver were significantly enlarged.

A biopsy of a posterior cervical lymph node and a bone marrow biopsy both confirmed diffuse poorly differentiated lymphocytic lymphoma. Subsequently, a lymphangiogram revealed suspicious nodes along the large arteries of the pelvis, including the aorta. Because of these findings, Patient #24 was diagnosed with widely metastatic, stage IV disease.

While still hospitalized, Patient #24 agreed to participate in an experimental chemotherapy program, the Eastern Oncology Group Protocol Study, in which lymphoma patients were randomly selected to receive one of several experimental drug regimens. In Patient #24's case, the assigned treatment consisted of the four drugs Cytoxan, Bleomycin, vincristine and prednisone.

In early February 1978, after completing his first cycle of chemotherapy as an outpatient, Patient #24 became extremely ill, improving only slowly over a three-week period. When in March 1978 Patient #24 reacted to the second round of drugs even more violently, he decided to discontinue therapy, although his doctors warned him the disease was not yet in remission.

At that point Patient #24 began investigating nutritional approaches to cancer, learned of Dr. Kelley, and soon after began the nutritional program in March 1978. Within months, the many swollen lymph nodes regressed completely.

Patient #24 followed the full program for approximately five years, before tapering down to a maintenance regimen. Today, nine years after his diagnosis, Patient

#24 is in good health with no sign of cancer, and by all standards he appears cured of his disease.

Currently, 32% of patients with diffuse poorly differentiated lymphocytic lymphoma aggressively treated with chemotherapy live five years.[1] Prolonged survival requires intensive therapy, usually multi-agent regimens combined with radiation. DeVita describes this form of lymphoma as "aggressive," reporting that only in a "minority" of patients does the disease regress completely, allowing for any hope of survival beyond two years.[2]

In summary, Patient #24 was diagnosed with stage IV diffuse poorly differentiated lymphocytic lymphoma, initially treated with only two rounds of a projected multi-course drug protocol. His brief trial of chemotherapy did not induce remission but on the Kelley program, his disease, by all clinical standards, resolved.

REFERENCES

1. Harvey, AM, et al. *The Principles and Practice of Medicine*, 20th Edition. New York; Appleton-Century-Crofts, 1980, page 562.

2. DeVita, VT, et al. *Cancer Principles & Practice of Oncology*. Philadelphia; J.B. Lippincott Company, 1982, page 1372.

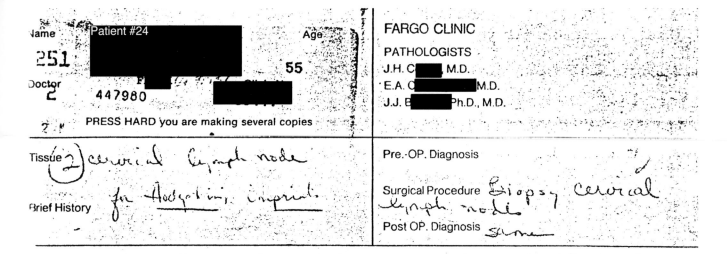

Name Patient #24   **Age** 55

251

Doctor 2   447980

PRESS HARD you are making several copies

FARGO CLINIC

PATHOLOGISTS

J.H. C███ M.D.

E.A. C███████ M.D.

J.J. B███ Ph.D., M.D.

Tissue cervical lymph node for Hodgkins, imprint.

Brief History

Pre.-OP. Diagnosis

Surgical Procedure Biopsy cervical lymph node

Post OP. Diagnosis same

GROSS:
The specimen consists of a smooth rounded lymph node measuring 2.5 x 1.5 cm.

MICOROSCOPIC:
Sections show the architecture of the node is completely effaced and no follicles or germinal centers remain. The sinusoidal pattern is no longer evident except in the very center of the node and here it is invaded by lymphocytes. A few remnants of the peripheral sinus can still be identified, also containing lymphocytes; and there is invasion of the capsule by lymphocytes. Higher magnification shows the principal cell is a rather poorly-differentiated lymphocyte with coarse nuclear chromatin and scant cytoplasm. Small numbers of cells contain nucleoli. Mitotic figures are rare. No Reed-Sternberg cells are seen.

DIAGNOSIS:
Malignant lymphoma, diffuse poorly-differentiated lymphocytic type, involving cervical lymph node.

James H. C███ M. D,sl   M.D.

Date

SURGICAL PATHOLOGY REPORT 2-1-78 ✓

2 84 FE

270

CONTINUATION SHEET

For Continuation of History, Physical Data, Consultation, Treatment, Progress

Name: Patient #24 ████████ Date: _____ Case No. ████████

DISCHARGE SUMMARY

Date of admission January 30th, date of discharge February 10th.

DISCHARGE DIAGNOSIS: Diffuse poorly differentiated lymphocytic lymphoma, stage IV.

REFERRING PHYSICIAN: Dr. Donald E████, Alexandria Clinic, ████████, Alexandria, Minnesota 56308

ADMISSION EVALUATION: Cervical adenopathy.

HISTORY: This 55 year old white ~~female~~ male was referred to Dr. B█████ for evaluation of right cervical adenopathy. He was well until mid December until he noticed the onset of pneumonia. He was treated but readmitted with midabdominal pain. At that time he had had some weight loss and history of swelling of the right posterior and anterior neck for about 5 weeks. On admission here physical examination revealed a well developed adult white male in no acute distress. There are multiple nontender 2 cm. hard rubbery lymph nodes in the right posterior cervical chain and one in the right anterior cervical change just beneath the right mandible. Chest was clear. There were also several palpable lymph nodes in the left axillary region as well as the right axilla and bilateral groin. Both the liver and spleen were felt 2 cm. below the costal margins. The remainder of his examination was unremarkable.

COURSE IN HOSPITAL: Patient was seen by Dr. F█████ of the ENT Service and a right sialogram was done which was essentially unremarkable. On February the 1st he had a biopsy of the posterior cervical lymph nodes which revealed diffuse, poorly differentiated lymphocytic lymphoma. He was seen by the Oncology Service and bilateral bone marrow aspirates and biopsies were performed which revealed malignant lymphoma in all bone marrow smears. Further evaluation in the hospital included a hemoglobin of 14.8, white count 10,300, platelet count 180,000. Throat culture was normal. Urinalysis was negative. ASO titer was 50 TODD units. The febrile agglutinins revealed a positive titer to paratyphoid A and a slightly positive H titer. Monospot test was negative. Panel 12 was entirely unremarkable except for a slightly elevated SGOT to a value of 69. The remainder of his liver function tests, renal tests, calcium and electrolytes were all normal. EKG normal. Skin tests for candida was positive. Skin test for lumps was negative. Indirect Coomb's test was negative. Quantitative immunoglobulins reveals a slightly decreased RTM level but the remainder were all normal. A serum protein electrophoresis was unremarkable and a serum immunoglobulin electrophoresis was within normal limits.

NSO 13

Name   Patient #24   Date   Case No. ▮▮▮

Patient had complete pulmonary function studies which revealed minimal obstructive
airway disease otherwise unremarkable.   X-ray examination included a negative chest.
Liver spleen scan revealed a mildly enlarged spleen otherwise normal.   Bone scan
negative, IVP negative, Lymphangiogram revealed grossly abnormal enlarged external
and common iliac nodes bilaterally, involvement of small periaortic and venous nodes.
Gallium scan was negative aside from some activity in the neck.   Upper GI
series and small bowel series were all negative.   It was felt the patient had stage
IV nonhodgkin's lymphoma.   He was eligible for protocol therapy and in that regard
The Eastern Cooperative Oncology Group Protocol was discussed thoroughly with him and
the patient agreed to participate in the study.   In that regard he was randomized to
receive a combination of Cytoxan, Bleomycin, Vincristin and Prednisone.   On February
9th he received Cytoxan 2,200 mg. intravenously as well as Prednisone 220 mg. orally
daily for 5 days.   He tolerated this well with no nausea or GI distress.   His blood
counts at the time of administration revealed a hemoglobin of 14, white count 6,600
and a platelet count of 180,000.   He was discharged on February 10th.   Condition
on discharge was feeling low with no complaints.

   PLAN OF FOLLOWUP: Patient will return to the clinic in two weeks with a CBC
and platelet count and at that time will receive Vincristin and Bleomycin.

   DISCHARGE MEDICATIONS: Prednisone 220 mg. daily x 2 with Maalox and Allopurinol
300 mg. daily.

                                        G. W. M▮▮▮▮▮   M.D./dm

Dictated 2-4-78, transcribed 2-6-78.

cc: Donald ▮▮▮▮▮, M.D.   **DS**
     Alexander Clinic
     ▮▮▮▮▮▮
     Alexandria, MN 56308

Patient #25

Patient #25 is a 63-year-old woman from Florida who has survived more than 11 years since her diagnosis of diffuse poorly differentiated lymphocytic lymphoma. In addition to lymphoma, she has a past history pertinent for early stage cervical cancer, discovered on routine Pap smear in 1967 and treated successfully with localized excision.

Patient #25 had been in good health when in May 1974 she first experienced "twinges" of pain in the left chest wall and breast, which she initially attributed to muscle spasms. Although she didn't seek medical attention at that time, a year later, in May 1975, after several cutaneous nodules suddenly appeared in the same region, Patient #25 consulted her gynecologist, who—suspicious of cancer—quickly referred her to Mt. Sinai Hospital in Miami.

After a preliminary examination, the attending surgeon at Mt. Sinai described the findings in his summary note:

> A firm nodule 1 cm. in diameter was noted in the left subacromial (shoulder) area, and an area of subcutaneous nodularity and thickening radiated from this area toward the breast.

Biopsies of two chest wall lesions on May 30, 1975 both confirmed "lymphoma cutis," a slow-growing cancer usually confined to the skin. The diagnosis of purely cutaneous disease seemed more certain when additional studies, including an ultrasound of the abdomen and a bone marrow biopsy, indicated no evidence of metastases.

Her doctors initially recommended no treatment because of the superficial nature of the malignancy. However, over the following months, Patient #25 developed multiple new nodules in the left shoulder region. She consulted her surgeon, who on September 24, 1975 excised two of the lesions, both identified as lymph nodes infiltrated by "diffuse malignant lymphoma intermediate cell type, left shoulder."

Patient #25 was then referred to the University of Miami Medical Center where, after review of all biopsy specimens, her disease was classified as diffuse poorly differentiated lymphocytic lymphoma, a very aggressive malignancy.

Her oncologist then suggested she proceed with both radiation and aggressive chemotherapy, but before agreeing to any treatment Patient #25 decided to seek out another opinion at Memorial Sloan-Kettering Cancer Center in New York. There, when she was seen in mid-October 1975, a review of the slides confirmed diffuse poorly differentiated lymphocytic lymphoma.

The Sloan-Kettering physicians strongly recommended a lymphangiogram and other tests, to be followed by radiation to the chest wall and surrounding areas. Although they warned the disease could be fatal if untreated, Patient #25 refused any further evaluation and returned home to Florida.

At the suggestion of her son, in early November 1975 Patient #25 set up an appointment with Dr. Kelley. Before her scheduled visit, Patient #25 went for a stay at a California health spa where she was in turn encouraged to pursue Laetrile therapy in Mexico. Despite a trial of the drug at a Tijuana clinic, her cancer continued to spread and when she was first seen by Dr. Kelley some weeks later, her disease involved a large area of the left chest wall.

But over the following months, as Patient #25 pursued her nutritional protocol, the numerous chest nodules gradually regressed. She eventually followed the full Kelley program for four years, before tapering to a maintenance program which she continued another five years. When last contacted in mid-1986, 11 years after her diagnosis, she was in excellent health, with no evidence of lymphoma.

This patient's cancer, diagnosed as diffuse poorly differentiated lymphoma limited to the skin, if untreated tends to metastasize rapidly, as DeVita reports:

> Although the disease may appear circumscribed at the time of diagnosis, progression to systemic disease is such a common feature that these patients are now treated in most centers with regimens similar to those for acute lymphoblastic leukemia of childhood.[1]

Since Patient #25 refused conventional treatment, her long-term disease-free survival must be attributed to the Kelley regimen.

REFERENCE

1. DeVita, VT, et al. *Cancer Principles & Practice of Oncology*. Philadelphia; J.B. Lippincott Company, 1982, page 1342.

RICHARD MARION F█████ M.D., F.A.C.S.
ENRIQUE B█████ M.D., F.A.C.S.

MIAMI BEACH, FLORIDA 33139

October 8, 1975

51 y/o
at ███

Memorial Hospital
New York, New York

Patient #25

Att: Dr. F███

Dear Dr. F███:

The above named patient has apparently contacted you and we are enclosing copies of the pathology reports, as well as the reports of consultations obtained here locally.

█████████ was first seen by me on May 23, 1975 because of a possible lump in the left breast. At that time a firm nodule 1 cm. in diameter was noted in the left subacromial area, and an area of subcutaneous nodularity and thickening radiated from this area toward the breast. There was rubbery nodularity in the other breast but no distinct mass was felt.

A xeromammogram taken on June 26, 1975 showed fibrocystic changes and mammary dysplasia of moderate degree but there was no radiographic evidence of malignancy.

A punch biopsy from the left subacromial area on May 30, 1975 was reported as Lymphoma Cutis.

█████████ was then referred to Dr. B█████ for a work up. I am enclosing a copy of his report. She was also seen by Dr. L█████ of the University of Miami, a copy of his report is enclosed.

On September 24, 1975 the left subacromial node was excised and grossly two lymph node like lesions were removed from the area.

If there is any further information you need please do not hesitate to call me.

Very truly yours,

Enrique B█████ M.D.
EB:m
Enc:

275

MOUNT SINAI MEDICAL CENTER
DEPARTMENT OF PATHOLOGY AND LABORATORY MEDICINE
TISSUE REPORT

LAB. NO. S-9235-75

Name of Patient: Patient #25

Adm no:

Room: —

Sex Female

Age 51

Date Specimen rec'd 9-24-75

Date of Report 10-1-75

Dr. F_____ & B_____

Nature of Specimen and Clinical Data: Nodule from left shoulder.

Clinical data: Subcutaneous left subacromial node for 2 years. Punch biopsy last May revealed lymphoma cutis. Bone marrow and complete workup negative. Subcutaneous nodule has increased since. Progressive changes of overlying skin.
Preop. diag.: Possible lymphoma, left shoulder area.

GROSS EXAMINATION:

The specimen consists of multiple rubbery, grayish-tan, fibroadipose tissue fragments, measuring in aggregate 6.5 x 2 x 1.3 cm. On each of the submitted specimens is a firm, irregular, rubbery, gray-tan, well circumscribed nodule, measuring from 0.7 cm. in greatest dimension to 2 cm. in greatest dimension. These nodules appear to infiltrate the adipose tissue. (3 ST)

DIAGNOSIS:

- DIFFUSE MALIGNANT LYMPHOMA INTERMEDIATE CELL TYPE, LEFT SHOULDER.

SC:bl

ROLANDO O_____ M.D.

MEMORIAL HOSPITAL

SURGICAL PATHOLOGY

SUBMITTED BY DOCTOR _R._____

SUBMITTED SLIDES ☑ _S-9235-75_ SUBMITTER BLOCKS ☐

(4) OUTSIDE SOURCE _Mt. Sinai Hosp._

Miami Beach, Fla.
_33140_

Patient #25

PATIENT NAME AND ADDRESS

DEPT
2
1
0
1

LABORATORY USE ONLY

☐ SMALL BIOPSY ☐ SPECIMEN ☐ SMEARS ☐ CLOT ☐ IMMEDIATE EXAM (F.S.)

0-1 _SSL. Biopsy (L) Chest wall_

2	5	8	11
3	6	9	12
		7	10

ANATOMIC SOURCE OF SPECIMEN _By. Left chestwall_

CLINICAL DATA _"Lymphoma Cutis"_

PREVIOUS ACCESSIONS IN THIS LABORATORY ☐ YES ☑ NO   PREVIOUS PATHOLOGY NUMBERS

SIGNIFICANT CLINICAL DATA (USE ANATOMIC STAMPS WHEN POSSIBLE) AGE _51_ SEX _F_

By. left chest wall 5/75 revealed
"Lymphoma Cutis"
Now has indurated area on chest wall in
region previous by - dk red pigmented
area 5x2 cms ~~~~~ skin of left chest
wall above breast - No palpable lymph
nodes LSK not palpable

DISPOSITION OF REPORT IF OTHER THAN TO CHART

DATE OF REPORT _10.13.75_ _MCM_

PATHOLOGY REPORT
(SEE REVERSE SIDE FOR GROSS PATHOLOGY)

ACCESSION DATE AND NUMBER

13 OCT 75 14754

MICROSCOPIC REPORT BY DR. _M.C.M_____ /P.H.L_____/ljs

Submitted Slides S-9235-75 (4 slides) : Malignant lymphoma, poorly
differentiated lymphocytic type, diffuse (lymphoma cutis). Cannot
predict behaviour of solitary lesion of this type.

PATH. REPORT

11

P-0965

F-U ☐

CHART COPY

277

DATE _____

Patient #25

MEDICAL ONCOLOGY B.

October 21st, 1975:   WT: 49.8   T.: 36.5

Record patient name and case number

████████ is a 51 year old white female which was reffered to the Lymphoma Clinic
from the Medical Diagnostic Clinic because of a biopsy-proven diagnosis of malignant
lymphoma poorly-differentiated lymphocytic diffuse-type from a skin biopsy in the
left pectoral area.

█████████ was well until approximately 1967 when a Pap-smear showed question of a
carcinoma of the cervix. She had cocaization done in St. Joseph's Hospital in
Florida and since then been followed in a 2-6 month interval with pap smears since
that period of time and has had no reccurence.

She did well until approximately 2 years ago when she started to notice achee
discomfort in the left petral area and upper breast region. This is approximately
stable until approximately April 1975 when she started to notice a slight enlargemen
in the area and therefore consulted a physician in Miami. A biopsy was done in
May 1975 which was read-out as a lymphoma cutis. She was reffered to a
Hematology-Oncology group there, where a work-up was performed including a bone
marrow aspiration which was negative, a normal CBC, a normal SMA-12, a normal
Chest X-Ray, Thiogram of the abdomen and an IVP.

She then reffered herself here for further evaluation and therapy. She does not
note any other evidence of nodularity or skin problems except a lession on her
right neck which was biopsied in May 1975. The diagnosis of which was basal cell
carcinoma. She has had several areas of hyperpigmentation, one on the right
axillary area and theother in the left buttock area which have not changed or
over the last 15 to 20 years. She denies fever, night sweats, weight loss, and
has continued to live an active life with no alterations in her normal routine
since these biopsies where taken. Past history, surgical history, ect... are in
reviewed well in the Medical Diagnostic's work-up.

P.E.:   HEENT.
         Pharynx is unremarkable.
         There are no palpable lymph nodes, there is a small hyperpigmented
         slightly raized area in the skin over the right maxilla approximately
         1 x 1 cm.
         Chest is clear to A.&P.
         Cardiac exam: No murmurs, rubs or gallops.
         Chest wall: The skin over the left petral area reveals some nodularity
         subcutaneously, this is very fine, there are no true discrete masses.
         There is no other nodularity noted over the entire remaining chest wall.
         Abdomen is soft.
         No liver, spleen or masses are palpable.
         There is a right lower quadrant scar.
         Bowel sounds are active.
         Extremities: There is no edema.
         Lymph nodes: There is no peripheral adenopathy.
         Skin: Well tanned. There is a 1.5 x 1.5 cm. nodular pigmented lession
         in the left buttock area.

FORWARD

278

In view of the histology here confirms the biopsy diagnosis of
Diffuse poorly differentiated lymphocytic lymphoma which apparently is
comfined to the skin.

We will obtain a lymphangiogram to rule-out retroperitoneal disease, but
I would not be surprissed if this was negative.

The case should be discussed at the stadium conference for definately
plan after therapy, if the lymphangiogram is negative.

She indeed may be under control at this point in time, with local
radiation to the involved areas and then to observe her for future
development of problems with disease.

This case was discussed with Dr. M▮▮▮▮ and it was felt that we will
get a lymphangiogram, see her in 2 weeks and then make decisions
regarding further therapy at that point in time.

The diagnosis was discussed with the patient at length as she had no
apparent knowledge of what her true problem was.

Notice that the fact that her VDRL is 2+ possitive.

She had intrasyphillis pain back in 1950 which it had been treated at
time in 1950 and also relatively recently and the patient states that
her VDRL has persisted to run possitive.

We will wait the confirmation by the Board of Health and ▮▮▮, but I don't
think this is something which needs therapy. It's probably a long
possive history of a possitive VDRL.

                                        Dr. H▮▮▮▮/lc.

10-13-75

DATE 10/13/75

Patient #25

Record patient name and case number

Problems

1. S/p bx. left chest wall
5/75 & 9/75 — revealed "Lymphoma Cutis"
2. S/p Conization Cf. 1967 - ? Ca - subsequent Paps. wnl.
3. 1 cm. pigmented area right infra orbital
area — R/o Hutchinson's Freckle

Plan
1. Rout. wfu c complete hemogram.
2. Serology
3. Submit Slides for review
4. Ref. to Lymphoma Clinic 10/21/75.
5. Cht. review 10/27/75.

J.O——— RN

RW Toude MD

10/28/75. Rout. wfu is wnl. VDRL is 2+
Slides of bx. left pectoral area read here
as lymphoma cutis. During "chance"
meeting c pt. outside of hospital, she
informed me that she had decided to
seek a "nutritional cure" for her disease
and did not wish to undergo further eval. or rx.
at M.H. I advised her to consult physician

FOLLOW
UP
NOTES

5

FORWARD

P-0635

280

in Symptoms Clinic before making final decision   J. B_____ R.N.

Patient #26

Patient #26 is a 45-year-old man from Pittsburgh, alive nearly ten years since his diagnosis of nodular poorly differentiated lymphocytic lymphoma.

In August 1977, Patient #26 first noticed a swollen, nontender lymph node in his left groin which enlarged over a six-week period. In October 1977, his family physician referred him for a biopsy which confirmed nodular poorly differentiated lymphocytic lymphoma.

In mid-October 1977, Patient #26 was admitted to St. Margaret's Memorial Hospital in Pittsburgh for further evaluation. At the time, he was noted to have swollen, tender lymph nodes in the right neck as well as in the groin. A liver-spleen scan and a bone marrow biopsy were both negative for metastatic disease, but a CT scan revealed many abnormal lymph nodes and tumors in the posterior retroperitoneal (abdominal) region. The discharge summary from that hospitalization describes the findings:

> left inguinal lymphadenopathy, left lymph node mass in the left adjacent
> ileo-psoas muscle, retroperitoneal lymph node mass obscuring the aorta,
> and the inferior vena cava and lymphadenopathy on the spleen.

Exploratory surgery to determine the precise extent of disease was then scheduled, but when Patient #26, a Jehovah's Witness, refused permission for blood transfusions, the procedure was canceled. In late October 1977, Patient #26 was then transferred to St. Francis Hospital in Pittsburgh, for additional non-surgical evaluation. There, a bone scan showed no evidence of skeletal metastases but a lymphangiogram on October 27, 1977 documented cancer throughout the pelvis and abdomen, reported as:

> marked enlargement of lymph nodes of the left inguinal, iliac and
> retroperitoneal areas, pelvic and retroperitoneal areas [sic] on the left.
> Some of the lymph nodes on the right side were also seen to be abnormal
> . . . At the level of L2-L3 (lower back) on the left, there appeared to be
> some partial filling of a large mass of lymph nodes . . . All the lymph
> nodes in the left chain are enlarged . . . it is believed that most of the
> visualized lymph nodes are affected by the disease . . .

A repeat CT on October 27, 1977 also confirmed extensive malignancy, described as "marked lymphadenopathy of the pelvic and retroperitoneal areas."

At St. Margaret's on November 7, 1977, a biopsy of a right cervical (neck) lymph node again revealed nodular lymphocytic lymphoma. After this complicated evaluation which included two biopsies, Patient #26's doctors could say with certainty that the disease extended from his neck to his groin.

His oncologist then recommended a 4000 rad course of radiation, to be administered at the St. Francis outpatient facility. Patient #26 agreed to the treatment, which he began in early November 1977, but after receiving only 1500 rads to the groin and retroperitoneal regions, he refused to proceed with therapy—even though his disease was not yet in remission.

In a letter written to another consulting physician, the attending oncologist on the case described Patient #26's limited treatment regimen:

> Tumor doses of approximately 1500 rads were delivered to these regions in twelve days. As you know, this dosage is not adequate to destroy lymphoma . . .

At that point, Patient #26 decided to seek out yet another opinion. In mid-November 1977, he travelled to Memorial Sloan-Kettering Cancer Center in New York, where the physicians agreed with the previous diagnosis and urged Patient #26 to resume radiation. But after returning to Pittsburgh, Patient #26 instead opted to investigate unconventional approaches to cancer, learned of Dr. Kelley, and in March 1978, began the full regimen. He reported to me that within months, all his enlarged lymph nodes regressed completely.

Patient #26 followed the Kelley regimen for three years, during which time he remained free of any evidence of his cancer. When last contacted, nearly ten years after his diagnosis, he was in excellent health, apparently cured of his once disseminated cancer—or at least in prolonged remission.

Although experts consider nodular poorly differentiated lymphocytic lymphoma (NPDLL) one of the less aggressive lymphomas—Owens reports a 72% five-year survival rate—the disease is considered ultimately incurable.[1] As DeVita writes:

> The series of Jones and colleagues from Stanford and the older literature, indicate that the average survival of patients with NPDL is 6 years, even when the treatment used is regional radiotherapy, or radiotherapy followed by single agent chemotherapy . . . The paradox of the 'good prognosis' lymphomas is that although NPDL is an indolent illness, all patients ultimately succumb to their disease.[2]

DeVita also reports a lack of "convincing evidence" that aggressive chemotherapy regimens benefit patients diagnosed with this particular subtype of lymphoma.[2]

Rosenberg and his colleagues at Stanford have followed a group of patients with NPDLL, many of whom survived beyond five and ten years without therapy.[3] DeVita, in his analysis of the Stanford data, emphasizes that these long-term survivors were carefully selected for study and may not be representative cases.[4] Nonetheless, these results indicate some untreated patients with NPDLL do live for prolonged periods.

I still believe Patient #26's course to be unusual. He was diagnosed with very extensive disease which regressed only after he began the Kelley program.

REFERENCES

1. Harvey, AM, et al. *The Principles and Practice of Medicine,* 20th Edition. New York; Appleton-Century-Crofts, 1980, page 562.

2. DeVita, VT, et al. *Cancer Principles & Practice of Oncology.* Philadelphia; J.B. Lippincott Company, 1982, page 1372.

3. Rosenberg, SA. "The Low-Grade Non-Hodgkin's Lymphomas: Challenges and Opportunities." *Journal of Clinical Oncology* Mar 1985; 3:299–310.

4. DeVita, VT, et al. *Cancer Principles & Practice of Oncology.* Philadelphia; J.B. Lippincott Company, 1982, page 1372.

NAME _____ Patient #26 _____   PATH. NO. _____ S-3083-77

CHART NO. _____   DATE _____ 10-11-77

WARD _____ Outpatient   AGE _____

TISSUE MARKED _____ Biopsy Lymph Node Lt. Groin   PHYSICIAN: _____ Dr. C▮
      F.S. Biopsy Lymph Node Lt. Groin

GROSS:

"A" This gross specimen consists of a glistening, gray to pinkish-tan, focally hemorrhagic, soft lymph node which measures 3 x 1.8 x 1.5 cm. Cut surfaces are smooth, glistening and finely granular. RSS "B" This gross specimen consists of a similar appearing portion of soft, glistening tissue which measures 1.2 x 1 x 0.3 cm. TE

MICRO:

Sections "A" and "B" are similar and show a lymph node with effacement of the architecture and infiltration by similar appearing cells of intermediate size with an irregular nuclear membrane, some of them cleaved. A few more immature cells have prominent nucleoli. Occasional mitotic figures are noted and a few scattered eosinophils. There is a tendency of follicular arrangement. The capillaries show prominent endothelial cells. The peripheral sinus is also obliterated with focal infiltration of the capsule and into the adjacent adipose tissue.

DIAG:

NODULAR LYMPHOCYTIC LYMPHOMA, POORLY DIFFERENTIATED - LYMPH NODE BIOPSY OF LEFT GROIN

_____ B.K.H ▮
PATHOLOGIST

SURGICAL PATHOLOGY   CHART COPY

285

ATTACH 3D REPORT ALONG HERE ↑ AND SUCCEEDING ONES ON ABOVE LINES

ATTACH 2D REPORT WITH TOP AT THIS LINE ↑

home

RADIOGRAPHIC REPORT

Drs. Mc████-O'█████-S█████

Patient #26

UNIT NO.	LOCATION
████████	6632D

CT SCAN OF ABDOMEN AND PELVIS
A repeat CT scan of the abdomen and pelvis was performed on this
patient following the injection of Ethiodol in the lymphatics of both
feet. Most of the masses that were previously described in the
pelvic area showed, in fact, to be enlarged lymph nodes filled with
contrast material. Some of the retroperitoneal masses seen in the
abdomen showed uptake of Ethiodol confirming the presence of lymphadenopathy of the retroperitoneum. Part of this mass did not show the
presence of contrast, but are still believed to be affected nodes
that even at the lymphangiographic study did not show contrast
uptake most likely because of excessive involvement by abnormal cells.

IMPRESSION: This study confirms the impression of the previous
lymphangiogram CT scan of marked lymphadenopathy of the pelvic and
retroperitoneal areas.

10/27/77   S. B█████, M.D.   bh-10/28/77

═══════════════════════════════════

ST. FRANCIS GENERAL HOSPITAL
PITTSBURGH, PA.

10-27

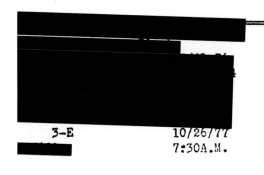

3-E   10/26/77
            7:30A.M.

ST. FRANCIS GENERAL HOSPITAL

RADIOGRAPHIC REPORTS

286

LYMPHANGIOGRAM

Following the injection of contrast material in the lymphatics of both feet, there was good visualization of the lymphatic channels of the pelvic and retroperitoneal areas. No obstruction or collateral circulation was noted. The take off of the thoracic duct was visualized. The cephalic end of the thoracic duct was also visualized. The supraclavicular node could not be seen.

Films exposed 24 hours after the injection of contrast material showed marked enlargement of lymph nodes of the left inguinal, iliac and retroperitoneal areas, pelvic and retroperitoneal areas on the left. Some of the lymph nodes on the right side were also seen to be abnormal in their intrinsic structure as shown by a speckled appearance of the contrast material. No enlargement of the nodes was noted on the right side. At the level of L2-L3 on the left, there appeared to be some partial filling of a large mass of lymph nodes that did not otherwise visualize. All/ the lymph nodes in the left chain are enlarged and mottled in appearance.

IMPRESSION: In view of the patient's history of lymphocytic lymphoma, it is believed that most of the visualized lymph nodes are affected by the disease, more markedly on the left side as above described.

CONTINUED..........

ST. FRANCIS GENERAL HOSPITAL
PITTSBURGH, PA.

Note is made of the fact that recently similar changes have been described in both patients with lymphoma and patients without proven lymphoma that were pathologically proven to be due to fibrotic hyperplasia rather than to lymphomatous infiltration. Still it is believed that in this case the changes are related to the patient's lymphoma.

10/27/77   S. B███████ M.D.   bh-10/28/77

RADIOGRAPHIC REPORT

287

COMMONWEALTH OF PENNSYLVANIA
DEPARTMENT OF HEALTH   St. Francis Memorial Hospital
CHRONIC DISEASES

CANCER REGISTRY ABSTRACT   (195.5)

1. PATIENT'S NAME AND ADDRESS (INCLUDE FIRST NAME OF SPOUSE)
Patient #26

2. TELEPHONE

3. OCCUPATIONAL HISTORY
Supervisor, A T & T Operations.

4. NAME AND ADDRESS OF RELATIVE, EMPLOYER OR OTHER CONTACT
W

5. REGISTRY NO.

6. BIRTHPLACE | **BIRTHPLACE OF FATHER** | **BIRTHPLACE OF MOTHER** | **7. DATE OF ADMISSION**
10-12-77, outpatient

8. DATE OF BIRTH (36) | **9. RACE** W | **10. SEX** M | **11. MARITAL STATUS** M | **12. PRIVATE ☐ CLINIC ☐ SEMI-PRIVATE ☐ WARD ☐** | **13. HOSPITAL NO.**

14. FAMILY PHYSICIAN'S NAME AND ADDRESS

STAFF PHYSICIAN'S NAME AND ADDRESS
Christopher D____, M.D.   Pittsburgh, Pa. 15221

15. FINAL DIAGNOSIS
Nodular lymphocytic lymphoma, poorly differentiated

Stage IIIA

16. PRIMARY SITE
LYMPHOCYTIC LYMPHOMA, LT GROIN
(195.5)

17. BASIS OF DIAGNOSIS
SURGICAL SPECIMEN ☐   BLOOD ☐   BONE MARROW ☐   BIOPSY ☒   AUTOPSY ☐
EXFOLIATIVE CYTOLOGY ☐   X-RAY ☐   CLINICAL ONLY ☐   OTHER (SPECIFY) ☐

18. HISTOLOGICAL DIAGNOSIS AND DATE (PATHOLOGY REPORT)
S-3083-77 (10-11-77) Nodular lymphocytic lymphoma, lymph node biopsy, left groin.

S-3368-77 (11-7-77) Lymphocytic lymphoma - biopsy, mass right neck.

19. STAGE OF DISEASE
LYMPHOMA, LEUKEMIA, HODGKIN'S, MYELOMA ☒   RECURRENT AFTER TREATMENT ☐
LOCALIZED ☐   REGIONAL INVOLVEMENT ☐   REMOTE METASTASIS ☐

20. IF PATIENT HAS BEEN PREVIOUSLY TREATED ELSEWHERE FOR THIS CANCER, SPECIFY DATE, TYPE OF TREATMENT, DOCTOR AND HOSPITAL

21. IS THERE A HISTORY OF CANCER IN THE FAMILY?   NO ☒   YES ☐   SPECIFY MEMBER AND SITE

22. PRIMARY TYPE
...ollowing discharge at SFGH   Allopurinol 100mg. tid
lt. node areas below diaphragm.

23. SURGERY ☐   RADIATION ☒   CHEMOTHERAPY ☐ (SPECIFY)

PALLIATIVE ☒   SURGERY FOR HORMONAL EFFECT ☐ (SPECIFY)   HORMONES ☐ (SPECIFY)

CURATIVE ☐   RADIOACTIVE ISOTOPES ☐ (SPECIFY)   STEROIDS ☐ (SPECIFY)

NONE ☐   UNKNOWN ☐   REFUSES TREATMENT ☐   OTHER ☐ (SPECIFY)

24. ALIVE
NO CLINICAL EVIDENCE OF CANCER ☐   NOT FREE OF CANCER ☒   UNKNOWN ☐

25. IF DEAD, DATE OF DEATH
NO CLINICAL EVIDENCE OF CANCER ☐   NOT FREE OF CANCER ☐   UNKNOWN ☐   AUTOPSY ☐   YES ☐ NO ☐

26. IMMEDIATE CAUSE OF DEATH | **CONTRIBUTING CAUSE OF DEATH**

27. DATE OF REPORT
2-13-78

INITIALS
ESR/xio

(OVER)

288

SUMMARY

MRL-2 (7/74)

This 36 year old white male presented to our office with a large left
inguinal node, this was biopsied as an out-patient and was shown to have
nodular lymphocytic lymphoma of the non-Hodgkin's lymphoma type. He
had a BE and procto on the outside which were normal and he was admitted
to the hospital for further evaluation and possible staging.

PHYSICAL EXAMINATION: At the time of admission showed HEENT normal. Neck
at the time of this admission was normal, since discharge from the hospital, patient has developed a neck adenopathy which has been biopsied
and which was positive for disease staging him as a III. Lymphatics
the left groin area was healing well. The remainder of the physical exam
was unremarkable.

LABORATORY: CBC, urinalysis, EKG were within normal limits. IVP was
normal. Liver-spleen scan was normal. Bone marrow biopsy showed active
bone marrow with no evidence of lymphoma. PAC-18 showed normal. RPR
was non-reactive. Sed rate was elevated, CT scan showed left inguinal
lymphadenopathy, left lymph node mass in the left adjacent ileo-psoas
muscle, retroperitoneal lymph node mass obscuring the aorta, and the
inferior vena cava and lymphadenopathy on the spleen.

COURSE: The patient underwent the above mentioned studies and then was
seen in consultation by the Drs. B████ and it was felt that staging
laparotomy would be helpful in that we could safely biopsy the spleen and
the liver and remove the spleen to eliminate the need for radiation to
the left kidney and left lower lung field. However, the patient was a
Jehovah's Witness and absolutely refused to have a transfusion of blood
even to save his life and under these circumstances both the Anesthesiologist and the Surgeons felt that this was an unacceptable risk to place
upon our shoulders and therefore this was discussed with the patient and
the patient was consulted with Dr. M█████████'s group to start radiation
therapy. The patient was discharged with an appointment to start his
radiation therapy as an out-patient the week following admission.

FINAL DIAGNOSIS: 1. LYMPHOCYTIC LYMPHOMA NODULAR STAGE IIIA

                                    C. D████, M.D.

Dict: 11/9/77
Trans:11/11/77
kac

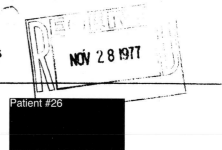

NOV 28 1977

Patient #26

DATE ___11/18/77___

Record patient name and case number

This 36-year-old man is seen because
he wishes an opinion regarding
treatment of his lymphoma.

PRESENT ILLNESS: One month ago he presented with a left groin
node which apparently revealed nodular
poorly differentiated lymphocytic lymphoma. Lymphangiogram was
positive. Cat scans revealed abdominal as well as hilar nodal
disease. IVP, barium enemia, upper GI, small bowel series and
marrow have all been negative. His only symptom has been some
low back pain which has been relieved since an inverted Y port
was started two weeks ago. Because he has developed a right
cervical node since the radiation therapy has started, he comes
here for another opinion.

PAST MEDICAL HISTORY, PERSONAL, SOCIAL & FAMILY HISTORY:
All negative.

PHYSICAL EXAMINATION: Wt. 85.6, PS 80 to 90, temp. 36.8, P 60
resp. 20, BP 150/80. He has some
induration under a well-healed scar on the left groin and the
same is true over the scar in the right cervical area. There
is some shotty axillary adenopathy of borderline significance.
I can find no other significant nodes. I can not feel a liver
or a spleen. No other masses in the abdomen and no other
abnormal findings.

IMPRESSION: NPDL stage III with disseminated nodal involvement
only.

PLAN: I am going to wait for the Path report to come back.
I see no need to do any further workup on this man. He
has had an excellent workup in Pittsburg. He is sent home and
I will be in touch with Dr. C████ and Dr. B████ regarding
treatment considerations.
Dr.B████ J. L██/np
cc: Dr. C█████
    Dr. B█████

FOLLOW UP NOTES

290

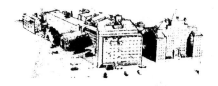

ST. FRANCIS GENERAL HOSPITAL

45TH STREET (OFF PENN AVENUE)   PITTSBURGH, PENNSYLVANIA 15201

DEPARTMENT OF RADIATION ONCOLOGY & NUCLEAR MEDICINE

JOHN D. M███████ M.D., F.A.C.R., DIRECTOR
JOHN P. O'████ M.D., F.A.C.O.G., F.A.C.S.
GEETA S████, M.D.

Administrative Assistant
MAUREEN L. HENRY, R.T.

Radiological Physics & Radiation Biology

KRISHNADAS B█████ Ph.D., DIRECTOR
JOHN G. F██, Ph.D.
MITCHELL J. J██████ JR., M.S.
LAWRENCE E. S██████ M.S.

November 22, 1977

Patient #26

RECEIVED NOV 2 9 1977

David P. C████████ M.D.
St. Francis Hospital
Pittsburgh, PA 15201

Dear Doctor C████████:

As you know, ██████████ has gone to Sloan-Kettering in New York. Prior to his leaving Pittsburgh, he received radiation therapy by means of the Betatron to both ilioinguinal-femoral regions as well as to the retroperitoneal lymph node chain. Tumor doses of approximately 1500 rads were delivered to these regions in twelve days. As you know, this dosage is not adequate to destroy lymphoma but the palpable nodes disappeared very quickly during the short course of treatment.

Thank you for having referred ████████ to us. I hope that he will do well.

Very truly yours,

John D. M████████, M.D.

JDM:slc

cc: Murray S██████, M.D.

291

Patient #27

Patient #27 is a 55-year-old man from Washington State alive ten years since his diagnosis of nodular poorly differentiated lymphocytic lymphoma.

In mid-1976, Patient #27 noticed painless swollen lymph nodes in his left groin that, over a period of several months, gradually enlarged. During that time he also experienced persistent fatigue, chronic insomnia, and occasional flu-like symptoms.

After consulting his family physician in early 1977, Patient #27 was admitted to Deaconess Hospital in Spokane for further evaluation. Biopsy of a left inguinal (groin) lymph node confirmed lymphoma, although the precise type could not initially be determined. The biopsy slides were then reviewed at Stanford University where the pathologist diagnosed nodular poorly differentiated lymphocytic lymphoma.

In late March 1977, Patient #27 entered the Sacred Heart Medical Center in Spokane for a lymphangiogram, which clearly revealed extensive disease, described in the official report: "The appearance is consistent with involvement of the peri-aortic, iliac and femoral nodes by lymphoma."

Both chemotherapy and radiation were then recommended, but Patient #27, who already knew of Dr. Kelley's regimen, refused all conventional treatment. Instead, after leaving the hospital, he consulted with Dr. Kelley and began the full program in the spring of 1977. Patient #27 reported to me that within months, the enlarged groin nodes regressed, and his persistent symptoms resolved.

Patient #27 followed his nutritional protocol for four years, all the while remaining in clinical remission, but in 1980, after discontinuing the prescribed supplements, the groin nodes swelled once again. Patient #27 consulted his former oncologist, who, assuming recurrent lymphoma, pushed for aggressive chemotherapy but Patient #27 chose instead to resume the Kelley regimen. As before, the enlarged nodes quickly returned to normal size.

Patient #27 says with confidence that he can regulate his disease at will. If he strays from the prescribed regimen, the nodes swell up within months; when he restarts the program, the nodes quickly regress. When I discussed this case with Dr. Kelley, he responded that he didn't find Patient #27's observations surprising.

Today, Patient #27, ten years after his diagnosis of lymphoma, continues on the Kelley program, remains clinically cancer-free, and reports excellent overall health. He has no plans at present to stop his nutritional protocol.

ADDENDUM

Pathology No. 77 - 3598 Medical Record No. 08C

A 45 year old man with a nine month history of left inguinal
lymphadenopathy. The patient is apparently otherwise healthy and
not taking any medication. Further workup has not been performed
at this time. Differential diagnosis includes reactive hyperplasia
and follicular lymphoma.

MICROSCOPIC:
I certainly favor the diagnosis of a follicular lymphoma, by
virtue of the extent of the nodules throughout the node, the
relative uniformity of the predominant cells, and their characteristic
cytologic features. They are atypical small lymphoid cells with
indented and angulated nuclear membranes. Phagocytosis is
conspicuously absent and many of the nodules show periperal fading
and coalescence.

DIAGNOSIS:
Lymph node, left inguinal, biopsy - Nodular lymphoma, poorly
                                    differentiated lymphocytic type
                                    - Rappaport 08-9693-9633
                                    (Follicular lymphoma, small lymphoid
                                    type-Dorfman).

Ronald F. D▮▮▮▮ M. D.
Stanford University Medical Center
Stanford, California

D▮▮▮▮:ih

▮vc:jw

CHART COPY

Ted E. L▮▮▮▮, M.D.   Edwin E. C▮▮▮r M.D.   Irby V. C▮▮▮▮ M.D.

293

NAME	Patient #27	45 yrs	3/28/77	AGE	X-RAY NO.

ADDRESS OP

PHYSICIAN DR. S. M_____   DATE

BILATERAL LYMPHANGIOGRAM

Multiple films of the pelvis, abdomen and chest immediately following
bilateral lymphangiography and at 24 hours demonstrate on the immediate
films relative obstruction to lymphatic flow in the left femoral
region with considerable holdup of contrast within channels at this
point and some collateral flow being directed laterally. There is
slight lateral displacement of multiple ectatic lymphatic trunks
at the L2 through L4 level on the right.

24-hour films show rather diffuse enlargement of all of the
visualized right periaortic nodes except for some nodes at the
L2-3 level which appear only partially opacified and are probably
largely replaced. Nodes in both femoral regions, particularly on
the right are considerably enlarged as are the external iliac
nodes bilaterally which have a foamy, reticulated appearance.
The
There is relatively poor fill of the left periaortic nodes although
very faint opacification is seen up to the level of L1-2 with these
nodes being displaced slightly toward the left. The faint
opacification is felt secondary to the obstructive process more
inferiorly.

The appearance is consistent with involvement of the periaortic,
iliac and femoral nodes by lymphoma.

DIAGNOSIS: ABNORMAL LYMPHANGIOGRAM COMPATIBLE WITH INVOLVEMENT
BY LYMPHOMA AS OUTLINED ABOVE.

            Edmund E. L____, M.D./bd

RADIOLOGIST

294

MELANOMA

Malignant melanoma is a potentially aggressive cancer of the melanocytes, the pigment forming cells of the skin, that claimed 5,800 lives in 1987.

Most melanomas can be cured if detected in the early stages, but once metastatic, the disease usually proves rapidly fatal. Overall five-year survival rates currently range up to 80%.

Pathologists categorize melanoma according to depth of skin invasion, using a system developed by Clark. "Clark's level I" includes melanomas confined to the epidermis, the outermost layer of skin. "Clark's level V" identifies cancers invading all layers of the skin as well as the underlying tissue. Melanomas of intermediate extent can be classified as Clark's level II, III, or IV.

Patient #28

Patient #28 is a 42-year-old man from Montana with a five-year history of recurrent malignant melanoma.

In February 1982, Patient #28 first noticed an inflamed, bleeding mole on his back. After consulting his family doctor, he was referred to a local surgeon who removed the lesion during the last week of February 1982. The nodule was classified as a Clark's level II (early stage) malignant melanoma, penetrating to a 4 mm depth in the skin.

Patient #28 was then admitted to Sidney Memorial Hospital in Sidney, Montana on March 1, 1982 for additional tests. A liver-spleen scan revealed a liver mass, described as a "space occupying lesion inferior portion right lobe of liver." For reasons that are not clear to me, the abnormality was not believed to represent metastatic disease.

The day after admission, as a precautionary measure, Patient #28 underwent wide local resection in the area of his previous melanoma surgery, but no additional cancer was identified. At that point, Patient #28's doctors pronounced him "cured."

But within weeks of the procedure, Patient #28's general health began to deteriorate, with onset of persistent fatigue, diminished appetite, and rapid weight loss. Then in May 1982 he noticed a new nodule in his left axillary region that his local doctors thought most likely represented recurrent melanoma. Patient #28 was referred to the Mayo Clinic, where on May 26, 1982, he underwent excision of the lesion along with axillary lymph nodes.

The superficial nodule was found to be malignant, with an area of active melanoma identified in the subcutaneous fat. In addition, of 16 lymph nodes removed at surgery, five were infiltrated with melanoma—a very ominous prognostic sign. Patient #28's doctors informed him his disease would mostly likely recur again and ultimately prove fatal; nevertheless, since he was clinically stable and showed no evidence of active metastases, they recommended no further treatment at the time.

Patient #28 subsequently reported back to Mayo at three month intervals for routine follow-up evaluations, and for a time he seemed to do well. However, in September 1982, after noticing a new subcutaneous mass in the area of his previous surgery, he returned to Mayo for removal of the lesion, which proved to be recurrent melanoma.

Once again, his physicians suggested no additional therapy. In a letter dated September 24, 1982 and written to Patient #28's Montana physician, the attending oncologist explained the Mayo position:

> We discussed these findings with [Patient #28] and his wife in some detail. With no evidence of other disease, there would appear to be no role for either systemic chemotherapy or for local radiation to the axilla at this time. We discussed the possibility or even probability of further recurrence with [Patient #28] and stressed the need for close observation.

After a brief respite, Patient #28 developed worsening fatigue and anorexia, although his local physician could find no evidence for active cancer. A liver-spleen scan performed at Sidney Memorial Hospital in November 1982 revealed the mass reported earlier, but no new lesions.

Subsequently, in March 1983, Patient #28 discovered a new nodule on his right forehead. At that point, Patient #28 decided to investigate unconventional approaches to cancer, and in April 1983, after learning of Dr. Kelley, he began the full nutritional program.

Patient #28 responded quickly to his unconventional regimen. He reported to me his fatigue lessened, his appetite improved, and within several months the nodule on his forehead regressed completely, as noted by Patient #28's Mayo physician in a note from September 1983. When last seen at Mayo in April 1986, he was in excellent health with no sign of cancer. Since that time he moved, and has been lost to follow-up after three years on the Kelley program.

Malignant melanoma, when metastatic to regional lymph nodes, usually kills quickly. In one study, Karaskousis reports a median survival of only 20.2 months in patients presenting with three or more positive nodes.[1]

In summary, Patient #28 experienced three bouts of melanoma within a seven month period, with a left axillary dissection documenting metastatic disease in five lymph nodes. Whatever the liver lesion noted on liver-spleen scan may have been, a nodule on his forehead regressed only after he began the Kelley regimen. Since Patient #28 received neither chemotherapy nor radiation, it seems reasonable to attribute his long-term disease-free survival to the Kelley therapy.

REFERENCE

1. Karakousis, CP, et al. "Prognostic Value of Lymph Node Dissection in Malignant Melanoma." *Archives of Surgery* 1980; 115:719–722.

X-RAY REPORT

Family Name Patient #28	First Name	Middle Name		Room No. B-5	Hosp. No.

☐ Treatment ☒ Examination of	Name—Part MELANOMA BACK		Sex M̶ F	Age—Years 37	X-ray No. 16503

Attending Physician J. D. M____, M.D.		Date 3-1-82	O.P.D. No.

Report:

LIVER-SPLEEN SCAN:
Following an intravenous injection of Technetium 99m labeled Sulfur Colloid, subsequent flow and static scans of the liver and the spleen were obtained. Flow scan is unremarkable. The liver and spleen are not abnormally increased in size and the re is no evidence of shift of the reticular endothelial function. A luscency along the inferior margin of the right lobe of the liver in the anterior projection is consistent with a gallbladder fossa. Within the inferior lateral most portion of the right lobe of the liver, there is suggestion of an area of decreased radioactivity which is bett delineated in the left anterior oblique projection. The possibility of a space occupying lesion in this area cannot be absolutely excluded.

CONCLUSION: 1. POSSIBLE SPACE OCCUPYING LESION INFERIOR PORTION RIGHT LOBE OF LIVER.

CHEST:
A Pa and lateral view is submitted. No prior chest films for comparison purposes. No abnormalities are discernible.

CONCLUSION: 1. NORMAL CHEST.

GF/jb
DD: 3-1-82
DT: 3-2-82

Signature of Roentgenologist
GREG F____, M.D.

FORM 745 BRIGGS. Des Moines. Iowa 50306   PRINTED IN USA   X-RAY REPORT

299

SURGICAL RECORD
MAYO CLINIC — ROCHESTER, MINNESOTA

No. ███████████ Age **37** Sex **M** Section **Monc-B** Date **1982**

Name **Patient #28** Address **Sidney, MT**

Name of Dr. _____ Dr's. Address _____

Operation advised by, Consultant **Medical** _____ **MONC-B** Surgical Consultant **P**██████

Preoperative Diagnosis **SUSPICIOUS NODES LEFT AXILLA, HISTORY MALIGNANT MELANOMA.**

Operation Indicated **LEFT AXILLARY LYMPHADENECTOMY.**
10-203B Meth. / Recorder **pike**

Date opr. **5-26-82(1)** Opr. Room **XXXI-1** Sur. **DJP**████████**(249) KWD**████████**(O)**
A.T.2:45(PS-2) O.T.1:40

Oper. Diag.: **Metastatic malignant melanoma left axilla.**
Intradermal nevus left shoulder.

Oper.: **Excision of subcutaneous nodule and axillary lymphadenectomy.**

Drainage **Jackson-Pratt drain**

Add. cond. to index:
Detail: Skin antiseptic: **betadine**

After the usual sterile preparation and draping with the patient lying with the left side propped up, an elliptical incision was made in the lower posterior shoulder(posterior axillary area) where there was a palpable sub-cutaneous lump. Just above this a pigmented lesion was present so this was included in the dissection. Skin and subcutaneous tissue was resected free and delivered to pathology. This wound was then closed after hemostasis was obtained. We then made the usual S-shaped incision in the left axilla beginning superiorly over the pectoralis major muscle, continuing into the axilla and then curving distally along the anterior edge of the latissmus dorsi muscle. Flaps were made in the usual manner. Fascia overlying the pectoralis major muscle was dissected and continued with the fascia over the pectoralis minor and in continuity with the node-bearing tissue along the lateral chest wall. The clavipectoral fascia was incised and all the node-bearing tissue was dissected in the apex of the axilla along the medial border of the axillary vein. The lateral thoracic vein was ligated and sacrificed. The nerve to the latissmus dorsi and serratus anterior muscles were protected. The entire blockk of tissue was dissected free and delivered to pathology. Hemostasis was checked. The wound was closed in layers over two Jackson-Pratt suction drains.

*closure

300

Path.report: Ellipse skin, 3 x 2.5 x 1 cm. from left posterior shoulder, and left axillary lymph nodes. Circumscribed nodule of metastatic malignant melanoma, 1 cm. in diameter, situated in the subcutaneous fat tissue. The skin excision shows an intradermal nevus, 0.8 x 0.5 x 0.2 cm. Multiple(5) of (16) axillary lymph nodes are involved by malignant melanoma. TAG

1982   DJP███████
        MELANOMA, ?RECURRENCE.
      . EXCISIONAL BIOPSY.
Out   Meth.
9-22-82(x)   XXXI-1   DJP███████████ 249)   *MGR███████   glf
OT :25 AT :50 PS-2   (0)
                        Recurrent melanoma, left axilla.
                        Excision of nodule, left axilla, for diagnosis.

Skin Antiseptic: GSI, alcohol, and betadine
        The patient was placed in the right lateral decubitus position. The skin was prepared and draped. Under local anesthesia, the small nodule was removed with the surrounding boundary of normal subcutaneous tissue. This was sent to pathology. The wound was thoroughly irrigated, and hemostasis was obtained. The subcutaneous tissue was approximated with 3-0 vicryl and steristrips applied to approximate the skin edges. A light dressing was applied, and the patient returned to the recovery room in satisfactory condition. . .Dr. B███████
        *excision of nodule, closure.

PATH. report: Specimen from left axilla. Circumscribed recurrent malignant melanoma forming a black nodule 0.9 cm in diameter, situated in subcutaneous fat tissue. All embedded. TAG.

September 24, 1982

3-618-196

J. D. M███, M.D.
███████████████
Sidney, MT 59270

Dear Doctor M██:

I saw ▓Patient #28▓██████████ recently during his evaluation at the Mayo Clinic for complaints of a recurrent subcutaneous nodule in the area of his left axillary node dissection. ████████ noticed this nodule last week, but has had no other complaints. He states that he feels well otherwise.

On examination his weight was 74.1 kg. He had a small 3 to 4 mm firm subcutaneous nodule above the lateral end of the left axillary scar. There were no other palpable nodules and no palpable lymphadenopathy. His chest was clear and his cardiac rhythm was regular at 70 beats per minute. His abdomen was soft and there were no palpable masses. A chest x-ray was unremarkable and a CBC showed a hemoglobin of 15.9 with a white blood cell count of 7,600 and a platelet count of 304,000.

Because of the concern that this nodule was recurrent melanoma, Dr. Douglas P████████ performed an excisional biopsy with the finding of recurrent malignant melanoma. █████████ tolerated the biopsy very well and had no complications from this.

We discussed these findings with █████████ and his wife in some detail. With no evidence of other disease, there would appear to be no role for either systemic chemotherapy or for local radiation to the axilla at this time. We discussed the possibility or even probability of further recurrence with ████ ████ and stressed the need for close observation. We plan to see him in late December, but I would be happy to see him sooner if problems should arise.

Thanks again for your help and for allowing us to be part of his care.

Sincerely yours,

Ronald L. R██████████, M.D.

RLR/brm

302

April 23, 1984

3-618-196

Ms. Beverly C████████
Employees of Churches of
  Christ Insurance Group
P.O. Box █████
Spring, TX 77373

Dear Ms. C███████:

Patient #28 ███████████ has asked me to write to you regarding his medical condition. ███████████ was first seen at the Mayo Clinic in May 1982 for evaluation of possible recurrent melanoma. He had noted some enlargement of a mole on his back in February 1982, and a biopsy of this showed malignant melanoma with a depth of penetration of 4 mm. Liver and bone scans were performed at that time and were negative. Shortly after this biopsy, he underwent a wide local excision of the area but no residual disease was found in the resected specimen. In May 1982 he was noted to have palpable left axillary nodes and was referred to us for further assessment. On May 26, 1982, ███████████ underwent a left axillary node dissection with the finding of metastatic melanoma in five of sixteen axillary lymph nodes. He also had resection of a small subcutaneous nodule adjacent to the previous scar from his wide excision, and this nodule likewise was found to have malignant melanoma. He was seen, subsequently, in September 1982 and was noted to have a small subcutaneous nodule near the lateral end of the scar from his axillary node dissection. This likewise was biopsied and was found to be malignant melanoma in a nodule 0.9 cm in diameter.

Since that time we have followed ███████████ at frequent intervals, and we are pleased to say that he has done quite well with no evidence of disease recurrence. I saw him on Monday, April 23, 1984, and at that time his physical examination was unremarkable, his chest x-ray was normal, and serum chemistries and a complete blood count were normal as well.

As you know, malignant melanoma is a malignancy which traditionally carries a rather grave prognosis. The behavior of this type of neoplasm is unpredictable, and I think we need to be concerned about the possibilities of further problems with disease recurrence despite the interval from his last excision in September 1982. It is difficult to accurately predict the behavior of this malignancy though realistically the odds of this recurring at some time in the near or intermediate future are quite high.

If you need additional information regarding ███████████ condition, please contact me.

Sincerely yours,

Ronald L. Ri███████, M.D.

RLR:djl

303

Patient #29

Patient #29 is a 50-year-old woman from New York with a history of metastatic malignant melanoma.

In 1975, Patient #29 noticed a new, small pigmented "mole" on her left calf. She consulted her family physician, who assumed the lesion to be a benign nevus. Four years later, in July 1979, when the "mole" suddenly enlarged and became tender to touch, she was referred to the Dermatology Clinic at New York University Medical Center in New York. There, a biopsy of the lesion confirmed malignant melanoma.

Patient #29 was then admitted to NYU Medical Center on November 11, 1979 for wide local excision in the area of the original cancer, as well as sampling of the left groin lymph nodes. As it turned out, two of the nodes were found to be infiltrated with melanoma, a very ominous finding that warranted, her doctors insisted, aggressive adjuvant treatment.

Patient #29 was discharged from NYU on November 24, 1979, with plans to begin chemotherapy as an outpatient, but once home, she decided to investigate unconventional approaches to cancer. After learning of Dr. Kelley, Patient #29 refused to proceed with chemotherapy despite strong pressure from her doctors, and in January 1980, began the full nutritional protocol.

Patient #29 followed her regimen for three years before tapering to a maintenance program which she still follows. Today, nearly eight years after her diagnosis, she is in excellent health, having remained cancer-free during this time.

Karakousis and his colleagues report a median survival of only 26.9 months for patients, such as Patient #29, presenting with two positive lymph nodes.[1] Since this patient refused all conventional therapy after surgery, her long-term, disease-free survival can be reasonably attributed to the Kelley program.

REFERENCE

1. Karakousis, CP, et al. "Prognostic Value of Lymph Node Dissection in Malignant Melanoma." *Archives of Surgery* 1980; 115:719–722.

NEW YORK UNIVERSITY
MEDICAL CENTER
UNIVERSITY HOSPITAL

REPORT OF EXAMINATION
OF TISSUE

PATHOLOGY
LAB NO.

9601-79

NAME OF PATIENT		UNIT NO.	ROOM
Patient #29		███████	1220

SEX	AGE	DATE SPECIMEN		DATE OF REPORT	COPIES
		TAKEN	RECEIVED		
F	42	Nov. 12, 1979	Nov.12,1979	Nov.21,1979	

DOCTOR

S. G███████ M.D.

NATURE OF SPECIMEN TAKEN

Wide and deep excision melanoma left calf

FINAL DIAGNOSIS

Wide and deep excision of melanoma, left calf:

a) Malignant melanoma superficial spreading type with extension to approximately the reticular dermis (Level III-IV), pigmented (See Dermatopath report 34416-79).

b) No residual tumor seen in dermal scar

c) Secondary malignant melanoma in two inferior nodes out of 19 inguinal lymph nodes.

M. R███████ M.D./ Q. V███████, M.D.

MACROSCOPIC EXAMINATION:

Received fresh is an ellipse of skin measuring 12 cm. x 6 x 2 cm. and an inguinal lymph node dissection specimen. A scar is seen in the middle of the ellipse measuring 5 cm. in length. Three sections are taken from the middle of the scar and labelled "A," "B," and "C." A section is taken from the superior margin and labelled "D" and inked on its outer and deep margin. A section is taken from the medial margin, labelled "E," and inked on its outer and deep margin. A section is taken from the lateral margin and labelled "F." A section taken through the lateral border and labelled "G" and inked on its margins. Nodes are dissected from the inguinal lymph node dissection. Cloquet's nodes are taken and labelled "H." Nodes are dissected from the inferior of the specimen and labelled "I" through "P." Nodes dissected from the superior part of the specimen are labelled Q-T.

nh
1

305

DISCHARGE ORDER AND SUMMARY

Patient #29

NAME
RM. NO.
UNIT NO.

DISCHARGE PATIENT ON: 11/24 (A.M.) P.M.

DISCHARGE DIAGNOSIS: list in order of cause for hospitalization (DO NOT ABBREVIATE)

1. Malignant melanoma of Left Leg. Superficial spreading Type Level III → IV.

2.

	OPERATIVE PRECEDURE: (DO NOT ABBREVIATE)	DATE
3.	1. Wide and Deep Excision Melanoma left leg č split Thickness	11/12/79
4.	2. Skin graft and Left Groin Dissection	
5.	3.	

ADMIT DATE: 11/11/79

CHIEF COMPLAINT: Melanoma of (L) leg.

HISTORY OF PRESENT ILLNESS: 4 yrs PTA pt 1st noticed pigmented lesion which began increasing in size 4 mo PTA. It was also elevated and tender to touch Bx → Malignant Melanoma

PERTINENT FINDINGS: Physical Examination _____ WNL

Lab/Xray/Diagnostic Studies_____ CXR, SMA6, CBC, ESR, LFT WNL
EKG significant for PVCs.
U/S Scan WN (L)
V/A WNL

TREATMENT COURSE (Include operative procedures and dates where appropriate): _____
To OR 11/12/79 for excision melanoma, skin graft and groin dissection.

#3359

306

Patient #30

Patient #30 is a 66-year-old man from New York alive 17 years since his diagnosis of recurrent malignant melanoma.

For many years, Patient #30 had been aware of a "benign" nevus on the instep of his right foot. In March 1970, a local dermatologist removed the mole as a precaution, although it had not previously been troublesome. However, the lesion proved to be a malignant melanoma, confirmed at the Department of Pathology, Wyckoff Heights Hospital in Brooklyn. The official report describes: "Multiple level sections of the entire specimen, show an exquisite example of malignant melanoma." Furthermore, the cancer penetrated to a significant depth, involving two-thirds of the dermis.

Two weeks later, in mid-March 1970, Patient #30 was admitted to Wyckoff Heights for wide local excision in the area of the original melanoma, as well as exploration of the right groin. All specimens, including lymph nodes, were negative for tumor, and a chest X-ray and liver scan showed no evidence of metastatic disease. At that point, Patient #30's doctors assumed him to be cured.

Thereafter, he did well until August 1970, when he noticed a new "pinkish" nodule in the area of the original malignancy on his right foot. Patient #30's dermatologist removed the lesion, which was classified as recurrent melanoma.

Since the disease was still believed to be localized, the patient's doctors recommended no additional treatment. However, a month later, after several new nodules appeared along the length of his leg, in mid-September 1970 the patient's dermatologist excised a right groin lesion, identified as metastatic malignant melanoma.

Patient #30 was then referred to the Memorial Sloan-Kettering Cancer Center in Manhattan, where he was first seen in early October 1970. A review of all previous biopsy slides confirmed recurrent, metastatic melanoma, and at the time, on physical exam multiple suspicious lesions were noted on Patient #30's right leg. But a chest X-ray as well as brain and liver scans were clear of disease.

The attending surgeon at Sloan-Kettering, Dr. Joseph Fortner, recommended a right hemipelvectomy (amputation of the entire leg at the hip) but even with such a radical procedure, Patient #30 was told he most likely would not live two years. Furthermore, the various consulting physicians advised that neither chemotherapy nor radiation would provide much benefit, and immunotherapy, still experimental at that time, was not even discussed.

Patient #30, reluctant to lose his leg, requested surgery be postponed. After several more discussions with his doctors, he was discharged from Sloan-Kettering on October 9, 1970, with plans to be re-admitted two weeks later.

Once home, Patient #30 began investigating a number of unconventional cancer therapies, including the Kelley program, but he did return to Sloan-Kettering as scheduled on October 18, 1970. A second surgeon who had reviewed the case strongly recommended hemipelvectomy, but Patient #30, after considering his options, decided to refuse all further conventional treatment.

In the medical records, Dr. Fortner, the physician in charge of the case and a respected melanoma expert, reported the final diagnosis as "Recurrent malignant melanoma in the right lower leg," with a prognosis described as "poor."

After leaving Sloan-Kettering, Patient #30 traveled to Chicago for a course of Krebiozen, an unproven cancer remedy extensively promoted during the 1950s. Although scheduled for a two-month regimen of treatment, after several days he experienced a severe reaction to the drug and returned to New York. Subsequently, Patient #30 pursued no therapy of any kind until early 1971, when he finally began the full Kelley program under the supervision of a counselor trained in the method. He reported to me that shortly after beginning the treatment, the remaining lesions on his right leg crusted over, then fell off.

Patient #30 continued his nutritional approach for one and a half years and today, 17 years after his diagnosis of metastatic disease, he still follows a "healthy" diet though he uses no supplements. He describes excellent health, now having been cancer-free for the past 17 years.

In summary, Patient #30 experienced three bouts of melanoma over an eight-month period. He refused the proposed hemipelvectomy at Memorial Hospital after his disease recurred, and received no chemotherapy, radiation, or immunotherapy. When he began his nutritional program, Patient #30 had evidence of active disease.

Amer reports a mean survival of 9.7 months and a median survival of only five months in a group of 83 patients with melanoma recurring in the skin or lymph nodes.[1] Clearly, Patient #30's long-term survival on the Kelley regimen is most remarkable.

REFERENCE

1. DeVita, VT, et al. *Cancer—Principles and Practice of Oncology*. Philadelphia; J.B. Lippincott Company, 1982, page 1137.

WYCKOFF HEIGHTS HOSPITAL - DEPARTMENT OF PATHOLOGY

SURGEON	ASSISTANTS	DATE	LOCATION
		3/6/70	

SPECIMEN & SOURCE			
Lesion, right foot		Patient #30 ███████	NA█
		48	DOCT█
OPERATIVE PROCEDURE		S█████	

CLINICAL DATA   Pt. clams to have had this pigmented lesion
on the dorsum of the right foot for many many yrs.
with supposedly no recent change and now wishes it to
be examined and removed.

PRE-OP. DIAGNOSIS

POST-OP. DIAGNOSIS

REPORT   DATE   3/6/70   ACCES. NO. PA70-448
GROSS: As   rs
Specimen consists of an irregular oval segment of skin, measuring
2.5x2 cm. with much of the surface occupied by a slightly irregular
partly raised, diffusely pigmented lesion and measuring about 2 cm.
in dimension. Sections show the surface lesion pigmented, but within
it, there are zones of depigmentation. Grossly the lesion appears to
be completely, but not radically or widely excised.   Ent. sp.   48

MICROSCOPIC:
Multiple level sections of the entire specimen, show an exquisite
example of malignant melanoma. There are contiguous nests of lesional
cells, situated within the mid and upper dermis and closely applied
to the overlying epithelium, often associated with junctional nests
and in addition, showing zones of atrophy of the overlying epithelium,
with penetration of lesional x cells, within the epidermis. Not
infrequently the dermal lesional cells are collected into alveolar
nests and there are varying gradations of atypia, not infrequently
including definite hyperchromasia, with prominent nucleoli and with a
goodly number of mitotic figures. In varying zones, there may be
slight and occasionally prominent melanin pigmentation. Infrequently,
in juxta position to the nests of cells, consistent with malignant
melanoma, there are other nests of smaller darker staining cells entirel
consistent with the coexhistant and prior benign nevus. The lesional
tissue extends to fully 2/3rds of the dermis, but does not appear to
definitely reach the resected margins in depth and the lateral margins
are likewise free of tumor; therefore the lesion appears to exceed
completely though not widely excised.

DIAGNOSIS: MALIGNANT MELANOMA, SLIGHTLY PIGMENTED, OF SKIN OF RIGHT
           FOOT, INFILTRATING.

Dear Sir   April 6, 1985
     Following ████████ for your information

310

SUBMITTED BY DOCTOR Joseph F_____
SUBMITTED SLIDES ☑ 70-448(1), 70-602(1), 70-2425(1) SUBMITTED BLOCKS ☐
OUTSIDE SOURCE ARNOLD L. S_____
Wyckoff Heights Hospital B-2031(1)
70-2031(1)
Brooklyn N.Y. 11737

PLEASE RETURN

Patient #30

PATIENT NAME AND ADDRESS

DEPT. 2 1 0 1

LABORATORY USE ONLY

☐ SMALL BIOPSY   ☐ SPECIMEN   ☐ SMEARS   ☐ CLOT   ☐ IMMEDIATE EXAM (F.S.)

01 Slingt leg

1	4	7	10
2	5	8	11
3	6	9	12

ANATOMIC SOURCE OF SPECIMEN _____ Right Leg

CLINICAL DIAGNOSIS MALIGNANT MELANOMA

PREVIOUS ACCESSIONS IN THIS LABORATORY ☐ YES ☑ NO   PREVIOUS PATHOLOGY NUMBERS

SIGNIFICANT CLINICAL DATA: (USE ANATOMIC STAMPS WHEN POSSIBLE)

| AGE | SEX |
| 49 | M |

DISPOSITION OF REPORT IF OTHER THAN TO CHART

PATHOLOGY REPORT
(SEE REVERSE SIDE FOR GROSS PATHOLOGY)

DATE OF REPORT 10/15/70

MICROSCOPIC REPORT BY DR. R. D_____ A. H_____ ck

ACCESSION DATE AND NUMBER
14 OCT70-11266

A 70-448, B 70-2425, B 70-2031: MALIGNANT MELANOMA WITH
JUNCTIONAL ACTIVITY AND SHOWING EXTENSIVE INVASION
INTO UPPER ONE HALF OF DERMIS.

B 70-2007: SCLEROSING HEMANGIOMA OF SKIN

B 70-602: SENILE KERATOSIS WITH HYPERPARAKERATOSIS

F-U ☐

CHART COPY

311

Date _____

Patient #30

Memorial Hospital

RECORD PATIENT NAME AND CASE NUMBER

ADMITTED: 10-18-70

DISCHARGED: 10-22-70

ADMITTING DIAGNOSIS: Recurrent malignant melanoma of the leg.

SUMMARY OF MANAGEMENT: This was the *second* first Memorial Center admission of
                         this 49 year old white male who was admitted
with a history of having had a lesion in the dorsum of his right foot
excised widely and skin grafted 8 months previously. This had been
combined with an ipsilateral groin dissection. Two months prior to
admission, he had a satellite nodule excised. This was found to be
histologically positive for melanoma. One month prior to admission,
another satellite nodule was found just below the groin scar and this was
histologically positive for melanoma.

                         Physical examination was essentially negative
                         except for the right extremity. Chest xray was
essentially negative except for some apical fibronodular lesions probably
old tuberculosis. EKG was normal. Hemogram was normal. Screening
profile was within normal limits; 5' Nucleotidase, 12.2; stools were
negative for occult blood. Urinalysis was negative; Serology was negative.
Skeletal survey was negative; Liver and brain scans were normal. A
hemipelvectomy was recommended to the patient which he refused. He asked
to be seen by Dr. Robert J. B██████ who saw the patient in consultation
and concurred in the recommendation. The patient declined these procedures and was discharged on 10-22-70 to be followed by Dr. Phillip
Z█████, his referring physician.

FINAL DIAGNOSIS: Recurrent malignant melanoma in the right lower
                         leg.

PROGNOSIS: Poor
OPERATIVE PROCEDURES: None

JOSEPH F█████, M.D.

DISCH.
SUMM.

12-21-70/bc

1B

312

MYELOMA

Multiple myeloma affects the antibody-producing plasma cells, a mature form of the B lymphocyte series that originates in the bone marrow. Once established, this disease can destroy large areas of the bony structures, leaving characteristic punched-out lesions evident on X-rays.

Multiple myeloma killed 8,000 Americans in 1987. Today, with aggressive treatment, approximately 25% of patients survive five years.

313

Patient #31

Patient #31 is a 74-year-old woman from California who has survived 11 years since her original diagnosis of advanced multiple myeloma.

In early 1976, Patient #31 first experienced severe lower back pain that gradually worsened over a period of several weeks. She eventually consulted her primary physician, who referred her to the Sansum Clinic in Bakersfield, California, for further evaluation. There, a bone scan revealed areas of deterioration consistent with multiple myeloma in the anterior skull, lumbar spine, and right foot. In addition, serum protein electrophoresis, a study of blood immune proteins, documented the classic "gamma spike" characteristic of the disease.

With the diagnosis established, Patient #31 began a proposed one-year course of chemotherapy with the drugs vincristine and prednisone. However, she tolerated the medication poorly, with persistent side effects including nausea, chronic nosebleeds and a peripheral neuropathy (deterioration of the nerves in her hands and feet). When after eight months of treatment she still showed signs of active disease, Patient #31 refused to continue with the regimen, choosing instead to investigate "nontoxic" approaches to cancer.

Patient #31 subsequently learned of Dr. Kelley, consulted with him, and began the nutritional program in early spring of 1977. Within months, her fatigue, back pain and other symptoms resolved, and X-ray studies confirmed that the formerly extensive bone lesions had healed.

Patient #31 discontinued her nutritional program two years later, in early 1979, because she felt herself cured. Thereafter, she did well until January 1981, when she developed recurrent lower back pain, associated with persistent fatigue and loss of appetite. Despite these symptoms, Patient #31 did not seek medical advice until September 1981, when she consulted her primary care physician, who referred her back to the Sansum Clinic. There, a bone marrow biopsy indicated that fully 60% of the marrow had been replaced by cancerous plasma cells. In addition, X-rays of the spine and pelvis clearly documented malignant lesions in all visualized bone, along with compression fractures in numerous vertebral bodies.

Patient #31 was admitted to the Loma Linda University Medical Center in Loma Linda, California, on September 28, 1981, for more aggressive management. An X-ray survey of her skeleton confirmed extensive metastatic disease, described as "Multiple small round lytic lesions of all the bones consistent with widespread metastatic multiple myeloma."

A repeat bone marrow biopsy revealed infiltration of the marrow by myeloma cells, and a serum protein electrophoresis study again demonstrated the myeloma "gamma spike."

Patient #31 then resumed chemotherapy, this time with the drugs Alkeran and prednisone. When she failed to enter remission after eight months, Patient #31 discontinued the drugs, choosing instead to resume the full Kelley program.

As before, her bone pain, fatigue, and other symptoms quickly improved. Even the multiple compression fractures of her spine, which have never been surgically treated, appeared to heal. Today, 11 years after her initial diagnosis and six years since her recurrence, Patient #31 still follows her nutritional protocol, and reports excellent health with no clinical sign of cancer.

Even with aggressive chemotherapy, the prognosis for multiple myeloma is bleak. Alexanian describes a median survival of only 30 months for all myeloma patients; for those with widely metastatic disease who fail to respond to chemotherapy, such as Patient #31, the median survival falls to less than one year.[1]

Patient #31's long-term survival is unusual, with her history of two episodes of multiple myeloma involving most of her skeleton. Each time, she failed to go into remission despite chemotherapy, and each time her disease regressed only after she began the Kelley program.

Dr. Kelley believes that had Patient #31 remained faithful to the regimen initially, she would not have suffered a recurrence. Furthermore, he feels that Patient #31, because of her history of aggressive cancer, should follow her protocol for life.

REFERENCE

1. Petersdorf, RG, et al. *Harrison's Principles of Internal Medicine*. New York; McGraw-Hill Book Company, 1983, page 365.

DATE OF ADMISSION: 9/28/81   DATE OF DISCHARGE: 10/3/81

REFERRING PHYSICIAN: Dr. Steven Y██████
                            Sansum Medical Clinic

DISCHARGE DIAGNOSIS: 1. Multiple myeloma, monoclonal gamma A
                                immunoglobulin.
                            2. Status post initiation of chemotherapy.
                            3. Nummular eczema, resolved.
                            4. Multiple compression fractures of the spine,
                                with generalized osteopenia and generalized
                                osteolytic lesions.
                            5. Bibasilar pulmonary atelectasis, etiology
                                undetermined.

HISTORY OF PRESENT ILLNESS:
This 68-year-old Caucasian female was referred here by a Dr. Steven Y██████
of Sansum Medical Clinic in Bakersfield. In 1976, the patient was having
lower lumbar pain and was diagnosed to have multiple myeloma. Bone scan
at that time demonstrated abnormalities in the anterior calvarium, lumbar
spine and right foot. She was treated with Prednisone and chemotherapy,
consisting of Vincristine. However, she did not tolerate the Prednisone
well, because of nausea and this was discontinued after several days. A
later attempt resulted in similar results. The patient quit taking the
Vincristine after eight months on her own due to side-effects, including
nose bleeds. She apparently did have follow up with several other physicians with x-rays demonstrating healing of the back and was told she was
in remission. The back in generally did well, except for discomfort on
over exertion or fatigue until January 1981. At that time she noted having increasing back pain and discomfort. Blood tests in March of 1981
were stated to be normal. Since May of 1981, the patient has had increasing back pain and weakness and decreasing appetite. She saw Dr. Steven
Y██████ on 9/10/81 at which time she also admitted to a weight loss of approximately five pounds in two months. A bone marrow demonstrated approximately 60% replacement of hematopoietic elements by plasma cells consistent
with multiple myeloma. X-rays of the lumbosacral spine and pelvis demonstrated multiple lytic lesions on all the visualized bone with central compression deformities of all the lumbar vertebral bodies and anterior compression of the vertebral body at L1 and several compressed lower thoracic
vertebral bodies. Other problems noted at that time were nummular eczema
and neurodermatitis, for which was treated with topical cream with improvement. The patient also has symptoms of an upper respiratory tract infection and was treated with oral Erythromycin.

The patient was referred to Loma Linda University Medical Center by Dr.
Steven Y██████ for chemotherapy.

PHYSICAL EXAMINATION:
VITAL SIGNS: Temperature 98.6, pulse 112, respirations 24, blood pressure
160/80, weight 4'11", weight 138 lbs. GENERAL: Moderately obese Caucasian
female, in no acute distress, alert and oriented. SKIN: Several large
areas of excoriating rash over the lower extremities, upper extremities,
and the back. HEAD: Nontender, normocephalic with no irregularities.

317

EYES: Pupils equal, round, reactive to light and accommodation, extraocular muscles intact, visual fields within normal, conjunctiva not injected, sclera nonicteric, funduscopic exam demonstrated sharp disks with melanosis bilaterally, no exudate or hemorrhage noted. EARS: Tympanic membrane with good light reflexes bilaterally. NOSE/MOUTH & THROAT: Unremarkable. NECK: No JVD, carotids ++ bilaterally, without bruit, thyroid not enlarged. Trachea midline. There is a soft 3x4cm mass on the right side of the trachea, lying over the right sternocleidomastoid muscle, approximately 5cm below the angle of the jaw, consistent with a lipoma. LYMPH NODES: No cervical, supraclavicular, axillary or inguinal lymphadenopathy palpated. BREASTS: No masses or discharge, nontender. CHEST: Ribs mildly tender to percussion at right 4th-5th anterior ribs and left 8th-9th ribs at the anterior axillary line. LUNGS: Bibasilar rales present, no wheezes or rhonchi. HEART: Tachycardic at rate of 104, Grade 2/6 systolic ejection murmur, best auscultated at the left sternal border. ABDOMEN: Obese, midline suprapubic scar, bowel sounds active. Right upper quadrant tender to palpation. Liver approximatley 9-10cm at midclavicular line. No splenomegaly. No masses appreciated. BACK: Tender to percussion at approximately L2 to L3 areas, but without obvious deformity. Spine: Limitation to movement, no cva tenderness bilaterally. EXTREMITIES: Mildly tender to palpation at the left mid humerus, right anterior iliac crest and bilateral femurs. Nails pink, without cyanosis, no edema noted. NEUROLOGICAL: Cranial nerves II through XII grossly intact. Sensation and strength symmetrical and equal bilaterally. Some ataxia of the right hand on finger-to-nose maneuvers without passpointing. Heel-to-shin maneuvers good and equal bilaterally. Gait normal. Reflexes equal bilaterally. Mental status: Patient is alert, oriented with appropriate affect.

DIAGNOSTIC DATA:
On admission WBC 7.1, hemoglobin 9, segs 50%, bands 7%, lymphocytes 34%, monos 8%. Platelets 435,000. Potassium 3.6, uric acid 7.5, calcium 2.4, total protein 9.6, albumin 4.5, alkaline phosphatase 146, SGOT 36, remainder of the random chem profile essentially benign. Potassium 5.3, 6, on discharge, 4.2. Bone marrow examination from slides obtained from Sansum Medical Clinic is consistent with multiple myeloma. Serum immunoelectrophoresis demonstrates the presence of a monoclonal IgA, having lambda light changes. Urine immunoelectrophoresis demonstrating no monoclonal immunoglobulin or light changes detected. Serum protein electrophoresis demonstrating paraprotein spike in the gamma region, Gamma 3.5gm/dl (normal 0.6 to 1.3), total protein 9.6gm/dl (normal 6.3 to 7.9). Urinalysis unremarkable. EKG demonstrating sinus tachycardia, rate 103, otherwise normal.

Chest x-ray demonstrating plate-like atelectasis in the right and left base. Probable calcified hilar lymph nodes. Mild elevation of the anterior portion of the right hemidiaphragm. Multiple scattered, small, round lytic lesions, consistent with the history of metastatic multiple myeloma. Severe osteopenia with multiple compression fractures of the thoracic spine.

Metastatic bone survery demonstrating severe diffuse osteopenia. Degenerative changes of the entire spine with multiple compression fractures. Multiple small, round lytic lesions of all the bones, consistent with wide spread metastatic multiple myeloma.

HOSPITAL COURSE:

On admission calcium level was within normal, 2.4 with total protein 9.6 and albumin 4.5. Due to the patient's disease she was placed on a low calcium diet without salt restriction, although she has a history of hypertension. Her blood pressure was noted to be elevated to 170 systolic and 105 diastolic, thus she was started on Dyazide 1 q a.m. On admission, potassium level was 3.6, following 80mEq of KCL it rose to a level of 6. Thus, 30mg of Kayexalate was given with the replacement of Dyazide by Minipress for control of the hypertension. During the hospitalization course, the patient was afebrile with vital signs stable and good control of her blood pressure. She was started on chemotherapy, consisting of Alkeran 15mg q day x4 days and Prednisone 125mg q day x4. She tolerated both the Alkeran and Prednisone well, without any side-effects. After the patient finished her four day course of chemotherapy, she was discharged home in a stable condition.

DISCHARGE PROGRAM:

Discharge Medications:
1. Minipress 1mg 1 po tid.
2. Colace 100mg 1 po bid.

Outpatient follow up with Dr. G██████ in one month, during which time she will receive another course of chemotherapy. Lab work consisting of CBC, platelet, random chem profile prior to clinic visit.

Pauline C█, M.D.(H)/dwrcc

THOMAS G████ M.D.
ATTENDING PHYSICIAN

cc: Dr. Steven Y████
       Sansum Medical Clinic

DISCHARGE SUMMARY

LOMA LINDA UNIVERSITY MEDICAL CENTER

CHART COPY

Patient #31

319

please
have done same
time as CXR today

LOMA LINDA UNIVERSITY MEDICAL CENTER
DEPARTMENT OF RADIOLOGY — RADIATION SCIENCES
DIAGNOSTIC RADIOLOGY, RADIATION ONCOLOGY

LOMA LINDA RADIOLOGY MEDICAL GROUP, INC.

AGE 68	DATE OF BIRTH 3-23-1913	SEX ☐ MALE ☒ FEMALE	PREVIOUS X-RAY HERE ☐ YES ☐ NO UNKNOWN	DATE EXAM TO BE DONE 9/28/81

X-RAY EXAMINATION(S) REQUESTED:	PROVISIONAL DIAGNOSIS, PERTINENT HISTORY, OR CLINICAL DATA:	BILLING CODE
1. Bone Survey	R/O Met	
2.		
3.		

☐ Portable X-ray Required ☐ Pt. is Ambulatory ☐ Guerney
☐ Stat Reading Desired ☒ Wheelchair ☐ Pt. is Diabetic

ATTENDING PHYSICIAN	RESIDENT	SERVICE

REPORT:
Patient #31

METASTATIC BONE SURVEY INCLUDING LATERAL SKULL AND CERVICAL SPINE, RIBS, LATERAL THORACIC SPINE, LATERAL LUMBOSACRAL SPINE, PELVIS, FEMURS, AND AP VIEW OF THE HUMERI: 28 September 81

There is marked osteopenia of the bones. The bony calvarium shows multiple scattered small round lucencies. The visualized cervical spine shows degenerative disc disease of C3-C7 with anterior oteophytic spurring and there are multiple round lucencies noted in the vertebral bodies and posterior elements. The ribs also show diffuse multiple small round lytic lesions scattered throughout. There is kyphosis of the thoracic spine and multiple compression fractures throughout the thoracic and lumbar spine, most marked at T4, T12, L1 and L5. The vertebral bodies of the lumbar spine demonstrate biconcavity of the endplates. There are degenerative changes with anterior osteophytic spurring throughout the thoracic and lumbar spine. There are also multiple small round lytic lesions scattered throughout the spine. The visualized pedicles are intact. The sacrum, pelvis and femurs demonstrate multiple scattered small round lytic lesions. No soft tissue abnormalities are noted. The humeri demonstrate occasional scattered small, round lytic lesions, with larger lesions suspected in the left humeral shaft.

IMPRESSION:

Severe diffuse osteopenia.

Degenerative changes of the entire spine with multiple compression fractures as described.

Multiple small round lytic lesions of all the bones consistent with widespread metastatic multiple myeloma.

RN/mf
RN
11.3452, 38.3452, 48.3452

CHRISTINE W M.D./mf/29
29 September 1981

PREGNANT	INITIAL	FLUORO TIME	INITIAL	GONADAL SHIELDING USED		REPORT CALLED	INITIAL
☐ Yes ☐ No				INITIAL		☐ Yes ☐ No	

PATIENT IDENTIFICATION

LOMA LINDA UNIVERSITY MEDICAL CENTER
RADIOLOGY CONSULTATION
Loma Linda, California 92354 • Tel. (714) 796-7311

05-0289 (5-81)

SPECIMEN NO.	81H290
DATE RECEIVED	9/30/81
REFERRING PHYSICIAN	G█████

Reason for Examination/Consult_____Slides from Santa Barbara_____

Site_____Unknown_____ Aspiration ( ) Biopsy ( ) Both ( )

PATIENT HISTORY: 68 year old lady with a diagnosis of
multiple myeloma made some 18-24 months ago. Was followed and
treated? for a short time and has been loss to followup for
last twelve months plus. Now admitted to Medical Oncology for
re-evaluation.

PERIPHERAL BLOOD SMEAR: Red cells are normochromic, normocytic.
Few target cells, no schistocytes. Rouleaux formation is moderate
in degree. Overall WB count is normal. Some atypical lymphocytes
are seen. Platelets are of normal number with a few large forms.

MARROW CLOT/BIOPSY SECTION: Cellularity is 30-80% with M:E ratio
about 3:1. There is a moderate increase in plasma cells which
become solid sheets in some areas. Eosinophils are mildly
increased.

MARROW SMEAR: Erythropoiesis is sparse as is granulo-
cytopoiesis. Sheets of only moderately well-differentiated
plasma cells are seen. There are some trilobed and bilobed
plasma cells. No other infiltrative lesion is noted.

ASSESSMENT:

CONCLUSION: CONSISTENT WITH MULTIPLE MYELOMA. CORRELATION WITH
                      URINE AND PLASMA PROTEIN STUDIES SHOULD BE REQUESTED

Hematologist Consultant _____ Date_____ 10/2/81 IK/ch
                        I. K███ M.D.

CONSULTATION REPORT

HEMATOLOGY

Previous Data	
WBC	_____
RBC	_____
Hgb	_____
Hct	_____
MCV	_____
MCH	_____
MCHC	_____
Lymph	_____
Mono	_____
Eos	_____
Baso	_____
Segs	_____
Bands	_____
Other	_____
Platelet	_____
Retics	_____
Serum Fe	_____
TIBC	_____
Iron Stain	_____

Patient Identification

Patient #31 █████████

OVARIAN CANCER

Cancer of the ovaries claimed the lives of 11,700 American women in 1987.

Surgery, often combined with radiation and aggressive chemotherapy, can cure this disease if localized, but even with intensive treatment only 38% of all patients survive five years after diagnosis.

Patient #32

Patient #32 is a 40-year-old woman from Oklahoma alive more than 13 years since diagnosed with ovarian cancer.

In April 1974, during a routine exam, Patient #32's gynecologist noted a painless 6 cm left ovarian mass, initially believed consistent with a benign cyst. When the lesion continued to enlarge over a four-week period, Patient #32 was admitted to McAlester General Hospital in Oklahoma on June 17, 1974 for evaluation.

The following day, during exploratory surgery tumors were evident on both ovaries, along with metastatic disease throughout the pelvis. After frozen section biopsy confirmed ovarian cancer, the attending surgeon proceeded with a hysterectomy and oophorectomy (resection of the ovaries). Review of the surgical specimens confirmed a papillary mucinous cystadenocarcinoma of the ovary, stage III.

The records clearly describe the extensive disease:

> At the time of laparotomy [surgery] she was noted to have mucin in her abdomen along with a 6–8 cm. left ovarian mass and a 4 cm. right ovarian mass . . . There were multiple small papillary areas of mucus secreting tumor on the pelvic peritoneum but exploration of the abdomen revealed no other evidence of metastatic disease . . .

The patient's physicians then recommended cobalt radiation to the pelvis, along with a course of the chemotherapeutic drug chlorambucil. Patient #32 agreed to the treatment regimen, which she began shortly after her discharge from the hospital. At the same time, she decided to investigate unconventional approaches to cancer, consulted with Dr. Kelley, and in early fall of 1974 began the full nutritional program. She also continued chemotherapy until the fall of 1975.

Patient #32 eventually followed her nutritional protocol for seven and a half years before tapering down to a maintenance regimen. Today, 13 years since her diagnosis, she is in excellent health and cancer-free.

Despite advances in therapy, the prognosis for metastatic ovarian cancer remains poor. Tobias describes a 5% five-year survival rate for patients, such as Patient #32, with stage III disease even when aggressively treated.[1]

In summary, Patient #32 was diagnosed with bilateral, metastatic ovarian carcinoma. Although she did complete a course of radiation and a full year of chemotherapy, her long-term, disease-free survival, now in excess of ten years, is nonetheless most unusual.

REFERENCE

1. Tobias, JS, et al. "Management of Ovarian Carcinoma; Current Concepts and Future Prospects." *New England Journal of Medicine* 1976; 294:818-822.

Patient #32

Admitted: 6-17-74   Dismissed: 6-24-74

The patient is a 27 yr. old Gravida I, Para I who was admitted on 6-17-74 because
of a left ovarian cyst which had been present since April 1974. The cyst was approximately 6 cm. in diameter at the first examination. She had regular menstrual periods with the last menstrual period 6-1-74. Pap smear was normal. History
was otherwise unremarkable.

Physical examination was within normal limits except for a 6-8 cm. cyst in the left
adnexal region.

Laboratory studies on admission revealed a hemoglobin of 13.5 gm., hematocrit 40%.
White count 10,200 with 74 polys and 26 lymphs. UA unremarkable. Blood type 0+,
Serology non-reactive.

She was taken to surgery the day after admission where examination under anesthesia
revealed a small mass in the right ovary. It was enlarged slightly above normal.
At the time of laparotomy she was noted to have mucin in her abdomen along with
a 6-8 cm. left ovarian mass and a 4 cm. right ovarian mass. She had a total abdominal hysterectomy and bilateral salpingo-oophorectomy. There were multiple small
papillary areas of mucus secreting tumor on the pelvic peritoneum but exploration
of the abdomen revealed no other evidence of metastatic disease clinically. Her
postoperative course has been essentially uncomplicated. She has been completely
afebrile. She had a chest x-ray which was normal and an IVP which revealed no abnormalities, only four lumbar vertebrae were noted.

Postoperative hemoglobin was 11.9 gm., hematocrit 36%.

She is being dismissed on 24 June 74 and arrangements are being made to have her
receive further care.

Dismissal medications include Premarin 1.25 mg. daily because of menopausal symptoms, Phenaphen #3 for pain and Valium 5 mg. for nervousness and a rash which she
developed with the nerves.

FINAL DIAGNOSIS: 1.   Stage III papillary mucinous cystadenocarcinoma of the ovary.
                   2.   Dermoid cyst of the right ovary.

Paul S███████, M. D.

'S:lg
c:Clinic
:6-24-74
:6-24-74
Copy sent along with copies of H&P and Op. report with patient per request of
Dr. S███████ 6-24-74.

326

ANATOMIC PATHOLOGY

Date   6/18/74   S 74-1094

Patient   Patient #32   P. S___ .M.D.   27   f   143-

Admission No._____ Doctor_____

Pre-Operative Diagnosis_____ frozen section left ovarian cyst

Post-Operative Diagnosis_____

Specimen   **cervix, uterus, bil. ovaries, bil. tubes**

Clinical History_____
        date of last menstrual :   6/1/74

Gross & Microscopic Examination

Specimen consists of an ovary measuring 5 x 5 x 4.5 cm. The surface is white and has a fibrous consistency. It is cystic with the wall averaging 2 to 3 mm in thickness. Internally the lumen is filled with papillary tumor consisting of innumerable cauliflower-like verrucous yellowish tan nodules which are embedded in nests of semitransparent mucoid material. A previous frozen section has been done.

B. Specimen is received in formalin and labeled cervix, uterus, bilateral tubes and bilateral ovaries. The gross specimen consists of a uterus, cervix, both fallopian tubes and ovaries. The uterus measures 8 x 6 x 3 cm. and weighs 92 gm. The external surface is moderately smooth and glistening with scattered fibrous areas along the right posterior wall. The myometrium averages 1 1/2 cm. in thickness and is uniform red-tan throughout. The endometrium measures 4 mm in thickness and is uniform red-tan throughout. Representative sections of each are submitted for microscopic examination.

The cervix has a 1 1/2 cm transverse external os lined by intact mucosa. The endo-ceriveal canal is intact. Two (2) representative sections of cervix are submitted for microscopic examination

The right ovary measures 5 x 4 x 4 cm. and reveals multiple cysts. The cut section reveals a cystic space 3 cm in diameter filled with whitish tan greasy material admixed with some hair fragments. There is a second cyst measuring 2 cm and is filled with clear fluid and a smaller cyst measuring 1 cm. in diameter which appears to have some papillary fragments protruding from the wall. There is a corpus luteum noted in the intervening stroma.

The fallopian tube measures 7 x 1 cm. and has a moderately uniform external diameter. One (1) representative section is submitted for microscopic examination.

The left ovary measures 3 x 2 x 2 cm. and has a 2 cm in length recent sutured incision.

white–Chart Copy   canary–File Copy   pink–Doctor's Copy   gold–Tissue Committee

327

ANATOMIC PATHOLOGY

6/18.74   S 74-1294

Patient.   Patient #32   Age   Sex   19

Admission No.   Doctor.   P. S   ,M.D.

page 2

The cut section of the ovary reveals a slightly hemorrhagic area. The remainder of
the ovary is basically unremarkable. One (1) representative section is submitted.

The fallopian tube measures 7 x 1 cm. The external surface is unremarkable. The
cut section is unremarkable. One (1) representative section is submitted.
MDBet

MICROSCOPIC EXAMINATION
... Microscopic slide contains sections of tissue which consists largely of papillary
projections covered by columnar epithelium. The epithelium shows pseudostratification
of nuclear atypicalities . The underlying stroma is edematous appearing ovarian
stroma .   There is a hemorrhagic corpus luteum cyst noted along one margin.

B . The first microscopic slide contains sections of endometrium and myometrium. The
endometrium is composed of glandular spaces lined by columnar epithelium which shows
pseudostratification of nuclei and an occasional mitosis. The surrounding stroma is
moderately dense. The underlying myometrium is unremarkable.

The next microscopic slide contains sections of cervix. The external squamous mucosa
is thin and uniform.   The squamo-columnar junction is basically unremarkable.
The endocervical epithelium is unremarkable.   The endocervical glands are unremarkable.

The next microscopic slide contains sections of right ovary and fallopian tube.
The external surface of the ovary is basically unremarkable. The ovarian substance
consists of corpora albicans and an occasional cystic space lined by flattened epithelium
One cyst contains tissue similar to that described in A. Another cystic space is
lined by stratified squamous epithelium.

The cross section of fallopian tube is unremarkable. The next microscopic slide
contains sections of left ovary and fallopian tube. The ovarian substance contains
corpora albicans and cysts. Some cysts are lined by flattened epithelum and other
cysts are lined by luteinized epithelium.

The cross section of the left fallopian tube is unremarkable.

328

ANATOMIC PATHOLOGY

Date: 6/18/74   Path. Specimen No. 3-74-1254

Patient: Patient #32

P. S_____ M.D.   Age____ Sex____ Room No. 143-1

Admission No. _____ Doctor_____

page 3

DIAGNOSIS:

Uterus, no pathological diagnosis T3200- m0001
Endometrium, proliferative phase Ts4Lo-
Cervix, no pathological diagnosis T8800
Ovary, left, T8701
   1. Papillary cystadenocarcinoma (mucinous) m 8463
   2. Corpus luteum cyst m3552
   3. Follicular cyst m3449
Ovary, right, T8701
   1. Papillary cystadenocarcinoma (mucinous) m 8463
   2. Dermoid cyst m9080
   3. Corpus luteum cyst - m 3552
   4. Follicular cyst m3449
Fallopis tube, right and left, no pathological diagnosis

MDBet

Patient #33

Patient #33 is a 46-year-old woman from Minnesota who has now survived 15 years since her diagnosis of metastatic ovarian carcinoma.

In early 1970, Patient #33 experienced an episode of severe lower abdominal pain, lasting only about one minute. Over the next two years, although the pain occasionally recurred, Patient #33 was otherwise asymptomatic until March 1972, when she developed a sensation of "fullness" in her pelvis. She consulted her physician, who noted, on physical exam, a large mass in the area of the right ovary.

On April 3, 1972, Patient #33 was admitted to St. Paul Ramsey Hospital in Minnesota for further evaluation. The following day, during exploratory surgery she was found to have carcinoma involving both ovaries, adjacent lymph nodes, and extending into most of the pelvis. When a frozen section biopsy confirmed cancer, the attending surgeon proceeded with a hysterectomy and oophorectomy.

The operative note describes the extensive disease in detail:

> Exploration of the pelvic cavity found a mass of matted tissue involving the entire cul-de-sac [area around uterus] and the ovaries and uterus were incorporated in an entire mass of adhesions. At first it was felt that the masses on the left and right lateral pelvic walls were lymph nodes and a biopsy was taken from the surface of one of these lymph nodes. The frozen section was reported as cystadenocarcinoma . . . The right ovarian mass measured 10 cm . . .

Final review of the surgical specimens revealed stage III disease, as documented in the pathology report:

> Bilateral serous cyst adenocarcinoma extending to peritoneal surface with peritoneal seeding and stromal infiltration . . . Intracanalicular tumor metastasis in the right [Fallopian] tube.

While still hospitalized, Patient #33 began a series of cobalt radiation treatments to the abdominal cavity, which she continued as an outpatient after her discharge on April 15, 1972. She tolerated the therapy poorly, experiencing a number of serious side effects including persistent nausea and vomiting, associated with rapid weight loss. When her white blood count fell to dangerously low levels, Patient #33 was re-admitted to Ramsey Hospital on April 26, 1972.

After several days Patient #33 stabilized to the point she could complete the planned 4,000 rad course of cobalt as an inpatient. Despite the treatment, her doctors detected a rapidly growing pelvic tumor shortly before her discharge from Ramsey Hospital in late May 1972. However, her physician decided to observe her progress for several weeks, before recommending additional therapy.

At a scheduled follow-up exam in early June 1972, the mass was still clearly evident. Although a complete re-evaluation was recommended, Patient #33 chose to refuse all further diagnostic tests and treatment as documented in her physician's notes:

> Pelvic exam on discharge from the hospital indicated a large pelvic mass which could be felt by vaginal exam as well as rectovaginal [rectal] examination which was smooth, firm, with no cystic tendencies and seemed to occupy the entire pelvis . . . It was recommended that the patient have an IVP and barium enema. However, the patient has refused this.

At that point, Patient #33 decided to investigate unconventional cancer therapies. In late June 1972, she learned of Dr. Kelley, consulted with him and began the full nutritional program. Only months after she began treatment, the large pelvic mass regressed completely.

In January 1973, Patient #33 returned to her physician for a routine follow-up evaluation. On pelvic exam only a small amount of residual fibrotic tissue, attributed to the earlier radiation therapy, was evident, as the record indicates:

> There are no masses felt, except in the right vaginal apex, there is a small firm area which is indiscrete and probably related to cobalt treatment.

Then in a later note dated May 30, 1973, the physician noted her obvious improvement once again:

> Bimanual and rectovaginal are entirely negative for masses. It appears that the patient has complete resolution of tumor.

Patient #33 followed the full Kelley program from 1972 until 1983, except for brief periods when she slacked off because she felt so well. Today, 15 years after her diagnosis, she is in excellent health and cancer-free.

So in summary, Patient #33 was initially diagnosed with metastatic ovarian carcinoma, affecting the entire pelvis and multiple lymph nodes. Despite a course of cobalt, the disease recurred with a vengeance, rapidly filling her pelvis, and then regressed completely after she began the Kelley program.

331

NAME Patient #33   DATE 4/4/72   WARD 514

OPERATION BY Dr.L▮   SPECIMEN Lymph node, R.hypogastric   AGE 32
retroperitoneal - uterus, fallopian tube &
ovaries, more tumor right ovarian site

GROSS:

The specimen is submitted in three parts:

Specimen (A) is designated "lymph node right hypogastric retroperitoneal" and consists of a segment of whitish tissue measuring 3 x 2 x 1 cm. A frozen section is reported as showing a papillary adenocarcinoma.

Specimen (B) is designated "uterus, fallopian tubes and ovaries" and consists of a resected uterus with right and left tubes and ovaries attached.   The right ovary forms a tumor measuring 7 x 6 x 6 cm. which includes the right ovary and ovarian tissue can be recognized at the marginal portion of the tumor. The tumor is cystic and multi-loculated, is filled by papillary masses which extend to the ovarian surface where they cover an area of apparoximately 8 x 6 cm. at the lateral aspect of the ovary and approximately 3 x 4 cm. at the medial aspect of the ovary. The right tube is present, measures $9\frac{1}{2}$ cm. in length. The peritoneal surface near the right ligamentum rotundum is roughened and seems also to show some papillary formations. It seems to represent tumor implant. The left ovary measures $2\frac{1}{2}$ x 3 x 2 cm. and on its surface carries a papillary tumor mass measuring about $2\frac{1}{2}$ cm. in diameter. On cut section the ovary contains a cyst filled with the same friable papillary tumor material as found in the right ovary. The tube is markedly dilated and seems to form a tubal ovarian mass. The uterus measures $8\frac{1}{2}$ x 4 x 3 cm. Its posterior surface is covered by adhesions and hemorrhagic material. Sections of the right tumor and ovary, as well as tube, are labelled (1), sections of the left tube, ovary, and tumor (2), sections of the uterus (3).

Specimen (C) is labelled "more tumor from right ovarian site" consists of several segments of papillary tumor tissue measuring up to 2 cm. in diameter.

(continued)

ST. PAUL-RAMSEY HOSPITAL, ST. PAUL, MINN.   SURGICAL NO. ▓▓▓▓

SURGICAL PATHOLOGY REPORT

FILE NO. ▓▓▓▓

NAME __Patient #33▓▓▓▓_____   DATE __4/4/72__ WARD __514__

OPERATION BY __Dr. Lu▓▓▓▓_____ SPECIMEN __Lymph nodes_____ AGE __32__

GROSS:

PAGE TWO:

MICROSCOPIC: Microscopic sections of Specimen (A) show a papillary tumor consisting of numerous irregular papillary formations lined by a cylindrical epithelium consisting of cells with large hyperchromatic nuclei of irregular, size, shape and chromatin pattern. Epithelial elements have lost their polarity and show in some areas piling up into several layers of neoplastic cells. Fibrous tissue stroma is cellular, consists of large and histologically benign fibroblast-like cells. Vessels are sparse. Sections of the right ovary with tumor (B1) show multicystic areas of the same papillary tumor as described above. The tumor is seen to extend to the ovarian surface and is found in subserosal location in tissue of the broad ligament. In some areas the tumor forms calcospherites. Sections of the right ovary show several cystic follicles. Section of the right tube shows in one location nests of calcospherites surrounded by a few atypical cells. This is interpreted as representing intracanalicular spread of tumor elements extending from the abdominal cavity.

Sections of the left ovary show an identical appearing tumor occupying several cysts within the ovary and extending from one of them to the serosal surface of the ovary; also the ovarian stroma appears infiltrated by some nests of tumor tissue, forming irregular papillary glandular structures. Sections of peritoneum, from the area of the round ligament show subserosal tumor implants with calcospherite formation.

Microscopic sections of the left tube show some dilated lymphatic channels with subserosal tissue and a moderate dilatation of the tubal volume. In the subserosal tissue there are some atypical glandular structures.

Microscopic examination of Specimen (3). In the area of the right round ligament there are numerous tumor implants in the subserosal tissue developing numerous calcospherites and surrounded by an inflammatory reaction and hemorrhage. Microscopic sections of the cervix show a severe inflammatory reaction in the area of the squamocolumnar junction with abundant amount of polymorphonuclear exudate filling several cervical glands, and infiltrating the fibrous tissue which in one circumscribed area shows local necrosis with abscess formation. The endometrium shows a proliferative pattern.

Microscopic sections of Specimen (C) show identical tumor tissue.

(Continued)

ST. PAUL-RAMSEY HOSPITAL, ST. PAUL, MINN.   SURGICAL NO. ____ Patient #33

SURGICAL PATHOLOGY REPORT

FILE NO. _____

NAME _____ DATE _____ WARD _____

OPERATION BY _____ SPECIMEN _____ AGE _____

=====================================

GROSS:

PAGE THREE:

IMPRESSION: Bilateral serous cyst adenocarcinoma extending
              to peritoneal surface with peritoneal seeding
              and stromal infiltration.   87-8443

              Acute and chronic cervicitis with abscess for-
              mation.   83-4174

              Intracanalicular tumor metastasis in the right
              tube.   86-8143

ERHARD ▉ M.D.
Pathologist

cs/pe

334

ST. PAUL-RAMSEY HOSPITAL - ST. █████████

RECORD OF OPERATION

Patient #33

NAME OF PATIENT ████████████████████████████████████ AGE _31_ A# _____

DATE OF OPERATION _4 Op 1972_   P# _677703-1_   CIRCLE # _5E_

OPERATION _Simple total abdominal hysterectomy - bil. salpingo-oophor___ SPECIMEN _____

ANESTHESIA _Gen_   ANESTHESIOLOGIST ██████████

ANES. BEGAN _7³⁵ A_   ANES. ENDED _11⁰⁵ A_   GROUND PLATE ① _Buttock_

STAFF SURGEONS _B_████████████   SURGEONS ██████████

ASSISTANT SURGEONS ████████, ███████, ███████

SERVICES _Gyn_   OPER. ROOM # _7_   OPER. BEGAN _8⁰⁰ A_   ENDED _11⁰⁵ A_

SCRUB NURSES _V. P_███████   CIRCULATING NURSES _M. E._ ████████

SPONGE COUNT (1) _Correct_   (2) _Correct_   (3) _____

         _M. E._████████   _M. E._████████

PREOPERATIVE DIAGNOSIS: Right ovarian mass.

POSTOPERATIVE DIAGNOSIS: Bilateral cystadenocarcinoma of the ovaries.

TITLE OF PROCEDURE: Total abdominal hysterectomy and bilateral salpingo-oophorectomy.

HISTORY AND DESCRIPTION: 32-year-old Para 1-0-0-1, LNMP 3 weeks, was noted to have an ovarian mass on routine pelvic examination, measuring 12x15x15 cm. Past medical history is noncontributory. She is a Jehovah's Witness and refused blood transfusions. She is being scheduled for an exploratory laparotomy.

The patient was prepped and draped in the usual manner under general anesthesia. A midline incision extending from the umbilicus to the symphysis pubis was made. The fascia was identified. The peritoneum subsequently identified and the peritoneal cavity entered. Serous fluid in the peritoneal cavity was collected and submitted for malignant cells. Exploration of the pelvic cavity found a mass of matted tissue involving the entire cul-de-sac and the ovaries and uterus were incorporated in an entire mass of adhesions. At first it was felt that the masses on the left and right lateral pelvic walls were lymph nodes and a biopsy was taken from the surface of one of these lymph nodes. The frozen section was reported as cystadenocarcinoma. With alternate blunt and sharp dissection the ovaries on both sides were freed of adhesions and mobilized into the abdominal wound. They had virtually rotated and incarcerated into the cul-de-sac as well as the lateral pelvic walls. The right ovarian mass measured 10 cm., was irregular, lobulated with numerous

-continued-

335

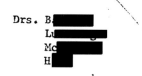

papillary growths on the surface. The left ovary was somewhat smaller in size, measuring 5 cm., also lobulated with multiple papillary growths on the surface. The remainder of the abdominal cavity was explored and no evidence of implants were noted in the bowels, in the omentum, liver, spleen or periaortic lymph nodes. Three papillary excrescences were lopped off by palpation of the ovaries and were collected from the cul-de-sac periodical The decision was made to do a total abdominal hysterectomy and bilateral salpingo-oophorectomy at this time.

The infundibulopelvic ligaments on both sides were identified, clamped, transected and ligated. The round ligaments on both sides were clamped with a Kocher, transected and ligated with #1 chromic. The reflection of the peritoneum was then identified, and the ureter identified on both sides and followed in its course in the pelvis. The uterine arteries on both sides were clamped, transected and ligated with #1 chromic size catgut. The peritoneal reflection over the anterior cervix together with the bladder was dissected downwards from the anterior cervix until the distal portion of the cervix was identified. The uterus was reflected anteriorly and a transverse incision was made in the posterior reflection of the peritoneum. Both uterosacrals were identified, clamped, transected and ligated with #1 chromic. Pericervical tissue on both sides was similarly clamped, transected and ligated with #1 chromic size catgut. The entire tissue was dissected off the cervix until it was completely free anteriorly, laterally and posteriorly. A right angle clamp was then placed on the vagina on both sides distal to the end of the cervix and the vaginal orifice opened and the entire specimen removed from the surgical field.

The angles of the vagina were ligated with figure-of-eight chromic catgut and the remainder of the vaginal vault was closed with #1 chromic catgut interrupted sutures. A defect was left in the middle of the vagina through which a drain was placed into the vagina. The peritoneum from one end of the base of the infundibulo-pelvic ligament was then sutured completely retroperitonealizing the pelvis space. There were no complications.

The patient was closed as follows: The peritoneum continuous #1 chromic catgut; the fascia interrupted #2-0 Tevdek; three transfixion sutures were placed with #1 Tevdek; the subcutaneous tissue was closed with #2-0 plain catgut; and the skin with interrupted #4-0 silk. The patient left the Operating Room in satisfactory condition.

Surgeon: Dr. Ismail B▮▮▮▮▮   Assistants: Dr. Gary L▮▮▮▮, Dr. Miriam Mc▮▮▮▮, and
                                              Dr. Patty H▮▮▮▮
                                  Staff: Dr. B▮▮▮▮▮

Dictated by Dr. B▮▮▮▮   7-13-72

SURGEON: ▮▮▮▮▮▮▮▮▮▮▮▮▮▮▮
         I. B▮▮▮ M.D., Staff

jm 7-26-72

NAME: Patient #33

NO:

This 31-year-old Jehovah Witness, Para 1-0-4-1 whose LMP was 4-1-72 was admitted on 4-3-72 for laparotomy to explore right adnexal mass.

HISTORY OF PRESENT ILLNESS: For the last 2 years the patient has felt 4 episodes of severe, transient, lower abdominal pains which last less than a minute. For a month prior to admission she complained of feeling pressure on her bladder, plus feeling that something was in the way, preventing bowel movements occasionally.

PAST MEDICAL HISTORY: In 1961 she had a cyst on her breast removed.

OB HISTORY: Noncontributory.

FAMILY HISTORY: Grandfather died of a stroke, father had cancer of the colon.

HOSPITAL COURSE: On admission physical a right adnexal mass, about 10 cm., was palpated, was firm and fixed to the uterus and non-mobile. Hemoglobin 13.4, WBC 7,700, VDRL negative, SMA-12 normal except for a slightly elevated albumin and protein, blood type O+, UA and UC were within normal limits. Exploratory laparotomy was done on 4-4 and revealed cancer in both ovaries which was hand dissected, both off the rectum and the right pelvic wall. A total abdominal hysterectomy and bilateral salpingo-oophorectomy were performed. There were implants on the peritoneal surface of the uterus, however, there were no obvious metastases to the bowel, liver or peritoneum or the lymph nodes. On the 6th postop day she was begun on Cobalt therapy to the abdomen with chimney up the aorta. She tolerated Cobalt poorly at first with nausea and vomiting, however, after 4 days vomiting was controlled with Compazine and she was able to take over 2000 cc. of fluid p.o. CBC on discharge showed hemoglobin of 11.8, WBC 5,000 and lytes within normal limits. She is to continue Cobalt as an outpatient and to be followed in Tumor Clinic weekly with hemoglobin, WBC and platelets. She was discharged on Fergon and Compazine.

PATHOLOGICAL DIAGNOSIS: (1) Bilateral serous cystadenocarcinoma extending to peritoneal surface with peritoneal seeding and stromal infiltration. Intracanalicular tumor metastasis in Rt. tu(2) Chronic cervicitis Papillary adenocarcinoma of the ovary, Stage 2-B.

FINAL DIAGNOSIS:
1. Papillary adenocarcinoma of the ovary, Stage 2-B.
2. Status post TAH and BSO.
3. Status post 1 week of Cobalt therapy.

RECOMMENDATION: Weekly follow up in Gyn Tumor Clinic with hemoglobin, WBC and platelets. She is to call if she begins vomiting or if she can't drink at least 8 glasses of fluid per day. She is to receive radiation therapy as an outpatient and take Fergon t.i.d. and Compazine 10 mg. prn. nausea.

Patty H.___ M.D., Intern
OB-Gyn Service
St. Paul-Ramsey Hospital

Ismail B.___ M.D.,
Attending Staff Physician

4-18-72/kjw

337

[handwritten] Patient to be admitted at SPRH on 4/3/72
[handwritten] discharged on 5/11/72

Patient will be seen on 3·27·72 Monday at
which time an admission note will be dictated

3·27·72 Wt – 132½
Same as admit note

6·1·72   6 June Barium – IVP 8⁰⁰
6·15·72 wt = 109   BP 108/70   Hgb 11.8   Eos 1%
get eff today   Leuk 4000/mm
                           N 78%
                           L 13%
                           M 9%

This is the first visit since discharge on May 25. Pelvic exam on discharge from
the hospital indicated a large pelvic mass which could be felt by vaginal exam as
well as rectovaginal examination which was smooth, firm, with no cystic tendencies
and seemed to occupy the entire pelvis. The upper limit of this mass was
not adequately palpated. It was recommended that the patient have an IVP and
barium enema. However, the patient has refused this.

At the present moment she is having a normal diet on vitamins and iron and she
is having regular bowel movements. She has no complaints and she is well.
General physical examination including chest was negative. Neck was negative for
masses. Breasts and axilla are negative.

Abdomen: Soft, somewhat moderately tender with no masses palpated. Groins are
free of nodes. There is no CVA tenderness.

Extremities are normal.

Pelvic: External genitalia: Normal.

             Vagina: Pale with small areas of ectasia and vaginal vault the angles
of which are somewhat hemorrhagic and the right angle shows a small
pyogenic granuloma.

Bimanual exam: shows two areas of induration, one in the right side which is
approximately 1 1/2 cm. in largest diameter, somewhat mobile and occupying the
angle of the vault of the vagina. The other mass is somewhat deeper in the pelvis on
the left side, less distinct, about 3 cm., tender hard, immobile.

338

11-22-72 cancelled.
12-6-72 Cancelled
1-24-3 wt=117.

no problems   This patient has missed several appointments and in interviewing
her she has pursued a certain course of management which the details
of which I am not familiar with. She states that she went to Mexico
and had some intravenous treatments for the cancer, the nature of
which are unknown to her except that they are enzymes. She has also
received several enzyme enemas. Have requested from her to have the
organization which has performed these therapeutic measures to send
me a copy of the details of her treatment.

As far as the patient is concerned, she feels very well. She is
eating well and has gained 7 pounds since her last visit in August
here.

General examination: Lymph nodes entirely negative in neck, arm pits,
              and groin.

                      Chest is clear.

                      Heart is negative.

                      Abdomen is entirely negative.

Pelvic examination: External genitalia, normal.

                      Vagina shows some atrophy with hemorrhagic spots.

Bimanual exam: There are no masses felt, except in the right vaginal
              apex, there is a small firm area which is indiscrete
              and probably related to cobalt treatment.

              Left adnexa is entirely negative.

Impression: No evidence of recurrence of disease.

              Patient will be followed here periodically at 3 month
              intervals, however, she has refused any diagnostic or
              therapeutic measures.

                                        Ismail B████████ M.D.

5-30-73   wt=128   BP=120/80   urine alb. 0
      Patient came in for routine check.   gl. 0
      Chest is clear.   Hgb 12.1
      Breasts are negative for masses, axilla negative for nodes.
      Abdomen negative for masses and organomegaly.
      Groin nodes are negative.
      Pelvic: External genitalia, normal.
              Vagina, normal.
              Vault is healed.

FORM NO. 679-1-270

339

5/30/73 con't: Bimanual and rectovaginal are entirely negative for masses.

It appears that the patient has complete resolution of tumor. I am
still awaiting details of her treatments in Mexico. She still is reluctant
about having tests done. Will follow at 3-month intervals.

MIsmail B██████, M.D.

11/28/73 wt 131 BP 120/86   CBC
                                                                12 Cl
This patient is coming in for routine checkup--post-operative serous   chest
cystadenocarcinoma of the ovaries done in March of 1972.   x-ray

The patient has been asymptomatic, has gained weight, and had no GYN
GYN complaints.

She looks very well and healthy.

A complete physical examination was done:

Neck--supple, no masses or nodes.

Breasts--negative for masses and axillæ are negative for nodes.

Chest is clear to percussion on auscultation.

Heart is negative.

Abdomen--no masses

Groin--no lymph nodes.

Pelvic exam: External genitalia, normal.

Vagina is somewhat hyperemic and constricted.

Vault is negative.

Pap smear was taken.

Bimanual and rectovaginal showed no evidence of tumor recurrence in the
pelvis.

Have obtained the following: 1. A 12-Channel and CBC.
                             2. Chest x-ray.

Patient is dubious about obtaining an IVP, and she will return at her
convenience for that.

Impression: No evidence of recurrence.

Will see in 6 months.

Ismail B██████, M.D.

1-8-75 Cancelled JC
1-22-75 Failed JC

340

PANCREATIC CANCER

The pancreas consists of two distinct tissue types, the endocrine islets and the exocrine acini, as they are known, with completely different functions. The islet cells secrete hormones such as insulin and glucagon directly into the bloodstream to regulate glucose and fat metabolism. The acinar cells synthesize the various digestive enzymes, which are released directly into the small intestine during meals. There, the various proteases, amylases and lipases break down respectively the proteins, carbohydrates, and fats present in food.

Though cancer can originate in either of these two tissues, the exocrine variety is most common, accounting for 95% or more of all pancreatic tumors. Overall, pancreatic malignancies claimed 24,300 lives in 1987, making the disease the fourth most common cause of cancer-related death, and the incidence seems to be increasing yearly. Experts consider malignancy of the exocrine pancreas one of the deadliest of all neoplasms, with fewer than 2% of patients alive five years after diagnosis despite intensive treatment.[1] The rarer tumors of the endocrine pancreas, though less aggressive, unless localized at the time of diagnosis eventually prove deadly.

REFERENCE

1. Harvey, AM, et al. *The Principles and Practice of Medicine*, 20th Edition. New York; Appleton-Century-Crofts, 1980, page 652.

Patient #34

Patient #34 is a 51-year-old woman from Wisconsin alive nearly five years since her diagnosis of metastatic adenocarcinoma of the pancreas.

Beginning in 1980, Patient #34 experienced occasional bouts of sharp mid-abdominal pain usually occurring after meals. Subsequently, over a period of two years, these episodes became more frequent and more intense, often persisting for hours at a time. However, Patient #34 did not seek medical advice until August 18, 1982, when she was awakened in the middle of the night with severe abdominal pain and nausea. After she vomited several times, her husband drove her to the emergency room at St. Elizabeth Hospital in Appleton, Wisconsin, where she was promptly admitted for evaluation. On exam her abdomen was extremely tender in the area of the pancreas. Initial laboratory studies were notable for a high white blood count and an elevated amylase level, a finding often associated with pancreatitis (inflammation of the pancreas).

The following day, an ultrasound study of the abdomen revealed numerous stones in the gallbladder, but no evidence of more serious disease. Although the bile ducts appeared patent, Patient #34's doctors diagnosed pancreatitis brought on, they assumed, by a gallstone blocking the biliary system.

After a course of intravenous fluids and antibiotics, Patient #34 stabilized and on August 26, 1982, underwent exploratory surgery and cholecystectomy (removal of the gallbladder). Though the gallbladder was as expected filled with multiple stones, the bile ducts seemed free of obstruction. However, the pancreas appeared distinctly abnormal, described in the operative note as:

> markedly enlarged throughout its entire length . . . There was induration
> extending into the base of the small bowel mesentery . . . When we lifted
> up the colon we found that the base of the small bowel mesentery and the
> base of the mesocolon were infiltrated.

The surgeon also discovered a 1 cm tumor in the right lobe of the liver, which on frozen section biopsy was classified as metastatic adenocarcinoma of pancreatic origin. Since the disease was clearly not localized, no attempt was made to resect the abnormal area of the pancreas or the liver lesion.

Postoperatively, further review of the liver biopsy confirmed metastatic adenocarcinoma from a pancreatic primary. Subsequently, a consulting oncologist informed Patient #34 that although chemotherapy might prolong her life slightly, it could not cure her disease. He didn't push any treatment, suggesting instead she get her "affairs in order." In his note he summarized the situation succinctly:

The patient's prognosis is judged to be between 9 and 15 months at most.

Patient #34 was discharged from St. Elizabeth's on August 31, 1982, and then readmitted two weeks later for additional diagnostic tests. A CT scan of the abdomen documented an enlarged head of the pancreas, though a barium enema and intravenous pyelogram (an X-ray study of the kidney) were both unrevealing. Patient #34 was discharged from the hospital on September 17, 1982 again with a diagnosis of pancreatic adenocarcinoma, with no further evaluation or treatment scheduled.

At that point, she decided to seek another opinion at the Mayo Clinic, where in mid-September, 1982 a CT scan confirmed an enlarged pancreas, and blood studies revealed an elevated SGOT, an indication of disordered liver function. At the conclusion of his work-up, the consulting Mayo oncologist wrote in the discharge summary:

I had a long discussion with her regarding treatment for her cancer. At the present time I would favor simply observation since we know of no known treatment that will necessarily prolong her life. Since she is feeling well at the present time I did not feel justified in making her symptomatic from the side effects of chemotherapy.

Patient #34 returned home determined to find another approach to her disease, and in a local health food store, she found an updated copy of Dr. Kelley's book *One Answer to Cancer*. After reading the book, she was convinced this was the approach for her, and in early December 1982, under the direction of a local chiropractor trained by Dr. Kelley and in consultation with Dr. Kelley directly, Patient #34 began her nutritional regimen.

Patient #34 responded very quickly to her protocol. Within six months, she was back to working 18 hours a day, seven days a week, running the family gas station, and today, nearly five years after her diagnosis, she is in excellent health. As she told me when I called her at her filling station, "I just don't have time to die."

Patient #34 never returned to her conventional physicians for follow-up testing, so I have no radiographic evidence of tumor regression, only her long term survival as proof of her response to treatment.

343

PATIENT NAME	ATTENDING PHYSICIAN	ROOM NO	DATE	CASE NO.	ADMIT DATE	DISCHARGE DATE
VAN STRATEN, Arlene	P. E. P███, M.D.	433W				

F(452 - 5/80

SURGEON: Dr. P███

ASSISTANT: Dr. B███████/Dr. Q█████

DATE OF SURGERY: 8/26/82

PRE-OPERATIVE DIAGNOSIS: Biliary tract disease with acute pancreatitis.

POST-OPERATIVE DIAGNOSIS: Cholelithiasis, acute pancreatitis, carcinoma of the pancreas, metastatic to the liver.

After the patient was suitably anesthetized with general endotracheal anesthesia by Merle M█████, the abdomen was prepped with Betadine and water and draped in a sterile fashion. A long right subcostal incision was made. The patient was extremely obese and difficult to work with surgically. The abdomen was entered and thoroughly explored. The stomach and proximal duodenum were normal. The spleen, both kidneys normal. Uterus, tubes and ovaries were surgically absent. No abnormalities were detected of the large/small intestine. The gallbladder was subacutely inflamed and contained multiple calculi, was not distended. The common duct was normal in caliber. The cystic duct was quite large. The pancreas was markedly enlarged throughout its entire length. There was induration of the entire head, body and tail. There was induration extending into the base of the small bowel mesentery. During the course of the exploration we ran across a small nodule high in the dome of the right lobe of the liver. This was eventually exposed and a portion was excised for biopsy purposes and measured 1 cm. in diameter. It was the only nodule palpable. Frozen section report was adenocarcinoma consistent with pancreatic or biliary tract primary.

The cystic duct was exposed and traced down to its junction with the common duct and cholangiogram needle was inserted. An operative cholangiogram was taken. This showed a normal sized biliary ductal system with no evidence of stones within it and free egress of dye entered the duodenum. The cystic duct was ligated, flushed with the common duct using two silver clips and the gallbladder was removed from the gallbladder bed by sharp dissection after the cystic artery and vein were ligated with clips. Bleeding was controlled with electrocautery.

The pancreas was then re-examined. When we lifted up the colon we found that the base of the small bowel mesentery and the base of the mesocolon were infiltrated. It was impossible to tell whether this was inflammation or tumor. It did suggest inflammation. There was some cloudy colored fluid in that location that was cultured. It almost looked like pancreatic juice. A large Jackson-Pratt drain was placed down to the Morrison's pouch and another Jackson-Pratt drain was placed beneath the mesocolon, both were let out through separate stab wounds in the right flank. All lap sponges were removed. Hemostasis was adequate. There was no evidence of obstruction of the duodenum or near obstruction of the duodenum and therefore, gastroenterostomy was not performed. Wound was closed using running 0 Vicryl in the posterior rectus sheath, running and interrupted sutures of 0 Vicryl in the anterior rectus sheath and midline fascia, 3-0 Vicryl in the subq. tissue and staples in the skin. Sterile dressings were applied to the wound.

cc Dr. B█████

		PHYSICIANS SIGNATURE	REPORT NAME	

CONTINUED ON BACK . . .

ST. ELIZABETH HOSPITAL

VAN STRATEN, Arlene
OP
Page 2

The patient was returned to the recovery room in satisfactory condition.

PEP/bek
T: 8/27/82   P. E. P█████, M.D.
D: 8/26/82

OPERATIVE REPORT

NAME	Van Straten, Arlene D. ▮	**AGE** 46	**LAB NO.** ▮
DOCTOR H▮/B▮/P▮ ROOM ▮	**DATE** 8-26-82	**HOSP. NO.** ▮

PREOPERATIVE DIAGNOSIS   Gallbladder Disease, Pancreatitis

SURGICAL PROCEDURE

POSTOPERATIVE DIAGNOSIS

SPECIMEN   A. Biopsy of Liver
                B. Gallbladder

TISSUES SUBMITTED (ENUMERATE)

GROSS: A. The specimen consists of a slender segment of tan tissue
8 mm. in greatest dimension. Frozen Section Diagnosis: Metastatic
Adenocarcinoma.
          B. The specimen is a gallbladder measuring 9 by 3.5 cm.
The serosal surface is not unusual. On section the lumen contains thin
green bile and multiple yellowish tan calculi, the largest of which is
8 mm. in greatest dimension. The mucosa of the gallbladder is trabeculated.
The wall measures 2 to 3 mm. in thickness.
(DCM/kg)

MICROSCOPIC: A. Sections of the liver biopsy reveal a small amount
of relatively intact normal liver along one margin. Most of the specimen
is composed of tumor which in turn is composed of irregular ductal structures
lined by columnar to cuboidal cells.
          Biliary tract or pancreas is suggested as a possible primary.
          B. Sections of gallbladder show, in some areas, a flattened
mucosa but in most areas the mucosa is eroded. The wall is considerably
thickened by relatively dense connective tissue.

DIAGNOSIS: A. Liver Biopsy--Metastatic Adenocarcinoma
              B. Gallbladder--Chronic Cholecystitis with Cholelithiasis
(DCM/kg)

☐ JAMES W. E▮ M.D.   ☐ ARMENIO C▮ M.D.   ☐ BRIAN P. M▮ M.D.

☐ PEARSE M▮ M.D.   ☒ DONALD C. M▮ M.D.   ☐
8-27-82 (D&T)

PAS Code: 1 2 3 4 5 6 7 8 9

SPECIAL ATTENTION DIAGNOSIS

CHART COPY

HISTOPATHOLOGY
(10)

346

PATIENT NAME	ATTENDING PHYSICIAN		DATE	CASE NO	ADMIT DATE	DISCHARGE DATE
VanStratton, Arlene	B.E K_____, M.D. P.E. P___, M.D.	4 W				

Medical oncology is asked to review the case of Arlene VanStratton and advise chemotherapy options.

Diagnostic Impression: 1. Pancreatic adenocarcinoma with liver metastasis.

Recommendations: I have had an initial discussion with the patient, I will return to talk to her husband. I believe the options are chemotherapy versus supportive care only, this will be discussed in detail with both the patient and her husband and we arrive at a final decision in the next week or so. If the patient has agreed to undergo an active treatment program, I would like to have a CAT scan of the abdomen. This will be ordered as appropriate.

History: This 46 year old white female was admitted to the hospital with a diagnosis of cholecystitis with accompanying acute pancreatitis. The patient had had occasional bouts of right upper quadrant pain and had suspected cholecystitis in the past. Prior to this episode she had been perfectly well. She had no change in appetite, no weight loss , was working 14 hours a day. The patient had no hint of back pain, no bone pain or symptoms suggestive of CNS metastasis, in short no symptoms.

This patient's past medical health has been excellent. She had a hysterectomy in the past. She has been hospitalized only for that and for her pregnancies. The patient is on no chronic medications. She is obese but does not have problems of hypertension, diabetes or heart disease.

PE: Shows a pleasant, moderately obese, middle aged white female. Vital signs are stable.

The skin is without evidence of jaundice. Pupils are equal and reactive to light. Mouth and throat are clear. The patient has no cervical or supraclavicular adenopathy. She has no spinal percussion tenderness or CVA tenderness. Breath sounds are equal bilaterally and are normal. Heart tones show normal S4 and @ without murmur or gallop. Abdomen shows a well healed shows a well healed surgical incision. There is no palpable liver or spleen, no other mass is detected. The patient has no calf tenderness, Hoffman's sign or pedal edema. The patient's deep tendon reflexes are 1+ and symmetric. There are no signs on neurologic exam suggesting focal or lateralizing deficit.

Review of the chest x-rays shows it to be within normal limits. On her screening chemistry battery she is seen to have a slightly elevated LDH. Other liver enzymes are within normal limits as are CBC. The patient has had an ultrasound of the gallbladder but has not had a liver and spleen scan or generalized abdominal ultrasound.

Histologic report is seen, documenting liver metastasis with adenocarcinoma. Gallbladder is not seen to be infiltrated with carcinoma. There is no histologic confirmation of cancer in the pancreas per se.

Discussion: The degree of involvement of the pancreas was difficult to determine at the time of surgery. The gland was diffusely indurated, but this could represent inflammation as well as tumor deposits. It appears that only 1 nodule was found in the liver, at least by surgical report, the liver was not grossly or diffusely involved with metastasis. With the liver metastasis it would appear that she has disease outside of a reasonable radiation port. I think chemotherapy would be her best mode of palliative treatment. The response rate for pancreatic carcinoma is low in the order of 20-30%. Combination chemotherapy seems to offer higher response than single agent, so this is what I would recommend. The patient's prognosis is judged to be between 9 and 15 months at most. If she is a responder to chemotherapy, these figures would be greater.

B.E. K_____, M.D.	< PHYSICIANS SIGNATURE	REPORT NAME >	Consultation
BEK/ebb			

ST. ELIZABETH HOSPITAL

347

Copy to Dr. B███.

SUMMARY: Mrs. VanStraten was initially admitted to the hospital because of severe abdominal pain and vomiting. The initial impression was that she had acute pancreatitis because an elevated amylase was detected on the examination in the emergency room. She had the past history of multiple attacks of upper abdominal pain that were consistent with gallbladder disease. She has been markedly overweight for a long period of time. Her appetite and energy have been normal.

On physical examination she was a markedly obese lady who did not appear to be acutely ill. Her pulse was 78 and regular. Skin was warm and dry and abdomen obese and generally soft. There was some tenderness in the epigastrium but no involuntary guarding, rebound or masses.

Laboratory data showed the serum amylase to be markedly elevated and white blood cell count was elevated with marked left shift. The remainder of the studies were within normal limits.

Hospital course: The patient was treated conservatively with intravenous fluids and antibiotics. She was seen in consultation with Dr. P███. An ultrasound of the gallbladder showed multiple biliary calculi. The patient's pain improved slowly and steadily, her amylase returned to normal and she was gradually advanced to a bland diet. When she seemed to be clinically well, she underwent elective cholecystectomy on the 26th of August. During the course of that operation, she was found to have a nodule in the right lobe of the liver that was 1 cm in diameter, biopsy of which showed it to be an adenocarcinoma consistent with pancreatic or biliary primary. The only other abnormality found on abdominal examination then were multiple calculi within the gallbladder and diffusely enlarged, irregular pancreas. There was a lot of inflammation of the pancreas and it was impossible to tell whether the inflammatory mass harbored a tumor or not. It was my suspicion that it did. Her postoperative convalescence was quite uncomplicated. She was gradually advanced to a 1,000 calorie bland diet, her wound healed primarily and she was eventually discharged home to be followed as an outpatient. Prior to her discharge, she was seen in consultation by Dr. Brian K███ regarding chemotherapy and the radiotherapy department was consulted regarding cobalt radiotherapy. It was felt that cobalt radiotherapy played no part in her future treatment. The recommendations from Dr. K███ were that chemotherapy would not be indicated until the patient became symptomatic. It was the impression of all the physicians taking care of Mrs. VanStraten that she should have a CT scan of the pancreas once the inflammation of the pancreas had a chance to subside, that is, several weeks after her discharge from the hospital. She requested a second opinion from the Mayo Clinic and arrangements will be made for that second opinion at the Oncology Department at that institution.

FINAL DIAGNOSIS:
    1. Symptomatic cholelithiasis.
    2. Acute pancreatitis.
    3. Probable carcinoma of the pancreas with a single metastasis to the right lobe of the liver.

OPERATION:
    1. Exploratory laparotomy.
    2. Cholecystectomy.
    3. Operative cholangiogram.
    4. Biopsy of a nodule on the right lobe of the liver.

PEP:kav
D&T: 9/15/82   cc: 3

P. E. P███ M.D.	███	< PHYSICIANS SIGNATURE	REPORT NAME >	DISCHARGE SUMMARY

ST. ELIZABETH HOSPITAL

348

PATIENT NAME	ATTENDING PHYSICIAN		DATE	CASE NO		
VAN STRATEN, Arlene	J. G. B█████, M.D.					

PRIMARY DIAGNOSIS: Carcinoma of the pancreas.

SUMMARY: The patient was admitted for diagnostic evaluation for sources
other than pancreas for her liver carcinoma metastasis. Prior to this
admission the patient underwent laparotomy and cholecystectomy. Liver
biopsy at that time revealed an adenocarcinoma. Also, physical findings
revealed an enlarged head of the pancreas. Impression at that time
was that the patient had carcinoma of the head of the pancreas with
metastasis to the liver. The purpose of this admission was to exclude
any other sources for metastatic carcinoma to the liver. The patient
was discharged after studies were completed. It was this patient's
intention was to seek another opinion from the Mayo Clinic after discharge.

JGB/bek
T: 11/02/82
D: 10/31/82

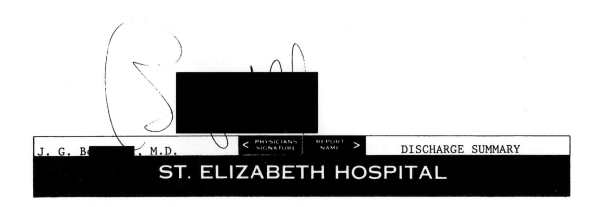

J. G. B█████, M.D.	< PHYSICIANS SIGNATURE	REPORT NAME >	DISCHARGE SUMMARY

ST. ELIZABETH HOSPITAL

September 24, 1982

████████

Phillip P███, M.D.
██████████████

Dear Doctor P██:

Thank you for referring Mrs. Arlene VanStraten to the Mayo Clinic for evaluation for her metastatic carcinoma. As you are familiar with her past history, I will not go into detail with it.

On physical examination she was obese and had a healing abdominal scar and the remainder of her physical examination was not remarkable. Chest x-ray was normal. Her hemoglobin was 12.7, leukocyte count 4,500 and platelet count 252,000. Serum chemistries revealed a slightly elevated SGOT of 44 (upper normal 31). Her blood sugar was 116 with the upper normal being 100. A CT scan was done of the abdomen and it showed the body of the pancreas to be somewhat larger than usual and its margins were ill-defined. These findings were unchanged from the examination done at home. Presently it was felt that this was more suggestive of pancreatitis, however, we could not rule out malignancy.

I had a long discussion with her regarding treatment for her cancer. At the present time I would favor simply observation since we know of no known treatment that will necessarily prolong her life. Since she is feeling well at the present time I did not feel justified in making her symptomatic from the side effects of chemotherapy. I have told her, however, that should she begin having complications from her cancer that we would begin chemotherapy then in the hopes of making her feel better. I believe she understands this rationale after much discussion.

We have set up a return appointment for her in two months and we will be looking forward to seeing her then. Should there be a problem before then or if I can be of any help, please let me know.

Sincerely yours,

Joseph R███, M.D.

JR:jed

Patient #35

Patient #35 is a 64-year-old man from Minnesota with a history of metastatic islet cell carcinoma of the pancreas.

During the summer of 1980, Patient #35 noticed a swelling in his abdomen, associated with the onset of fatigue and intermittent fevers. In late July 1980, Patient #35 consulted his family doctor, who, suspecting gallbladder disease, admitted Patient #35 to District One Hospital in Faribault, Minnesota for further evaluation. On physical exam, his physician noted a tender, palpable mass below the right rib cage, and X-ray studies revealed a significantly enlarged liver.

Several days later, at exploratory surgery Patient #35 was found to have an infected gallbladder. The surgeon drained one large abscess, but because of the extensive inflammation, decided to forgo removal of the gallbladder itself. In addition, a biopsy of a small tumor discovered along the liver edge revealed only a benign hamartoma.

Postoperatively, Patient #35 completed a course of intravenous antibiotic therapy before his discharge from the hospital on August 9, 1980, with plans to return for cholecystectomy (removal of his gallbladder) when the abdominal infection cleared completely. The slides of the liver biopsy were then sent to the Mayo Clinic for further study, where the tumor was once again classified as a benign lesion, specifically a hepatic adenoma.

Patient #35 was then re-admitted to District One Hospital in mid-January 1981 for the planned gallbladder surgery. During the procedure, the surgeon discovered multiple new tumors in both lobes of the liver, as described in the records:

> At the time of his surgery the liver was found to be virtually studded with tumors which were one to two, up to three centimeters in size, round, nodular in shape and covering the anterior surface, the inferior surface, and all the way over into the left lobe of the liver.

A biopsy of a liver lesion this time indicated not a benign process but metastatic islet cell carcinoma of the pancreas. Subsequent blood studies showed no evidence of the hormones normally associated with islet cell tumors such as insulin—an important finding, since non-functional pancreatic endocrine malignancies tend to be quite aggressive.

The biopsy slides were sent for review to the Mayo Clinic, where a consulting pathologist confirmed the diagnosis of metastatic islet cell carcinoma. Then in late January 1981, Patient #35 was referred for treatment to the Oncology Department at Mt. Sinai Hospital in Minneapolis. There he was deemed eligible for an experimental chemotherapy protocol consisting of the drugs streptozotocin and 5-fluorouracil, as part of the Eastern Oncology Group Study of islet cell carcinoma.

Before beginning treatment, Patient #35 was evaluated to document the extent of disease. At that time, a CT scan of the abdomen revealed, as described in the radiology report, "multiple intrahepatic metastases present throughout both lobes of the liver."

Patient #35 completed his first round of chemotherapy in February 1981. Despite treatment, his liver, along with his abdomen, continued to enlarge, and in June 1981, after his third course of drugs, a CT scan indicated further worsening of his disease. The official radiology report, dated June 18, 1981, describes:

> multiple metastases in the bed of the liver that seemed to have increased
> in number and slightly in size since the last examination of Jan. 27, 1981.

Since his cancer appeared resistant to the aggressive chemotherapy, Patient #35 decided to investigate unconventional approaches to cancer, including the Kelley program. When admitted to Mt. Sinai for a fourth round of chemotherapy, Patient #35 raised the subject of nutritional therapy with his oncologist, who apparently became enraged. Patient #35 explained to me:

> He threw a temper tantrum, and told me to leave the hospital which by
> that time I was really quite happy to do. And that was the end of my
> experience with chemotherapy.

In the official discharge summary, the attending oncologist makes no mention of his anger, although he does discuss Patient #35's decision to pursue an unconventional option. The doctor wrote:

> He [Patient #35] is talking about nonorthodox approaches to this disease. In attempts to educate him more, a full discussion was undertaken about these problems, and the hoax of the unconventional medications at this time.

Nonetheless, Patient #35 began the full Kelley program in late June 1981, never again contacting his oncologist and pursuing no further standard therapy of any kind. Subsequently, he did well, with apparent regression of his once extensive disease. In a note dated January 13, 1984, after Patient #35 had followed his nutritional regimen some two and a half years, his primary physician documented the improvement:

> Our office was contacted by the local cancer society regarding the status of the patient's health. He continues to function on his farm and is on a partial disability basis as far as working. His cancer remains in remission and he has a primary diagnosis of islet cell carcinoma of the pancreas with multiple metastatic lesions in the liver.

Patient #35 followed his nutritional regimen for five years during which time he did extremely well. But thereafter he became careless, gradually dropping off therapy, thinking himself cured. When last contacted in late spring of 1987, six years after his original diagnosis, he intended to resume his nutritional regimen.

Although the prognosis for islet cell carcinoma is somewhat better than that for tumors of the exocrine pancreas, few patients with metastatic disease survive five years. The Eastern Cooperative Oncology Group Study, in which Patient #35 briefly participated, followed 40 patients with the disease receiving streptozotocin and 5-fluorouracil. The investigators report a median survival for this group of only 26 months, compared to 16.5 months for patients receiving streptozotocin alone.[1]

In summary, Patient #35 was diagnosed with widely metastatic islet cell carcinoma that failed to respond to a course of experimental chemotherapy. In fact, he worsened considerably on the treatment. However, while Patient #35 pursued only the Kelley program, his cancer regressed, apparently completely.

REFERENCE

1. Moertel, CG, et al. "Streptozotocin Alone Compared With Streptozotocin Plus Fluorouracil in the Treatment of Advanced Islet-Cell Carcinoma." *New England Journal of Medicine* 1980; 303:1189–1194.

DISTRICT ONE HOSPITAL
FARIBAULT, MINNESOTA

DISCHARGE SUMMARY
Patient's Name: Patient #35
Hospital Number:

ADMISSION: 1-18-81
DISCHARGE: 1-24-81

The patient is a 58 year old white male who is admitted to the hospital for a cholecystectomy. The patient had a past history of having an empyema of the gallbladder
drained earlier last summer and at that time was found to have a tumor in the liver.
The operating surgeon biopsied this and the consense of the Mayo Clinic pathologist
and our pathologist was that this was a hamartoma. The patient was therefore electively
scheduled to come in now for cholecystectomy and the remainder of the hamartoma.

His physical examination was otherwise unremarkable and the patient was basically
feeling well except for tiredness. He came into the hospital and underwent cholecystectomy. At the time of his surgery the liver was found to be virtually studded
with tumors which were one to two, up to three centimeters in size, round, nodular
in shape and covering the anterior surface, the inferior surface, and all the way
over into the left lobe of the liver. The gallbladder was removed with no difficulty.
Two of the tumors were biopsied separately and this tissue was submitted to pathology.
The patient's pathology report showed that the tumor cells were metastatic islet cell
carcinoma in the liver. The remainder of the pathology report showed chronic cholecystitis and cholelithiasis. The patient really tolerated the procedure very well
and had no postoperative or post anesthetic complications. He was up and about and
was ambulatory at the time of discharge from the hospital. His surgical drains
had been removed. The sutures are probably not ready for removal until about Tuesday
of next week.

LABORATORY DATA: His laboratory data while in the hospital revealed an elevation of
his glucose but this was with IV running. His serum sodium was a bit low at 133.
He has had blood drawn to test for serum gastrin and serum insulin levels, but these
are not available at the time of discharge from the hospital. They should be back,
however, shortly. His white count and differential were normal with a white count of
8,000 and a hemoglobin of 14.8 grams. He is blood group A Rh positive. His serum
gastrin and serum insulin levels were sent to Mayo on the 23rd. Pathology report was
metastatic islet cell carcinoma of the liver and gallbladder showing chronic cholecystitis and cholelithiasis. The operative cholangiogram showed free flow of the
contrast into the duodenum without evidence of filling defect. The common duct is
larger than average, although it is not clear from this study why the common duct is
large. The chest x-ray revealed calcification and mild tortuosity of the aorta. The
chest is otherwise negative.

The patient is going to be discharged to home for two days and he is then going to
Mount Sinai Hospital on Monday of this week to see oncologist, Doctor S   in
consultation for institution of chemo therapy for his malignancy. The patient has been
given a full explanation of the fact that he does have a
malignancy in the liver which is extensive and that it is
felt to be extensive and that it is felt to be firm
metastasis from the pancreas. He also understands that
chemo therapy is planned for this.

BWGsb

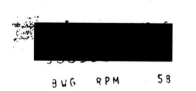

BWG   RPM   58

continued.

354

DISCHARGE MEDICATIONS: None

DISCHARGE DIET: As tolerated.   Activity as tolerated with no strenuous lifting.

DISPOSITION: The patient is to be referred to Doctor S███████ on Monday for oncology consultation as noted.

DISCHARGE DIAGNOSIS:
    1. Chronic cholecystitis and cholelithiasis.
    2. Islet cell carcinoma of the liver, metastatic, extensive.

SURGERY:
    1. Cholecystectomy.
    2. Biopsy of the liver tumors.

BWGsb
D: 1-24-81
T: 1-24-81

B. W. G██████, M.D.

cc Dr. S█████

TISSUE REPORT

Clinical Diagnosis:

Macroscopic Examination:

The specimen is submitted in four portions. The first is submitted
as liver biopsy of a large liver nodule which on previous biopsy
appeared to be adenoma (080-808). This on frozen section shows
tumor almost totally replacing the liver fragment which appears
to most closely resemble primary liver cell carcinoma. Section will
be labeled "A". The second nodule from the liver shows a similar patte
and will be labeled "B". The second is submitted as gallbladder and
consists of a partially opened gallbladder measuring 9 x 2.5 cm.
with a somewhat thickened appearing wall. The gallbladder was
previously drained with calculi present. The gallbladder contains
a small amount of inspissated bile and two 5 mm. diameter spherical
dark green calculi. The mucosa appears somewhat trabeculated.

Microscopic Examination:
Sections of the gallbladder will be labeled "C". The last portion
of the specimen consists of a 16 x 1 cm. fragment of grossly normal
appearing skin and soft tissue submitted as scar tissue.

D: 1-19-81
T: 1-20-81

Pathologic Diagnosis:

The liver tissue is almost totally replaced by tumor which shows
uniform appearing smaller cells showing no prominent nucleoli,
slightly eosinophilic cytoplasm with evidence of ribboning in some
areas. Some hemorrhage into the tumor is present and slight
necrosis is seen. The slides were reviewed again at Mayo Clinic
and it is the consensus that this represents an Islet cell carcinoma.
It is suggested that serum gastrin and insulin studies be performed
to ascertain function of the tumor. T

The gallbladder shows partially denuded mucosa with moderate
fibrosis of the wall.

Remarks:
AGNOSIS: Metastatic islet cell carcinoma - liver
Chronic cholecystitis with lithiasis
Scar tissue

D & T: 1-21-81

BWG   RPM   53

_____ M.D.
SIGNATURE OF PATHOLOGIST
Dean T. C██████, M.D./mc

CHART COPY

Name
Patient #35
Case No.
Dr.   DR S   MN CHA

Address Y28
Maiden Name
Age 58 Exom. Date 1-27 Wid. Div.

Room/Bed No.   Birth Date
Bd. Pt. Mt. Sinai room # 359
Request Date

CLINICAL DATA:
Ca Liver
tumor
isolate cell cancer

X-RAY REQUESTED:
CT of Abd & Pelvis

X-RAY FILE NO. NEW 220-223

RADIOGRAPHIC REPORT

CT SCAN OF THE ABDOMEN AND PELVIS WITHOUT AND WITH ORAL
CONTRAST AND INTRAVENOUS CONTRAST ENHANCEMENT: There are
multiple intrahepatic metastases present throughout both
lobes of the liver. No definite splenic metastases seen.
There is bilateral renal function. Cuts through the
pelvis are unremarkable.
IMPRESSION: Multiple intrahepatic metastases, etiology
not clear from scan.

1-27-81   J.S. M████, JR., M.D./pb

DATE_____

RADIOLOGIST_____
ST. JOSEPH'S — ST. PAUL, MINN

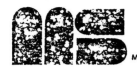

MOUNT SINAI HOSPITAL

2215 PARK AVENUE,

MINNEAPOLIS, MINNESOTA 55404

Dr. R.P. M██████
██████████████
Faribault, 55021

Dr. B. S██████████
Dr. Bruce G██████████
Faribault   55021

Date: ██████████

Discharged 2-8-81

REASON FOR ADMISSION: Chemotherapy for a Islet cell tumor
which had metastasized to the liver.   The reason chemotherapy was given now
was the rapid progression of this process.

Physical examination on admission essentially unremarkable.

HOSPITAL COURSE: The patient underwent chemotherapy
with Streptozotocin day one through day five, 5-FU day one through day five
and this will be repeated again in 6 weeks from now.

He should have a set of liver functions and kidney functions as well as
CBC, platelet count in about 2-3 weeks in Dr. G██████'s office.

The patient tolerated chemotherapy OK even though he had so me nausea and
some vomiting.

Hemoglobin 12.6 on admission, 13.8 on discharge, white count was 10,600,
8,200 respectively, platlet count 630,000, 559,000, M-12 was completely
normal.   Repeat BUN and creatinine was OK.   Electrolytes were alright.
Sugar was normal.

Chest x-ray was normal.   Cardiogram was OK.

FINAL DIAGNOSIS:

          1. Islet cell carcinoma of the pancreas, non-functioning
             tumor with metastases to liver.

Discharged improved, prognosis is guarded.

Discharged on a regular diet.   He should be having a set of liver function,
kidney function, SMA-12 and some lytes and CBC and platelet count in about
3 weeks in Dr. G██████'s office.

We will try and see him again when I come down to Faribault and will readmit
him again in 6 weeks from start of chemotherapy, namely, around 3-16-81 for
a repeat cycle if his laboratory work is OK.

                              B. S██████ M.D.

al
N7
2-9-81

MMC-102-69
00211-3 Rev. 12/69

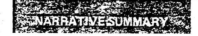

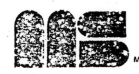

MOUNT SINAI HOSPITAL

2215 PARK AVENUE,

MINNEAPOLIS, MINNESOTA 55404

Date:

Discharged 3-27-81

HISTORY OF PRESENT ILLNESS: This is the 3rd Mount Sinai hospital
admission for this 58 year old patient, farmer from Faribault, Minn.
The patient was admitted 3-22-81.   The patient was admitted for chemotherapy
for islet cell tumor of the pancreas which had metastasized to the liver.
It was the second course of chemotherapy. January, 1981 while undergoing
cholecystectomy the patient was noted to have a liver studded with tumor.
Biopsy indicated that the tumor was islet cell cancer of the pancreas.   It
has been characterized as non-functioning type and the patient has no other
areas of metastasis.   He has been randomized on ECOG protocol drawing
the arm of Streptozotocin and 5-FU 5 days out of every 5-6 weeks.   The
first course of chemotherapy was in 2-1981.   He has completed his second
course of chemotherapy.   He tolerated the treatment well and is anxious
to go home.

The hospital course was unremarkable. He received 5 treatments of
Streptozotocin 1200 mgs. and 5-FU 900 mgs. per day for 5 days.   The
patient experienced some nausea and vomiting especially in the period
just following chemotherapy.   He found some relief with Compazine.

CBC, electrolytes and M-12 essentially normal, slight thrombocytosis
of 415,000.   Normal urine, urine culture, normal chest x-ray.
Urine, CBC, BUN, glucose were repeated and found to be normal, the 2nd hospita
day.   24 hour urine creatinine clearance collected and the results are
pending.

DISCHARGE DIAGNOSIS:

      1. Pancreatic islet cell tumor with metastases
      to the liver.

No medications.

The patient is to be seen in Faribault by Dr. S███ in 3 weeks with
CBC, lytes, BUN and glucose.   The patient will be returning to Mount Sinai
in 6 weeks for further course of chemotherapy.

B. S█████ M.D.

al
3-30-81
N7

MMC-102-69
00211-3 Rev. 12/63

dictated by Dr. J. Weber

359

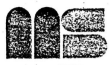

MOUNT SINAI HOSPITAL

2215 PARK AVENUE,

MINNEAPOLIS, MINNESOTA 55404

SEWELL S. G▓▓▓ M.D. & ASSOCIATES

RADIOLOGICAL CONSULTATION

CT SCAN OF ABDOMEN 6-18-81 Multiple transverse cuts were taken through the liver and the bed of the pancreas with oral contrast and both with and without intravenous contrast. Study shows multiple metastases in the bed of the liver that seemed to have increased in number and slightly in size since the last examination of Jan. 27, 1981. The pancreas is well visualized and appears to be normal. No other metastases are seen.

IMPRESSION: Slight progression of metastatic disease of the liver. IW/smc

360

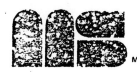

MOUNT SINAI HOSPITAL

2215 PARK AVENUE,

MINNEAPOLIS, MINNESOTA 55404

Dr. Neil H███████

Date: ADM: 6/28/81
DIS: 7/3/81

Fifty-nine-year-old man with an islet cell carcinoma of the pancreas, with liver metastases. He was admitted to Mount Sinai Hospital for protocol chemical therapy, with Streppozotozin and 5-Fluorouracil. Patient tolerated his chemical therapy well, with some minimal nausea.

LABORATORY STUDIES show a white blood count on admission of 9.4 and discharge 13.5. Hemoglobin is 15.3 on admission, discharge 17.5. UA is negative, 12-channel screening test is essentially normal, sodium and potassium are normal. Chest x-ray shows no evidence of metastatic disease, and no active disease.

Patient has some difficulty in accepting, I think, the chemical therapy of his disease at this time. He is talking about nonorthodox approaches to this disease, with Laetrile and other vitamin therapy. In attempts to educate him more, a full discussion was undertaken about these problems, and the hoax of the unconventional medications at this time. He is also concerned about his health insurance, and an attempt was made through Social Service to see if that could be straightened out with him. Basically, there were no problems with the hospitalization. He is going to be discharged. Follow-up will be with my associate, Dr. S███████.

DIAGNOSTIC IMPRESSION: Carcinoma of the pancreas, with liver metastases.

NEIL H███████, M.D.

mjk 7/7/81
PL

361

Date	
4-9-82 Continued	DX: GI bleeding and islet cell carcinoma of the pancreas with widespread metastasis to the liver. BWG:al
11-11-83	Refilled Percodan. #40. . BWG/dlh
12-7-83	Refilled Percodan #40 BWG/dms
1-13-84	Our office was contacted by the local cancer society regarding the status of the patient's health. He continues to function on his farm and is on a partial disability basis as far as working. His cancer remains in remission and he has a primary diagnosis of islet cell carcinoma of the pancreas with multiple metastatic lesions in the liver. . BWG:al

362

Patient #36

Patient #36 is a 59-year-old man from Vermont alive nine years since his diagnosis of metastatic pancreatic carcinoma.

In late 1977, Patient #36 experienced persistent fatigue and chronic abdominal pain, usually more severe after meals, associated with passage of frequent black, watery stools. When his symptoms worsened, in February 1978 Patient #36 was evaluated as an outpatient at St. Barnabas Hospital in the Bronx, New York. After a liver scan and abdominal ultrasound both revealed a mass in the left lobe of the liver believed consistent with malignant disease, Patient #36 was admitted to St. Barnabas on March 13, 1978. Two days later, during exploratory surgery a frozen section biopsy of a mass in the tail of the pancreas confirmed adenocarcinoma. At that point, the surgeon resected as much of the pancreatic tumor as possible, but only biopsied the liver.

On subsequent evaluation, the pancreatic tissue was thought consistent with islet cell carcinoma, with metastases evident in two adjacent lymph nodes. However, the liver lesion was classified as a benign hemangioma.

At that point, Patient #36's doctors informed him the lymph node involvement portended a very poor prognosis, suggesting he might live six months and recommending no further treatment. After his discharge from the hospital on March 21, 1978, Patient #36 subsequently pursued his follow-up care in his home state of Vermont, at the Vermont Regional Cancer Center. There, doctors agreed with the dismal prognosis, but offered a course of immunotherapy with the tuberculosis vaccine BCG, though no evidence supports this approach in patients diagnosed with pancreatic cancer.

After completing a series of BCG inoculations, Patient #36 then decided to investigate unorthodox approaches to cancer, learned of Dr. Kelley, and began the nutritional program in April 1977. He subsequently continued the full protocol for over a year before tapering to a modified regimen which he still follows. Today, nine years after surgery, Patient #36 is in excellent health with no sign of disease.

Since there was some confusion about the precise histological diagnosis, Dr. Good, with me watching, examined all biopsy and surgical slides. Dr. Good, who was Head of the Department of Pathology at the University of Minnesota before assuming the Directorship of Sloan-Kettering, found the cancer consistent with a very primitive, aggressive adenocarcinoma. In some of the specimens, the malignancy does mimic a variety of cell types including endocrine, an indication, he believed, of a particularly virulent tumor.

Obviously, Patient #36's prolonged survival is indeed an unusual outcome for such a deadly disease.

ST. BARNABAS HOSPITAL

BRONX, N. Y. 10457

FINAL SUMMARY

Patient's Name: Patient #36

Hospital Number: ███████

Admitted: **3/13/78**

Discharged: **3/21/78**

This 50-year old male was readmitted to St. Barnabas Hospital because of a liver scan which had been repeated several times in this institution and in other institutions as well as echo and sonogram all showing the presence of a mass in the left lobe of the liver. Malignancy could not be ruled out. Exploratory laparotomy and possible hepatectomy were planned.

Exploratory laparotomy was done. Chest x-ray, EKG and urinalysis were within normal limits. Liver scan was done. Exploratory laparotomy showed a hemangioma in the liver, section sent for biopsy. There was also a tumor in the tail of the pancreas. There was also swelling of the lymph nodes.

Partial pancreatectomy was performed and a specimen was sent for histology. This showed the presence of adenocarcinoma. At the same time a lipoma of the right forearm was removed. The postoperative course was completely uneventful. The patient was discharged after ten days without any complications.

FINAL DIAGNOSES:
1. Adenocarcinoma of the pancreas   157.9
2. Lipoma of the right arm   214.9

dictated by _____
                T. H█████, M.D., Attending

D: 3/31/78
T: 4/3/78wwt

365

ST. BARNABAS HOSPITAL
BRONX, N. Y.

REPORT OF OPERATION

Family Name	First Name	Middle Name	Age	Date	Room No.	Hosp. No.
Patient #36 ▓▓▓			50	3/15/78		▓▓▓

SURGEON: Dr. H▓▓▓   ASSISTANTS:

OPERATION: Resection of tail of pancreas, removal of lymph node; liver biopsy; removal of the lipoma of the right forearm.

PREOPERATIVE DIAGNOSIS: tumor of the liver   ANESTHETIST:

POSTOPERATIVE DIAGNOSIS:

hemangioma of the liver; lipoma of the right forearm; cancer of the tail of the pancreas, adenocarcinoma.

Under general anesthesia the patient was placed on the operating table in the supine position. The entire abdomen was prepped with ioprep and draped properly.

A midline incision was made from the xiphoid to 2" below the umbilicus. This was made on the left side, and the linea was opened. The Balfour retractor was placed, and the entire abdomen was explored. There were noted the hemangioma in the right lobe which was cavernous, and a liver biopsy was taken placing the 4-0 chromic catgut stitches surrounding the hemangioma.

An elliptical incision was made, and a good biopsy was obtained. The cut edge was approximated with #4-0 chromic catgut for the hemostasis. After the biopsy was taken, and the exploration was continued there was a mass in the tail of the pancreas and also the lymph nodes were swollen. These were removed by ligating the splenic artery and veins, and part of the pancreatic ducts. One surface of the pancreatic tissue was removed with the pancreatic tumor which was found out to be adenocarcinoma. Two Penrose drains were placed in the abdomen, which were drained through a separate incision through a stab wound.

The abdominal wall was closed in three layers using #1 chromic catgut in the posterior fascia and the peritoneum, and the anterior fascia was closed with #1 chromic catgut interrupted stitches. The skin was closed with #00 silk interrupted stitches. The patient left the O.R. A longitudinal incision was made in the right forearm, and two lipomas were removed which were sent out for histology. The skin was closed with #00 silk interrupted stitches. The patient left the O.R. in good condition. No blood transfusions were given.

D: 3/16/78
T: 3/17/78wwt

_____ M.D.
Signature of Surgeon

dictated by Dr. H▓▓▓, Attending

366

Department of Laboratories

Gerald Ka██████ M.D., Director

PATIENT: Patient #36
AGE: 5(\
SEX: M
ROOM: 1└8 A

SURGICAL # **78-370**
DATE OF OPERATION: **3/15/78**
HOSPITAL # ██████████████
ATTENDING PHYSICIAN: **Dr. H.**

CLINICAL HISTORY:

PRE-OPERATIVE DIAGNOSIS: **Hepatoma**

POST-OPERATIVE DIAGNOSIS: **Same**

SPECIMEN:
**A. Biopsy of liver, ? Hemangioma
B. Peripancreatic lymph node
C. Pancreatic tumor
D. Lipoma of anterior abdominal wall
E. Lipoma of right arm**

GROSS DESCRIPTION:

B. D██████, M.D.:

A. The specimen received fresh for frozen section consists of a
    minute piece of pink-white, soft tissue measuring 0.4 cm. in
    greatest dimension. The entire specimen is submitted following
    frozen section.

B. The specimen received fresh for frozen section consists of a
    pink, nodular mass measuring 1.5 cm. in diameter. On cut
    section it is partially pale-yellow and granular. The entire
    specimen is submitted, following frozen section.

C. The specimen received fresh consists of a segment of lobulated,
    pink-white pancreatic tissue measuring 4.5 x 3.0 x 2.0 cm. At
    one edge of this pancreatic tissue there is a hard, pale-brown,
    nodular mass with ill-delineated margins measuring 1.5 cm. in
    diameter. On cut surface it is glistening and somewhat lobulated.
    The adjacent pancreatic tissue is unremarkable. Adherent to this
    segment of pancreas with hemorrhagic, fibrous tissue, is a round,
    nodular mass measuring 3.0 cm. in diameter. On cut section
    it is pale-brown and granular and about half of this nodule is
    occupied by a pale-yellow, granular tissue. Representative
    sections are submitted.

D. The specimen received in formalin consists of a fairly-delineated,
    lobulated, pink-yellow adipose tissue mass measuring 3.0 cm. in
    greatest dimension. Its surfaces are mostly covered with a thin,
    fibrous capsule. On cut section grossly it is unremarkable.
    Representative section is submitted.

E. The specimen received in formalin consists of two flattened, firm,
    pink-white, nodular masses measuring 3.0 and 2.5 cm. in greatest

-continued-

367

Patient #36

SURGICAL #78-370

Dr. H.

- CONTINUED -

GROSS DESCRIPTION: (cont'd)

E.(cont'd)

dimension. Their surfaces are covered with a thin, fibrous capsule and on cut section they are pink-yellow and lobulated. Representative sections are submitted.

MICROSCOPIC: Sections on file

FROZEN SECTION DIAGNOSIS: A. BENIGN
B. METASTATIC ADENOCARCINOMA, LYMPH NODE

DIAGNOSIS: A. HEMANGIOMA, BIOPSY OF LIVER
B,C.=SEGMENT OF PANCREAS, SAID TO BE TAIL
=ISLET CELL CARCINOMA WITH METASTASIS TO PERIPANCREATIC LYMPH NODES, TWO
D. LIPOMA, ANTERIOR ABDOMINAL WALL
E. FIBROLIPOMAS, TWO, RIGHT FOREARM

Code #6

B D   M D
Bhakti D   , M.D.
Associate Pathologist

BD:lg,
ms

368

Patient #37

Patient #37 is a 62-year-old man from Missouri who has survived nearly ten years since his diagnosis of inoperable pancreatic carcinoma and carcinoid.

In 1975, Patient #37 developed mild adult onset diabetes, treated effectively only with oral medication. Thereafter he did well until early 1977, when he first experienced chronic upper abdominal pain that worsened particularly after meals of fried or fatty foods. Patient #37's family physician, initially suspecting gallstones, ordered an oral cholecystogram, but this dye study of the gallbladder was unrevealing.

In the spring of 1977, after a period of declining appetite and weight loss, Patient #37 became acutely jaundiced. At that point, he was admitted to Christian Hospital Northeast in St. Louis on June 22, 1977 for further evaluation of what was thought to be an obstructed biliary system.

A series of tests including a repeat cholecystogram, an upper GI series, an ultrasound study of the abdomen, a liver-spleen scan, and a barium enema were all clear. But when his symptoms, including his jaundice, worsened, Patient #37 underwent exploratory surgery on June 30, 1977 during which time a large inoperable pancreatic tumor, with metastases to the small intestine, was evident. The surgeon performed a palliative biliary bypass procedure to circumvent the area of obstruction, but made no attempt to resect the pancreatic tumor itself.

The medical records summarize the findings:

> There was a large mass in the head of the pancreas measuring some 5 by 3 cm. There were several nodes present in the distal portion of the porta hepatis [area of the liver adjacent to the gallbladder]. Abdominal exploration revealed the two areas of metastasis present in the small bowel mesentery . . . Biopsy of this vicinity was obtained . . . Pathologic report returned metastatic adenocarcinoma.

The formal diagnosis, as it appears on the operative note reads:

> Carcinoma of the pancreas—unresectable, incurable.

After further study, the lesion resected from the wall of the small intestine was thought to be more consistent with carcinoid than adenocarcinoma, although

Patient #37 had never reported the symptoms of flushing, diarrhea and sweating usually associated with this particular malignancy. The patient reported to me that his doctors thought he might have two distinct cancers, pancreatic adeno-carcinoma and carcinoid.

Postoperatively, both chemotherapy and radiation were strongly recommended, but Patient #37's physicians informed him the treatment most likely would offer little benefit. Consequently, he decided to refuse both options, instead choosing to seek out alternative care. After his release from the hospital in July 1977, he traveled to Mexico for a brief course of Laetrile, and then in August 1977 he consulted Dr. Kelley and began the full nutritional program.

Patient #37 responded quickly to his treatment, with significantly improved appetite and weight gain. Within a year, as he told me, he felt better than at any other time in his life, and a follow-up CT scan confirmed that the once large pancreatic tumor had completely regressed.

Patient #37 subsequently did well until early 1983, when he developed intermittent cramping abdominal pain associated with anorexia and a gradual 20-pound weight loss.

A CT scan performed in September 1983 was inconclusive, but when his symptoms worsened in early October 1983, Patient #37 was admitted to Christian Hospital Northeast. After a barium enema revealed an incomplete small bowel obstruction, a potentially life-threatening condition, Patient #37 was promptly taken for exploratory surgery.

A mass of scar tissue, apparently forming after the first operation, and a small residual carcinoid tumor were found blocking the small intestine. However, the surgeon could not find the pancreatic mass evident in 1977, as documented in the operative note:

> Peritoneal cavity was entered and explored with the liver, peritoneum, omentum, pancreas all appearing normal.

The obstruction was corrected, and after recovering from surgery, Patient #37 was discharged from the hospital on October 18, 1983. He then resumed the Kelley program and today, ten years after his original diagnosis, Patient #37 follows a maintenance protocol and is in excellent health with no sign of his disease.

I asked Dr. Kelley why he thought the carcinoid tumor had recurred in 1983. In response, Dr. Kelley said that even in compliant patients, sometimes tumors can regrow in areas of scar tissue, where poor circulation provides protection from the circulating enzymes.

In summary, Patient #37 was diagnosed with inoperable metastatic pancreatic cancer, obvious at surgery in 1977. He refused all conventional therapy, choosing to follow only the Kelley program after a brief trial of Laetrile. Eventually, the large pancreatic tumor regressed, as documented by sequential CT scan studies as well as exploratory surgery in 1983.

CHRISTIAN HOSPITAL NORTHWEST
Corporate Offices
11133 Dunn Road, St. Louis, Missouri 63136
314-355-2300

Patient's Name: **Patient #37**　　　　　　　　　Patient No.

Doctor's Name: Robert V. C██████, M.D.　　☐ NE DIV　☐ NW DIV

Type of Report

OPERATIVE REPORT:　　　　　　　　Room 518

Preop Dx:　　Choledocholithiasis

Postop Dx:　　Carcinoma of the pancreas--unresectable, incurable

Operation:　　Exploratory laparotomy with cholecystojejunostomy and biopsy of small
　　　　　　　bowel mesenteric metastatic implants

Findings:

After the patient had undergone adequate endotracheal anesthesia, his anterior abdominal
wall was prepped with Betadine, and he was draped for an abdominal exploration. Right subcostal incision was made with bleeders being controlled by the electrocautery. The rectus
muscle and the lateral muscle groups were transected using cutting current with some of
the larger bleeders being tied with 2-0 silk. The peritoneal cavity was entered and explored. The gallbladder was distended, thin-walled, and did not appear to have stones.
There was a large mass in the head of the pancreas measuring some 5 by 3 cm. There were
several nodes present in the distal portion of the porta hepatis. Abdominal exploration
revealed the two areas of metastasis present in the small bowel mesentery in different
position with marked thickening and foreshortening of the mesentery in this part. Biopsy
of this vicinity was obtained with bleeders being controlled with 3-0 silk suture ligatures.
Pathologic report returned metastatic adenocarcinoma.

The patient's liver was free of disease. There was no evidence of disease elsewhere in
his abdomen other than the previously mentioned places. Due to the patient's preoperative
jaundice and his incurable, unresectable state, a cholecystojejunostomy was performed after
an appropriate length of jejunum had been placed into the right upper quadrant. A posterior row of sutures were used to approximate the wall of the gallbladder and jejunum. After
the posterior row of sutures had been placed, the jejunum itself was opened after it had
been clamped on each side with atraumatic vascular and intestinal clamps. The gallbladder
was then opened and decompressed with aerobic and anaerobic cultures being taken. Interrupted seromucosal sutures of 3-0 chromic catgut were then placed and tied individually
until the anterior row of the anastomosis had been complete. An anterior row of interrupted 3-0 seromuscular silks were then placed. The right upper quadrant was then irrigated copiously with saline. A fashioned sump drain consisting of a multi-holed 18
red catheter placed through a large Penrose drain which also had several holes in it and
was brought out lateral to the incision site, and was directed inferior to the cystic duct
and inferior to the porta hepatis. The drain itself was fixed in place at skin level with
two 2-0 silk sutures. The small bowel was then replaced in orderly fashion after the
biopsy site had been ascertained to be non-bleeding, and it was covered then with omentum.
The linea alba was approximated with an interrupted figure of eight 0 Prolene suture. The
peritoneum and posterior rectus sheath was then closed with a running suture of 0 Prolene.
Further lateral the area was closed with figure of eight interrupted 0 Prolene. The area
was then irrigated well with saline, and the anterior fascia was approximated with interrupted 0 Prolene. Subcutaneous tissue was irrigated well with saline, and the skin edges

Patient's Name: Patient #37   Patient No.

Doctor's Name: Robert V. C████, M.D.   ☐ NE DIV ☐ NW DIV

Type of Report

OPERATIVE REPORT CONTINUED:

Findings.

were approximated with interrupted 3-0 nylon. Estimated blood loss was 100 cc. Sponge counts were correct times two. The termination of the procedure, a sterile dressing was applied to the incision site. The patient was awakened and extubated and transferred to the recovery room having tolerated the procedure well with no complications.

RVC:df
D: 6-30-77
T: 7-2-77

Robert V. C████, M.D.

cc: A. V████, M.D.

373

	Male	Age 58	Date 6/30/77
Doctor A. V___ M. D.	Female		

Source of Tissue
Small bowel mesentery for frozen section

Surgeon's Name DR. C___

Date Reported 6/30/77

FROZEN SECTION:

Undifferentiated tumor. (small bowel mesentery)

JHA

CH 309 R 12/75

GROSS:

The specimen consists of a previously bisected rubbery, yellowish white mass of tissue approximately 1 cm. in greatest dimension. Both pieces are submitted in their entirety.

JHA/aew

MICROSCOPIC:

Masses of uniform cells with round nuclei and eosinophil cytoplasm are seen as well as ribbons and trabeculae having columnar shaped cells of similar description. Argentaffine positive granules are present in cytoplasm in large and small size.

COMMENT: The pattern is that of carcinoid. Islet cell adenoma could not be ruled out in view of the presentation as pancreatic mass. These two entities can not be distinguished microscopically.

DIAGNOSIS: MESENTERY, SMALL BOWEL IMPLANT BIOPSY - CARCINOID TUMOR (SEE ABOVE DESCRIPTION).

LANDY W___, M. D.

LW/aew
D: 7/5/77
T 7/5/77

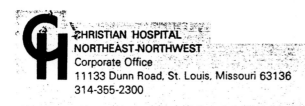

PATIENT NAME: Patient #37

PATIENT NO.:

DOCTOR:

REPORT OF OPERATION

DATE OF PROCEDURE:	10-10-83
SURGEON:	R. C_____, M.D.
PREOPERATIVE DIAGNOSIS:	Incomplete small bowel obstruction.
POSTOPERATIVE DIAGNOSIS:	Incomplete small bowel obstruction, secondary to recurrent carcinoid tumor.
OPERATION PERFORMED:	Exploratory laparotomy with massive adhesiolysis, small bowel resection, appendectomy.
ASSISTANT:	S. V_____, M.D.
ANESTHESIA:	General, Dr. K___/Dr. H___

DESCRIPTION OF PROCEDURE: The patient was brought to the Operating Room and placed supine on the operating table and had his abdominal wall shaved, prepped with Betadine and draped for the above operative procedure. Incision was made half way above and below the umbilicus for total distance of approximately 14 cm. with subcutaneous bleeders being controlled with electrocautery. Peritoneal cavity was entered and explored with the liver, peritoneum, omentum, pancreas all appearing normal. There was a massive ball of small bowel---some dilated, some collapsed---in the mid-abdomen. A massive adhesiolysis was then carried out with a great deal of difficulty due to vascularity of the adhesions. Eventually, at what seemed to be the root of the small bowel mesentery, there was a very firm mass that did appear to be tumor. This was biopsied and sent our for frozen section, returning as malignant, with some type of endocrine producing tumor present. Further adhesiolysis was then carried out and it was found at this point that the small bowel that was involved and the portion of the mesentery involved was resectible without compromising the remaining part of the small intestine or its blood supply. The small bowel was then clamped circumferentially in a proximal and distal fashion and stapled with the GIA stapler. The mesentery was incised, sequentially divided between clamps, and tied with 2-0 silk suture ligatures. A side-to-side anastomosis was then achieved after proper alignment had been obtained, with the GIA stapler and with the rent, being then closed in two layers, with a running continuous seromucosal 3-0 chromic catgut and an outer seromuscular interrupted 3-0 silk. The rent and the small bowel mesentery was closed then with mattress sutures of 3-0 silk. Attention was then re-directed to the right lower quadrant where the appendix, which had not been removed, due to the patient's expected prognosis after the first operation, now full of barium, not having emptied after upper and lower G.I., was freed up after some degree of difficulty. The mesentery to the appendix was divided between clamps and tied with 3-0 silk. The appendix was clamped and spaced with a straight clamp, removed and the stump inverted by placing interrupted seromuscular 3-0 silk and tying the sutures after the straight clamp was removed. This inverted the stump nicely and properly. The cecum was replaced in the right lower quadrant and the abdominal cavity was irrigated then with copious amounts of warm saline. Hemostasis was adequate and contamination had not been present. The small bowel was replaced in orderly fashion, covered with

(CONTINUED)

375

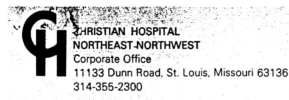

PATIENT NAME: Patient #37

PATIENT NO.:

DOCTOR:

REPORT OF OPERATION - PAGE TWO

omentum, and the midline fascia approximated with interrupted figure of eight
0-Prolene sutures. After fascia closure had been completed, the wound was
irrigated with saline and hemostasis was adequate. Skin edges were approximated
with the skin stapling device. Estimated blood loss during the operative procedure
had been one unit, blood replaced---none. Sponge, instrument and needles counts
correct times two. Nasogastric tube was placed during the operative procedure and
was present in the stomach during closure. The patient had been given two grams of
Mefoxin I.V. piggyback during the operative procedure. The termination of the
procedure was done and sterile dressing was applied to the incision site. The
patient was awakened, extubated and transferred to the Recovery Room, having
tolerated the procedure well, with no undue difficulties.

Robert V. C_____ MD

ROBERT V. C_____, M.D.

RC:45:849
DD:10-10-83
DR:10-12-83
DT:10-24-83

CC: Dr. R. C_____
      Dr. D. M_____
      Dr. D. L_____

Patient #38

Patient #38 died of Alzheimer's disease at age 77, 12 years after being diagnosed with unresectable carcinoma of the pancreas.

In mid-1973, Patient #38 first developed chronic fatigue and depression that both worsened over a several month period. In late 1973, he experienced episodes of nausea, abdominal pain, and anorexia that persisted throughout the first half of 1974. During that period, he lost a total of 50 pounds. Then, after becoming jaundiced in August 1974, Patient #38 was admitted to Halifax Hospital in Daytona Beach, Florida for evaluation.

The attending physician documented Patient #38's striking appearance in the records:

> The skin was grossly yellow, and sclera [whites of the eyes] were icteric [jaundiced].

Blood studies revealed abnormal liver function tests, including an elevated bilirubin level of 6 mg/dL (normal less than 1.0). A urinanalysis was positive for bilirubin, indicating a possible obstruction in the bile duct system.

Patient #38 subsequently underwent exploratory surgery on August 20, 1974, during which he was found to have a large, inoperable tumor of the pancreas extending into the common bile duct, with evidence of metastatic disease in the liver. His surgeon made no attempt to resect the tumor, nor did he—thinking the diagnosis obvious—wish to risk biopsy.

The operative note describes the findings in detail:

> On opening the abdominal cavity, immediately noted was a large nodular lesion occupying the head of the pancreas and extending and going downwards . . . pancreatic body was also felt and was grossly enlarged and nodular and firm . . . The liver was smooth, there was evident metastatic spread . . .
>
> The mass, itself, occupied most of the C-loop of the duodenum and the mass extending downward overlying the posterior mesenteric muscles . . .
>
> No attempt at pancreatic biopsy was deemed necessary because of the obvious findings and because of the dangers associated with this procedure.

Postoperatively, Patient #38's doctors informed him he most likely would not live beyond several months, and that additional therapy would be useless. But Patient #38, already aware of Dr. Kelley, had other plans. After leaving the hospital on August 29, 1974 and despite his unstable condition, he traveled with his wife to Texas to consult with Dr. Kelley. Days later, Patient #38 began the full nutritional regimen.

Subsequently, over a period of months his many symptoms completely resolved. His appetite improved, he gained weight, and within a year he felt well enough to return full-time to his work as a professional photographer.

Patient #38 remained in excellent health until 1985, when after a period of cognitive decline, he was diagnosed with Alzheimer's disease. He gradually deteriorated, eventually succumbing in April 1986, nearly 12 years after his original terminal diagnosis. At the time of death, he was, according to his wife, completely cancer-free.

Despite the lack of biopsy confirmation in this case, the clinical history and obvious findings at surgery are consistent with pancreatic carcinoma. I think by any standards of medical science, this patient's progress and long-term survival are unusual.

HALIFAX   HOSPITAL

DISCHARGE SUMMARY

DATES:	ADMITTED: 8/11/74	DISCHARGED: 8/28/74

PROVISIONAL DIAGNOSIS:

Obstructive jaundice.

FINAL DIAGNOSIS:

Obstructive jaundice due to carcinoma of the pancreas.

BRIEF HISTORY:
(reason for hospitalization:).

This is a 65 year old male who was admitted on 8/11/74 with a history of having pains in the abdomen and gradual development of jaundice.

Pertinent in his past history is that previously he underwent a left inguinal hernia repair. He is allergic to Penicillin. He smokes one pack of cigarettes a day. Otherwise he has been relatively healthy.

PERTINENT FINDINGS:
(physical examination, laboratory, etc).

Most pertinent findings on admission revealed a fully developed, nauseated male, not in acute distress, temperature 98, pulse rate 70, respirations 20, BP 160/70. The skin was grossly yellow and sclera were icteric. There was no neck vein distention noted. Heart and lungs were clear. Abdomen was tender in the right upper quadrant with no definite masses palpable. Rectal shelf was negative for any evasion or carcinoma. Stool was brown.

COURSE IN HOSPITAL:
(consultations, operations, treatment, complications).

He was then admitted and workup was accomplished. Dr. C   did the preliminary studies and chemistry survey initially showed marked elevation of total bilirubin to almost 6mg.%, alkaline p'tase was 240, LDH up slightly to 240 and the SGOT up to 175mg.%. Hb 15.5, hct 46.9, white count 12,600. ICD was 28 units and urine showed positive bile and the other studies were normal. Urobilinogen was 1.8, normal being 0.1 to 1.5 units for two hours. The repeat chemistry survey three days later showed an improvement in his normal liver functions and showed bilirubin down to 3 units, alkaline p'tase down to 175mg.% and the LDH and SGOT were normal. Preliminary studies of the chest showed normal chest findings and the barium enema showed no lesion in the colon, upper GI series was normal with normal loop. EKG on 8/11/74 showed it to be normal.

CONDITION ON DISCHARGE:
(improved, unimproved, same, expired).

With this, impression was an obstructive form of jaundice and I saw him in consultation subsequently and discussed the case with him and it was my impression that he was suffering from obstructive jaundice, most commonly due to stones.

FOLLOW-UP CARE and MEDICATION:
(transferred to, date and place of follow-up visits by Physician.)

Gall bladder series done on 8/17/74 showed nonvisualization on double dose study. On 8/19/74 a chemistry survey showed a bilirubin of 1.8, alkaline p'tase 140 and LDH and SGOT were normal. He was then subsequently prepared for surgery for exploration of his obstructive jaundice and this was done on 8/20/74.

(OVER PLEASE)

379

Findings at that time consisted of a rather large pancreatic CA involving the head and also the entire body of the pancreas. A biliary bipass procedure with cholecysto-jejunostomy and jejunostomy was accomplished.

Post operatively he was placed on VI fluids and Cleocin 600mg. bid was instituted,IPPB treatments and his course was essentially benign. He did not develop a fever and did quite well from that standpoint. The dressings were changed subsequently. The wound has been healing without any complications, drains were finally removed on the 7th postoperative day and he is discharged today on 6/29/74. Skin sutures are removed and he has retention sutures in place which will be removed in the following week.

His jaundice has practically disappeared and he is eating fairly well. The wife is madeaware of this finding and supportive treatment as much as possible was explained to the wife.

Condition on discharge: Improved.

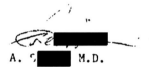

A. C████ M.D.

cc

Date 8-20 19 74   T CR- 8/29/74

Operator, Dr. ████████

Assisted by Dr ████████

Anesthetist Dr M ████████

Anesthetic General

Instrument Nurse ████████ W ████████ C████████

Sponge Nurse Mildred Jung RN

Operation Exploratory Lap - Cholecystectomy - Jejunostomy c̄ Jejunojejunostomy   Began 8 06 PM   Closed 9 56 PM

~~Exploratory laparotomy, cholecysto-jejunostomy with jejunostomy.~~

Preoperative Diagnosis: Obstructive jaundice.

Obstructive Jaundice

Postoperative Diagnosis: Same secondary to carcinoma of the pancreas.

Same 2nd to CA of pancreas

Gross Pathology: On opening the abdominal cavity, immediately noted was a large nodular lesion occupying the head of the pancreas and extending and going downwards. After the performance of the Kocher maneuver, palpation of the entire head of the pancreas was made and this was rather large nodular lesion and going posteriorly and superiorly towards the left side, pancreatic body was also felt and was grossly enlarged and nodular and firm. It was adherent to the posterior area on the left side, especially near the tail and distal part of the body of the pancreas itself. ~~The stomach and duodenum were grossly normal to inspection and palption.~~

Description of Operation:

The liver was smooth, there was evident metastatic spread and no gross lesions of the hepatoduodenal ligament was noted except for slight enlargement of the common bile duct. The GB was slightly enlarged, tense, and dull in appearance probably indicating some form of chronic mild infection. Both kidneys were in their usual anatomic areas and no abdominal aneurysm was noted. The rest of the abdominal viscera were all found revealing no obvious gross abnormaliti

PROCEDURE: and

The patient was given satisfactory general endotracheal anesthesia and the lower chest/ abdom were prepped wi th Betadine and draped as a sterile field. The abdominal cavity was entered through a rt. Kocher incision. Bleeders were cauterized for hemostasis. Fascia was then incis and rectus muscle bluntly elevated from its bed and alternately cut and clamped and tied with 3/0 silk ties. Transversus abdominis and oblique muscles were incised to expose the peritonea cavity. Balfour retractor was placed in position and exploration of the abdominal cavity was accomplished. With packs on the small intestine and a Kocher maneuver was performed and at th stage better palpation of the large pancreatic lesion was accomplished. The mass, itself, occupied most of the C-loop of the duodenum and the mass extending downwards overlying the posterior mesenteric muscles. It was also encroaching close to the ligament of Treitz (OVER

Sutures: PL3/0 ② OS 7/0 ① OS3/0 ① OS4/0 ②   PLEASE)
Cw ① CL3/0 ② PA#3 BS4/0 ②

Drains:
5/8" Penrose

Sponge Count: Needle { L W ████████ C ████████
{ M. O ████████ RN

Immediate Postoperative Condition:
Satis

Supportive Therapy and Comments:
See Record

.... M. L
Signature of Operator

OPERATIVE RECORD

381

medially and below this level also there was mesenteria. The whole mass was very large and going posteriorly, the body was felt and was also grossly enlarged, very firm and somewhat nodular. It was adherent to the distal part of the body and tail could not be elevated with the hand. When this was noted then, the other exploratory findings were noted.. With this I then proceeded to perform the bypass procedure by first localizing the proximal jejunum to the ligament of Treitz and bringing a loop of proximal jejunum close to the fundus of the GB. A posterior layer was started with 3/0 silk ties suturing the serosa of the small intestine to the serosa of the GB. Respective incisions into the GB fundus and the small intestine were then made and the next layer on the posterioraspect of the anastamosis was completed with 3/0 chromic catgut. Going anteriorly, the same procedure was done and a seromuscular suture, a second layer on the anterior anastamosis was accomplished with interrupted 3/0 silk sutures. The distance from the ligament of Treitz to the anastasmosis was over 18 inches atleast. About 6 to 7 inches below the gallbladder, the intestine anastamosis, a complimentary jejuno-jejunostomy was constructed with a two-finger stoma. Posterior seromuscular sutures on the each side of intestine were applied and intestine incised and a posterior layer completed within terrupted 4/0 silks. Going anteriorly from mucosa-to-mucosa approximation was also accomplished in the same manner and the serosal sutures applied with the use of interrupted 3/0 silk sutures. The anastamosis was very adequate and no leakage was noted on testing this area of anastamosis. When this was accomplished, then, two Penrose drains were inserted in the rt. subhepatic space and exited through a separate stab wound incision below the Kocher incision. A pre-closure check was accomplished and fluid removed by suction. No attempt at pancreatic biopsy was deemed necessary because of the obvious findings and because of the dangers associated with this procedure. Packs and retractors were now removed and the rest of the bowel returned into the abdominal cavity and greater omentum laid anteriorly over the small intestine. Closure of the incision then proceeded utilizing 0 chromic catgut for the peritoneum. A retention suture of #3 silk was first applied. Two such sutures were applied and placed in position. The peritoneum was finally reclosed with 0 chromic catgut. The fascia and oblique muscles were closed respectively utilizing figure-of-8 3/0 silk interrupted sutures. Subcutaneous tissue was cleared of debris and approximated with interrupted 3/0 plain catgut. Skin was closed with interrupted 4/0 silk sutures. Retention sutures were now tied i place. The drains were anchored at skin level with sutures and safety pins. Dressings were applied. Blood loss during the entire procedure wasvery minimal; patient tolerated the procedure well without any complications. Sponge and instruments counts were reported as correct. The patient subsequently transfered to the R. R. in satisfactory condition.

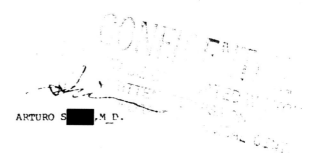

ARTURO S█████,M D.

bb

PROSTATE CANCER

In 1987, prostate cancer, a major cancer killer, claimed 27,000 lives.

For patients with prostate cancer, experts describe the extent of disease on an A-D staging scale: Stage A signifies malignancy limited to the prostate that cannot be palpated on rectal exam; B indicates the disease, though still restricted to the prostate, can be felt on digital probing; C correlates with local extension beyond the prostate into the surrounding tissues; and D defines prostate cancer that has spread to distant organs, such as the bone or lung.

If detected early, the disease can be cured with surgery or radiation. For metastatic disease, oncologists employ chemotherapy, and often, since the disease is thought to be hormone dependent, treatments to block testosterone production such as orchiectomy (removal of the testes) and female hormones. However, these approaches have not been proven to extend life.

At present, approximately 70% of all patients diagnosed with prostate cancer survive five years.

Patient #39

Patient #39 is a 67-year-old man from California alive eight years since first diagnosed with metastatic prostatic carcinoma.

In January 1979, Patient #39 experienced symptoms consistent with a partial urinary tract obstruction that worsened over a several week period. After consulting his family physician, he underwent an intravenous pyelogram, a dye study of kidney function, which revealed an enlarged prostate blocking the urethra. The findings were attributed only to a prostate infection, for which Patient #39's doctor prescribed a course of antibiotics. Though he initially improved on medication, within weeks his symptoms recurred.

In early April 1979, Patient #39 was referred to a urologist at the University of California at Los Angeles Medical Center. Despite the large prostate noted on physical exam, the physician decided to monitor Patient #39 for a month before recommending additional testing. When Patient #39 worsened, he returned to UCLA on May 18, 1979 for a needle biopsy of the prostate, which confirmed a moderately differentiated grade II adenocarcinoma. Additional radiographic studies, including chest X-rays and a bone scan, showed no evidence of metastatic disease.

At that point, Patient #39 was scheduled for a prostatectomy (surgical removal of the prostate), but before proceeding, he decided to investigate unconventional approaches to cancer. After learning of Dr. Kelley in late May 1979, he called his physician to defer surgery. His doctor wrote:

> [Patient #39] has called stating that he'd rather postpone surgery scheduled for Monday which we will happily do. He [is] going to see some Dietician in the Washington area which [sic] is supposedly treating cancer by dietary supplements and flushes [sic]. I have cautioned [Patient #39] against the possible 'quackery' involved in this form of therapy and strongly recommended against him seeing these people.

The warnings were effective. Patient #39 cancelled his visit with Dr. Kelley and in June 1979, travelled to the Scripps Clinic in La Jolla, California for a second opinion. After physicians there confirmed the diagnosis, he underwent exploratory surgery on June 7, 1979, during which he was found to have extensive, stage D1 disease throughout the pelvis. His surgeon excised several cancerous lymph nodes, but chose not to remove the prostate since the disease had already metastasized. Five of the excised lymph nodes, including one at the highest level of the iliac chain, were subsequently found positive for malignant disease.

The Scripps doctors then proposed an intensive treatment regimen consisting of radiation, chemotherapy, and estrogen, but Patient #39 decided to refuse all further conventional treatment. Instead, after leaving the hospital he consulted with Dr. Kelley in Washington State and in late June 1979 began the full nutritional program. Within months, all his symptoms resolved.

He subsequently remained in good health until 1984, when he again developed a urinary tract obstruction, requiring surgery for correction of what proved to be a ureter blocked by scar tissue. During the procedure, no evidence of the previously noted metastatic cancer could be found.

Patient #39 recovered quickly, resumed his nutritional protocol, and today, eight years after his diagnosis, he is in excellent health and cancer-free.

Untreated prostate cancer is usually rapidly fatal. Harnett, in his classic paper, reported a mean survival of only 19.5 months in 43 patients with the disease who refused all therapy.[1]

Paulson and colleagues studied 12 patients with stage D adenocarcinoma of the prostate treated with radiation only, all of whom died within three years.[2] Paulson writes:

> Although the potential for cure in the occasional patient with an isolated nodal metastasis exists, the accumulated data would support the statement that nodal involvement presents a patient at enhanced risk for treatment failure.[3]

Kramer and his associates described a median survival of only 31.6 months in a group of 44 patients with prostate cancer who, like Patient #39, initially presented with regional lymph node metastases but negative bone scans. All patients were either dead, or had evidence of active cancer within five years of diagnosis despite aggressive treatment with surgery, radiation and/or hormones.[4]

In summary, Patient #39 was initially diagnosed with prostate cancer that had metastasized to multiple pelvic lymph nodes. Since after his initial surgery he refused further conventional treatment, it seems only reasonable to credit the observed regression of this patient's cancer as evident during his 1984 surgery, and his long-term disease-free survival—now in excess of eight years—to the Kelley regimen.

REFERENCES

1. Harnett, WL. "The Relation Between Delay in Treatment of Cancer and Survival Rate." *British Journal of Cancer* 1953; 7:19–36.

2. DeVita, VT, et al. *Cancer—Principles and Practice of Oncology*. Philadelphia; J.B. Lippincott Company, 1982, page 762.

3. DeVita, VT, et al., page 764.

4. DeVita, VT, et al., pages 763–764.

ADDRESS:	DIVISION OF SURGICAL PATHOLOGY UCLA CENTER FOR THE HEALTH SCIENCES LOS ANGELES, CALIFORNIA 90024

PATIENT SERVICE
(MED, SURG, PED, OB/GYN, ETC.)   *urology*

LOCATION
(TUBE, WARD, CLINIC)   *OPJU*

PHYSICIAN COPY OF REPORT WILL BE SENT TO NAME AND ADDRESS BELOW

79S- 5163

CLINICAL DATA IS ESSENTIAL
FOR PROMPT, ACCURATE REPORTING

PHYSICIAN (WITH NECESSARY INITIALS)
R. B. J▓▓▓▓

DATE REC'D IN PATHOLOGY *5/▓▓-79*

PATHOLOGY ACC. NO.   79S 5163

ADDRESS OR HOSPITAL LOCATION   *66 - 118*

MAY 1979 14 26

Patient #39

SPECIMEN *Needle bx prostta*

ANATOMICAL LOCATION *Prostto*

PERTINENT CLINICAL DATA (INCLUDE HISTORY, P-E, ABNORMAL LAB RESULTS, DRUGS, RADIATION THERAPY, AND PAST SURGICAL PROCEDURES)

Rot bx.

CLINICAL DIAGNOSIS *R/o CaP Prostatic Hypertrophy*   SIGNATURE ▓▓▓▓ M.D.

GROSS: /specimen is received labelled "needle . . . bx prosth". It consists of three cylindrs of translucent tan tissue each measuring 2.5 cm in length and 0.1 cm in diameter. They are entirely submitted in Cassette A. MS/gm

MICROSCOPIC: Sections of prostate gland show numerous tiny glands infiltrating the stroma in a haphazard fashion. Some of these glands are clustered around a blood vessel, and there is perineural invasion. The adenocarcinoma is acinar and moderately differentiated (Grade II of III)

DIAGNOSIS: Prostate gland (needle biopsy)
          -Adenocarcinoma

M. S▓▓▓▓ M.D.
J. W▓▓▓▓ M.D.

cms/5-22-79

UCLA ███████████

May 25, 1979: ████████████ came in to talk about therapy for his carcinoma of the prostate. We have discussed the surgical approaches to the prostate as well as radiation therapy both external beam and interstitial radiation. I've explained to him the advantages and disadvantages of each approach. We've also talked about the importance of node dissection should he consider radical prostatectomy as a treatment of choice. We have scheduled a bone scan for next Wednesday. He will have an acid phosphatase, liver function tests performed today. He will call tomorrow or the next week regarding his decision regarding therapy.

Robert B. S████, M.D.
RBS:js

June 1, 1979: ████████████ has called stating that he'd rather postpone surgery scheduled for Monday which we will happily do. He going to see some Dietician in the Washington area which is supposedly treating cancer by dietary supplements and flush I have cautioned ████████████ against the possible "quackery" involved in this form of therapy and strongly recommended against him seeing these people. If he would desire to have radiation therapy or some other form of therapy which is proven, I would have no arguement. He states that he almost certainly will return here for radical prostatectomy but just feels that he would like to investigate this avenue. I have told him to feel free to call in the future should he desire to do a radical prostatectomy.

Robert B. S████, M.D.
RBS:js
xc: Les D██████, M.D.

FORM 210 (REV SEP 76) (REP JUN 77) 71431-452   PHYSICIAN'S NOTES – GREEN STRIPED – UNLINED

388

CHIEF COMPLAINT: ███████████████ is a 59-year-old accountant for the Filtrol Corporation, who is admitted to this hospital with prostatic cancer.

In February of 1979, the patient noted some minor blockage in the passage of urine. There was minor irritation when voiding but the main sensation was one of incomplete bladder emptying. A local physician treated him with antibiotics which improved the situation somewhat, but did not totally alleviate it. The symptoms came on rather abruptly, and the patient was referred to Dr. Robert Smith at UCLA Medical Center. A cystoscopy and prostatic biopsy was performed, which showed a Grade II adenocarcinoma of the prostate. Other pertinent data included a bone scan which was negative and a chest x-ray which did not show any metastatic disease.

As a result of several different factors, ████████████ came to see me for an opinion. I agreed in essence with that one allegedly submitted by Dr. S██████, namely that the best treatment in a man 59 years old with no other significant medical history was one of radical lymph node dissection, followed by radical prostatectomy if the lymph nodes failed to show any tumor. In addition, Mr. ████████ and I discussed at length radiation therapy. We also discussed dietary therapy which is being administered by the Kelly Foundation. During this discussion I outlined the pros and cons, complications and problems with all the treatment modalities. At the end of this discussion, Mr. ███████ went home and then called me back. He in essence had made a decision to go ahead with surgery, and asked me if I would perform the procedure.

The patient has been in excellent health. He can swim up to one mile and has really never had any cardiopulmonary problems. The patient also denies any musculoskeletal pain, hematuria or costovertebral angle pain.

MEDICATIONS: Macrodantin 50 mg. a day.
ALLERGIES: PENICILLIN, SULFA.
SURGERIES: Previously tonsillectomy and adenoidectomy.
MEDICAL HISTORY: No history of cardiopulmonary disease, hepatitis or tuberculosis.
FAMILY HISTORY: The patient's father died in his 90s of natural causes. His mother died at age 76 from digestive problems. Four brothers and sisters are alive and well. There is no history of any neoplasia in the family.
SOCIAL HISTORY: The patient and his wife live in Anaheim, California. They have no children. The patient was born in Vancouver, B.C., and worked for a period of time in Niagra, New York, before coming to the West Coast.
REVIEW OF SYSTEMS: HEENT: No syncopal episodes, chronic headaches, double vision. CP: No shortness of breath, dyspnea on exertion, orthopnea, chronic cough, hemoptysis, chest pain, angina or lower extremity edema. GI: No digestive problems, change in stool habits, history of melena. GU: See HPI. MS: No known bone or joint disease. No history of skeletal pain. DERMATOLOGY: The patient has a minor rash effecting his face and forehead for which he received some treatment from dermatologist intermittent.

PHYSICAL EXAMINATION:

GENERAL: The patient is a red haired, slender, alert man, who appears to be in excellent physical condition.
VITAL SIGNS: BP 106/60. Pulse 60 and regular.
HEENT: The pupils are round, regular and equal. They are reactive to light and accomodation.
NECK: The carotid pulses are 3+ bilaterally. There is no evidence of increased jugulovenous pressure. There are no palpable cervical or supraclavicular lymph nodes.   SIGNED _____ MD

SPECIMEN NO   3-79-1291

ROOM   602   PATIENT   Patient #39

DATE   6/7/79   DOCTOR

UNIT NO   064793

SPECIMEN: (A) RIGHT PELVIC LYMPH NODES
             (B) LEFT PELVIC LYMPH NODES

GROSS:

THE SPECIMEN CONSISTS OF:

(A) an elongated branching piece of fatty soft tissue identified as the
right pelvic lymph node chain. It includes the common and external iliac
nodes as well as the obturator nodes. The soft tissue is dissected at the
time of surgery. There are multiple nodes present ranging between 0.5
and 1.5 cm in size. The larger ones appear to be partially replaced by
fat. There is no gross evidence of metastatic tumor. A representative
sample of nodes is submitted for frozen section and reported, "no evidence
of tumor" (MLE). The remainder of the nodes are submitted.

(B) identified as left pelvic lymph nodes is a similar branching piece of
adipose tissue like that described above in A. It measures 12 x 6 x 1 cm
in overall dimensions. Various areas within the soft tissue are identified
including the common iliac nodes, external iliac nodes and hypogastric nodes.
These are examined and dissected at the time of surgery. There are grossly
suspicious and positive nodes in both the hypogastric and the common iliac
regions. A frozen section is reported, "metastatic adenocarcinoma in multiple
nodes" (MLE). The remainder of the nodes are submitted and are sublabeled
as follows; common iliac, BC; hypogastric, BH; and external iliac, BE.
MLE:tn

MICRO:

(A) A total of sixteen lymph nodes are present in the right iliac chain.
Grossly these all appeared normal. On microscopic examination there is
one small node that contains a micro deposit of well differentiated adenocarcinoma. Otherwise the nodes are typical pelvic nodes containing zones
of fibrosis and calcification.

(B) On the left side a total of 24 lymph nodes are present. Four of these
show evidence of metastatic tumor, and in most of these nodes this is gross
disease and not micrometastases. The involved nodes are present in the
common iliac chain and hypogastric areas. The external iliac nodes are not

(Continued on Page 2)

SURGICAL PATHOLOGY REPORT

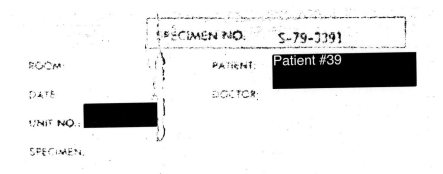

involved. The tumor is as previously described a well differentiated adenocarcinoma consistent with prostate origin.

DIAGNOSIS: (A) ADENOCARCINOMA, WELL DIFFERENTIATED, MICROMETASTASES TO
                 ONE OF SIXTEEN RIGHT PELVIC LYMPH NODES.
            (B) ADENOCARCINOMA, WELL DIFFERENTIATED, METASTATIC TO FOUR OF
                 TWENTY-FOUR LEFT PELVIC LYMPH NODES, PELVIC LYMPHADEN-
                 ECTOMY.

MLE:tn

——————— PATHOLOGISTS ———————
PHILIPS L. GAUSEWITZ, M.D. • GEORGE E. MEADOR, M.D. • KAI A. B. KRISTENSEN,
MAX L. ELLIOTT, M.D. • MICHAEL KAM, M.D. • BRIAN DATNOW, M.D. • EDWARD J. SCHLENK,

SURGICAL PATHOLOGY REPORT

CHART COPY

391

Patient #40

Patient #40 is a 65-year-old man from Colorado alive nearly nine years since his diagnosis of metastatic prostatic carcinoma.

In early 1978, Patient #40 experienced symptoms consistent with a partial urinary tract obstruction that gradually worsened over a period of several months. Though initially he did not seek out medical advice, in the summer of 1978 he finally consulted his family physician, who detected an enlarged prostate on physical exam. In addition, routine laboratory studies were significant for an elevated acid phosphatase, a marker for prostatic cancer. On two separate occasions, the reported values were 2.5 and 5.0 (normal less than 2.0).

On September 18, 1978, Patient #40 was admitted to Aurora Community Hospital in Aurora, Colorado for further evaluation, and a week later he underwent transurethral resection of the prostate (involving excision of tissue via the urethra). Review of the surgical specimens confirmed an "Adenocarcinoma of prostate, moderately differentiated." Furthermore, a bone scan on September 29, 1978 revealed evidence of metastatic disease, clearly described in the official radiology report:

> Multiple abnormal areas of uptake are identified. They are seen in the sternum, ribs, lumbar spine, pelvis, and cervical spine . . . The findings are highly suggestive of bony metastasis.

The patient's physicians then recommended orchiectomy as well as aggressive radiation therapy, though they informed him that even with such treatment, he most probably would live only a year. After considering his options, Patient #40 agreed only to Stilbestrol (oral estrogen, also called DES), and a brief course of radiation to his breasts to prevent the enlargement often associated with the hormone therapy.

After leaving the hospital in October 1978, Patient #40 decided to investigate unconventional approaches to cancer. After learning of Dr. Kelley, he began the full nutritional regimen in early 1979, after which time he pursued hormonal therapy only intermittently before discontinuing the medication for good.

Patient #40 responded rapidly to his nutritional protocol. Within months, his urinary symptoms resolved, and bone scans over a two-year period at the University of Utah documented healing of his multiple lesions. Thereafter, Patient #40 continued the Kelley program for two and a half years, before tapering down to a maintenance protocol which he still follows. Today, nearly nine years after his diagnosis, he is in good health and appears cancer-free.

Prostatic carcinoma, once metastatic to the bone, is a deadly disease. Kane describes a median survival of only 45.6 weeks in patients presenting with skeletal involvement even when aggressively treated.[1] Although Patient #40 did pursue a course of Stilbestrol, estrogen therapy has not been shown to prolong life once the disease invades bone.[2]

In summary, Patient #40 was diagnosed with biopsy-proven prostatic carcinoma with clear evidence of metastatic disease to multiple bones. After the initial diagnostic studies, he refused all conventional therapy other than oral DES, which he took only sporadically and briefly. Furthermore, this patient's extensive disease regressed, as documented by bone scan, only after he began the Kelley program.

REFERENCES

1. Kane, RD, et al. "Multiple Drug Chemotherapy Regimen for Patients With Hormonally-unresponsive Carcinoma of the Prostate." *Journal of Urology* 1977; 117:467–471.

2. DeVita, VT, et al. *Cancer—Principles and Practices of Oncology.* Philadelphia; J.B. Lippincott Company, 1982, page 765.

AURORA COMMUNITY HOSPITAL

P.O. BOX 31779 • AURORA, COLORADO 80011 • TELEPHONE: (303) 751-5353

Patient's Name: Patient #40   Hospital No:

Attending Physician: M   Room No: 436-2

Pathology No: 78-AP-2326   Age & Sex: M-56

CLINICAL DIAGNOSIS: BPH

GROSS:

Specimen is designated as "prostate" and consists of 14 grams of multiple somewhat nodular and lobulated portions of rubbery yellowish-pink-tan tissue. Entire specimen is submitted into 6 cassettes. PBV/d   9/25/78-9/26/78

MICROSCOPIC:

Multiple portions of prostatic tissue have a dense fibromuscular stroma heavily infiltrated by nests of closely spaced glandular acini giving a cribriform pattern and composed of cuboidal to low columnar cells with vacuolated eosinophilic cytoplasm and ovoid vesicular nuclei containing small nucleoli. In some portions there are scattered benign appearing prostatic glands with scattered surrounding chronic inflammatory cells. However, many of the portions of tissue are involved by the neoplasm. In some portions the neoplastic cells form lobular aggregates where glandular acini are not as evident and the cells are ballooned with vacuolated clear cytoplasm.

DIAGNOSIS:

PROSTATIC TISSUE (TUR), ADENOCARCINOMA OF PROSTATE, MODERATELY DIFFERENTIATED

PBV/d
9/16/78-9/26/78
(6-1)

P. B. V   M.D.

394

RADIOLOGY REPORT

AURORA COMMUNITY HOSPITAL 1501 S. POTOMAC AURORA, COLORADO 80012 AREA CODE (303) 751-5353

X/R ORDER

9/28/78 12:32PM TOMORROW WALK ███████████████████ 9/24/78

9-29-
8:00AM   Patient #40

BENIGN PROSTATIC HYPERTROPHY   056 M M█████, WILLIAM

████████ BONE SCAN   ITEM 03017 QTY : 1

(AS OUT PATIENT)
CDWS

FROM : 4NS
RAY [ ] NUCLEAR [X] ULTRASOUND [ ]

MA   TIME   COMMENTS:

RAY NUMBER 27244   REPORT:

9-29-78
BONE SCAN: 20mCi Tc-99m Diphosphonate administered I.V.
Multiple abnormal areas of uptake are identified. They are seen in the
sternum, ribs, lumbar spine, pelvis and cervical spine.

IMPRESSION:
The findings are highly suggestive of bony metastasis.

395

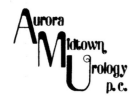

LOUIS N. A███████, M.D.
WILLIAM N. M███████M.D.
THOMAS B. W██████ M.D.

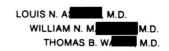

• AURORA, COLORADO 80011 •
DENVER, COLORADO 80218 •
AURORA, COLORADO 80012 •

UROLOGY AND GENITOURINARY SURGERY

October 12, 1978

Richard P████, M.D.
████████████████████
Aurora, Colorado   80012

Re: Patient #40

Dear Dick:

This is regarding █████████, who as you know, presented with
symptoms of prostatism and an elevated phosphatase, which was
noted by you. His prostate was suspicious. He underwent a TURP
on 9-25-78. This showed as adenocarcinoma, Grade 2. A subsequent bone scan revealed multiple metastatic lesions (Stage D).
Because of the marked spread of the disease we had a lengthy
discussion regarding the therapy and radiation. Following the
DES treatment he is to return for follow up. He was asked to
return to you for further care. I don't feel that the prognosis
is very good.

If I can be of further help, please let me know.

Sincerely,

Bill

William N. M██████s, M.D.

396

RADIOLOGY REPORT

AURORA COMMUNITY HOSPITAL 1501 S. POTOMAC   AURORA, COLORADO 80012   AREA CODE (303) 751-5353

X/R CHARGE

6/05/79   9:53AM   001 R   ████████   6/05/79

XRAY   057 M P███, RICHARD

463-03017 BONE SCAN   ITEM 3017 QTY : 001

FOLLOW UP PROSTATE   KJW
AY [ ]   NUCLEAR [X]   ULTRASOUND [ ]
/   MA   TIME   COMMENTS: _____
FROM : X/R   2214   REPORT:
AY NUMBER _____

6-5-79
BONE SCAN: 20mCi Tc-99m Diphosphonate administered I.V.
The study is compared with the previous study of 9-29-78.

Abnormal areas of uptake are identified in sites previously identified
as abnormal; however, the new areas of uptake do not show as much uptake
as on the previous study, and this may be due to healing. One wonders
if the patient is on chemotherapy. I do not identify any new areas of
abnormal uptake.

IMPRESSION:
There does appear to be some improvement.

D-6-5-79   **RADIOLOGY REPORT**
T-6-6-79jw
                  PHYSICIANS COPY   SIGNATURE OF RADIOLOGIST
                                                          A. R███████, M.D.

397

UNIVERSITY OF UTAH HOSPITAL
50 NORTH MEDICAL DRIVE
SALT LAKE CITY, UTAH 84132

1. Name Patient #40 ████████   Sex **M**   Age: **57**   Hospital No. ██████
                                                                          Referral Date **3/10/80**

2. Address █████████████████████████

3. Ref. Physician **Richard P██**, **M.D.**   Address: ████████████   **Aurora, CO**

4. Follow-up Physician   Address:

5. Final Diagnosis & Extent.

Adenocarcinoma of the prostate metastatic to bone.

6. Pertinent Hist. & Findings (Including Prev. Treatment, Lab. & X-ray findings.)

The patient underwent evaluation for prostatism in October 1978, and TURP revealed adenocarcinoma of the prostate. Acid phosphatase was elevated and bone scan, which has been
reviewed at UUMC, revealed multiple foci of metastatic disease in the spine, skull, ribs
and pelvis. He was asymptomatic from his metastatic disease, however. He was placed on
1 mg. of DES per day, after a prophylactic course of radiotherapy to the breast tissue.
At that time he received 900 rads in three fractions with 11 MeV electrons to each breast.
From that time to the present he has done very well, with acid phosphatase reported to have
returned to normal and bone scan having shown marked improvement. Prostate exam has also
become normal. He has continued to take 1 mg. of DES per day, and in the past few months
has noticed progressive gynecomastia. He was referred for consideration of further radiotherapy in attempts to prevent further breast enlargement. Physical examination was entirely
unremarkably, including no lymphadenopathy, no bony tenderness and no prostate abnormalities;
except for significant bilateral gynecomastia with mild tenderness in the subareolar areas.

7. Course and Condition at Conclusion of Treatment (Effects, Medications, Etc.)

He tolerated treatments with no difficulty, and at the conclusion of treatment reported no
itching or increased tenderness of his breast tissue

At the conclusion of treatment he underwent another bone scan which shows clearing of several
areas of uptake demonstrated on the September 78 scan, though mildly increased uptake is
noted in several of the other regions.

8. Advice to Patient at Conclusion of Treatment (Medication, Referral, Etc.)

He will return for follow-up in three months or call if any problems should arise earlier.

UH-MC-1126-3/75   REFERRING PHYSICIAN   SHEET 1

398

Patient #41

Patient #41 died at age 83 after surviving nearly nine years with widely metastatic prostatic carcinoma.

Patient #41 had been in excellent health when in early 1978, he experienced symptoms of a partial urinary tract obstruction. Although he did not initially seek medical advice, when the symptoms persisted over a several-month period, he eventually consulted his family physician, who noted an enlarged prostate on physical exam.

Patient #41 was subsequently admitted to Des Moines General Hospital on May 16, 1978 for further evaluation. After a bone scan and X-ray studies revealed abnormalities in the eighth thoracic vertebral body consistent with metastatic disease, on May 18, 1978, Patient #41 underwent a transurethral resection of the prostate. Evaluation of the tissue specimens confirmed a grade II adenocarcinoma.

With the diagnosis established, Patient #41 agreed to a course of the synthetic estrogen Stilbestrol. Despite the therapy, a follow-up bone scan in August 1978 showed that the metastases had not improved, and in early fall of 1978, his urinary symptoms recurred. His physicians recommended orchiectomy followed by radiation and chemotherapy, but Patient #41—believing himself too old for such an assault—refused all further conventional treatment.

In early November 1978, Patient #41 decided to investigate unconventional approaches to cancer. After learning of Dr. Kelley, he consulted with him, began the full nutritional program, and at the same time discontinued Stilbestrol.

Within months on his unconventional treatment and off hormones, all his symptoms resolved, but after a year on the program—against Dr. Kelley's advice—Patient #41 strayed from the prescribed diet and supplements. Although he did well for a time, in early 1980 Patient #41 developed chronic abdominal pain, and once again, a urinary tract obstruction. He was subsequently admitted to Des Moines General Hospital on February 17, 1980, for re-evaluation.

Laboratory studies confirmed an elevated acid phosphatase level, indicating active prostatic cancer. A repeat bone scan revealed a new lesion in the thoracic spine, described in the radiology report as "Increased activity . . . may represent either trauma or metastasis. Clinical correlation is recommended."

During a second transurethral prostate resection, Patient #41's surgeon discovered that the tumor had extended beyond the prostatic capsule into the surrounding tissues. All biopsy specimens were positive for cancer.

After surgery, Patient #41 again refused orchiectomy, radiation and chemotherapy, although he did agree to restart oral Stilbestrol. And, after his discharge from the hospital on February 29, 1980. Patient #41 resumed the full Kelley program. Six months later, he discontinued the hormone therapy, thereafter pursuing only the Kelley regimen for treatment.

Patient #41 followed his nutritional protocol for another six years, during which time he enjoyed excellent health, with a series of X-rays and bone scans confirming gradual healing of the previously noted metastatic lesions. After stopping the program in mid-1986, his disease recurred within several months and he eventually died in February 1987—at a time Dr. Kelley was no longer seeing patients—nearly nine years after his original diagnosis.

This patient's prolonged disease-free survival is remarkable, since prostate cancer, once metastatic to the bone—as reported in the case of Patient #40—usually kills quickly. Furthermore, Patient #41 refused orchiectomy, chemotherapy and radiation, the standard treatments for this disease. Although he did pursue two abbreviated courses of oral Stilbestrol, numerous studies have shown that hormone therapy by itself does not extend life in patients with metastatic prostate cancer.[1]

Dr. Kelley believes in retrospect this patient should never have discontinued his nutritional program. Evidently, his disease was well-controlled only as long as he remained on the full Kelley regimen.

REFERENCE

1. DeVita, VT, et al. *Cancer Principles & Practice of Oncology*. Philadelphia; J.B. Lippincott Company, 1982, page 765.

Patient #41

Attending Physician: Roger S█████ D.O.

REFERRING PHYSICIAN: Tom G█████ D.O.

DATE OF ADMISSION: 5-16-78

DATE OF DISCHARGE: 5-20-78, transfer of care.

This 74 year old, white male was admitted by me to the hospital on 5-16-78. I seen him previously in my office with history of slow urinary stream. It was my impression when I examined the patient that he had an adenocarcinoma of the prostate.

After admission to the hospital the following tests were performed. Bone scan with increased radioactivity at D-10 consistent with metastatic involvement of the bone. Ultrasonic examination of the prostate revealed hypertrophy of the prostate, also nodular area in the posterior wall. Postvoiding film showed poor evacuation. IVP had a possibility of a small obstructive situation in the distal right ureter, however, no calculi could be seen. Chest x-ray showed atheromatous changes within tortuous aorta. Uroflometry was performed on this patient revealing bladder outlet obstruction. Postvoid film showed marked postvoid retention.

It is my impression that this patient has probable diagnosis of adenocarcinoma of the prostate.

Metabolic profile: Glucose is elevated to 109. Creatinine was normal. Alkaline phosphatase 10 international units. BUN 25.9.

I took the patient to surgery on 5-18-78, TUR of prostate was performed, Foley catheter was removed the second postoperative day.

Patient was informed of his cancerous condition. I staged the tumor as a Stage D, Grade II, type adenocarcinoma of the prostate. I began treating him with Stilbesterol 3 mg, daily. Total care to Dr. L█████ in my absence after the 20th of May.

Dr. L███ will discharge this patient. I have recommended that he be rechecked in about three weeks in my office. I want to do a repeat bone scan in about three months to determine if there is more neoplastic involvement. If this disease progresses at this point, orchiectomy might be a procedure to consider in the future.

ROGER S█████ D.O.

RS:gw
cc: Dr. G█████
    Dr. Se█████
    Dr. L█████
DD: 5-20-78
DT: 5-30-78

401

X-RAY REPORT

Family Name	First Name	Middle Name		Room No.	Hosp. No.
Patient #41				324b	

☐ Treatment	Name—Part		Sex	Age—Years	X-ray No.
☐ Examination of	BONE SCAN		M F	76	

Attending Physician		Date	O.P.D. No.
DR. H.		2/18/80	

Report:

Total Body Bone Scan:
Total body bone scan demonstrates uptake of the nuclide mid portion of the spine at approximately the level of T-9. The remainder of the study is unremarkable.

Impression: Increased activity at what is believed to be T-9 consistent with metabolic bone disease. This may represent either trauma or metastasis. Clinical correlation is recommended.

LWBjr/mm

_____
Signature of Roentgenologist

REPORT OF OPERATION

Family Name	First Name	Middle Name	Attending Physician	Room No.	Hosp. No.
Patient #41			Roger S___, D. O.	324B	
	Resident		Intern	Date 2-21-80	

Preoperative Diagnosis: Adenocarcinoma of the prostate.

Postoperative Diagnosis: Adenocarcinoma of the prostate.

Surgeon: Roger S___, D. O. **Assistants:** Herber R___, D. O.
  Jan H___, D. O.

Operation: Transurethral resection of the prostate. '

GROSS SURGICAL FINDINGS: Patient had a marked resistance on calibration of the urethra, proximal area, in the area of the prostatic urethra. On direct visualization there was increased vascularity throughout the bladder wall. Both ureteral orifices were visualized. I could see no bladder neoplasia. The prostate had definite enlargement, typical of neoplasm when the cut surface was noted. It was very difficult to really adequately visualize the verumontanum, thus was unable to definitely appreciate the location of the external sphincter. Bimanual evaluation: Prostate was very hard, indurated, appeared to extend out from the side of the capsule, infiltrating the prostatic area into the hypogastric area.

PROCEDURE: Patient was prepped and draped. Dilatation was performed to 30 French. Resectoscope was inserted in the bladder. After gross visualization urethroscopy was performed. After urethroscopy, resection of the bladder neck and continuous prostate going toward the apical portion was carried out, starting at 6 o'clock, again starting at the bladder neck back to the apical portion, going around the left side to about 12 o'clock. Adequate tissue was removed, similar procedure was performed on the right side. Larger bleeding points were cauterized with fulguration. All pieces of tissue were removed. Foley catheter was left in place. Patient to postanesthetic recovery room in satisfactory condition.

RS:mb
D. 2-21-80
T. 2-25-80
cc: Dr. S___, Dr. R___
0241

ROGER S___, D. O.   Signature of Surgeon

Des Moines General Hospital

(OSTEOPATHIC)

DEPARTMENT OF PATHOLOGY

Case No [redacted]

Room 324 B

DATE RECEIVED ON REQUISITION:

Name Patient #41 [redacted] Age 76 Sex M Date of last Menses

Tissue Specimens to be Examined: Prostatic tissue

Clinical Diagnosis Possible prostate carcinoma

Exact Location of Biopsy NS

Dr. S[redacted] Dr. H[redacted] Spec. Received 2-21-80
Surgeon   Referring   Spec. Reported 2-22-80

Lab Specimen No. 80-P-710 Froz. Sec. Study Photo: Gross

MACROSCOPY: Numerous irregular portions of pinkish-white and grayish-white tissue are submitted, aggregating a combined weight of 8.0 gm. (All the specimen has been utilized in three containers.)   RMI

MICROSCOPY: Sections of the prostatic fragments show most infiltrated with anaplastic malignant epithelium. In most areas the tumor cells appear well differentiated, consisting of a columnar epithelium with the cells proliferating in areas with a cribriform pattern in a back-to-back manner. In small areas the lesion appears less differentiated, infiltrating in small groups.

SUMMARY: Prostatic curettings are submitted. Most of the fragments show infiltration with moderately well differentiated tumor.

DIAGNOSIS: Adenocarcinoma of the prostate, Grade II   T-77 M-8143

LWF:mh
CC:
Dr. S[redacted]
Dr. H[redacted]
Dr. G[redacted]
Dr. K[redacted]
Tumor Pty

[signature] D.O.
Pathologist

TISSUE STUDY

404

Family Name First Name	Attending Physician	Room No.	Hosp. No.
Patient #41	B. A. H████, D.O		████

Date of Admission: 2-17-80   **Date of Discharge:**   2-29-80

Admitting Diagnosis: Possible prostatic carcinoma

Final Diagnosis: Adenocarcinoma of the prostate
Urinary tract infection

Operations: Prostatectomy - transurethral

Consultants: R. S████, D.O.   L. B████, D.O.

Chief Complaint: This 76-year-old, white male is admitted to the hospital afer he was seen on an outpatient basis. He has a history of previous adenocarcinoma of the prostate. He was seen in my office complaining of abdominal pain with some difficulty on urination. Prostatic urination revealed a hard, nodular prostte and it was felt that this may be a recurrence of extension of his prostatic CA and he should be admitted to the hospital for evaluation and treatment as appropriate.

Laboratory Work: Sed rate was found to be 4 on admission. Urine reveals 1 to 2 WBCs, 0 to 1 RBCs, trace of bacteria per high powered field. CBC reveals 6.3 thousand white count. RBCs 4.64, hemoglobin 15.7, hematocrit 45.0. MCV was found to be 97. Colony count of the urine was 1.5 times 10 to the 6th organisms per cc. Cultured organisms were proteus mirabilis, Klebsiella pneumonia with multiple sensitivities. Surgical profile and potassium were found to be within normal limits. Blood type was found to be 0 Rh positive. CBC on 2-22 was basically within normal limits. Serum acid phosphatase is 0.37 which is slightly elevated. Metabolic profile reveals a gamma globulin of 9%. Other indices all within normal limits. Total body bone scan reveals increased activity at T-9 consistent with metabolic bone disease which is either trauma or metastasis. Colon x-ray and IVP revealed chronic bladder disease and prostatic hypertrophy with evidence of diverticular disease of the sigmoid colon. X-ray of the dorsal spine revealed spondylitic lipping anteriorly of many of the bodies. Chest x-ray was found to be normal. CT sccan of the prostate reveals benign prostatic hypertrophy with slight enlargement of the right superior lobe of the prostate with inability to prove any neoplastic changes. EKG reveals prolonged AV conduction with left bundle branch block.

After the patient was admitted to the hospital and workup was initially obtained, Dr. S████ was asked to see the patient. He felt that the patient in view of his symptoms and previous history shoulder undergo transurethral resection of the prostate for followup and treatment as appropriate. This was done and the final diagnosis came back adenocarcinoma of the prostate, Grade II. Consultation was then obtained with Dr. Loren B████ regarding possible chemotherapy and/or orchiectomy. The patient was advised that his best changes for survival would be to undergo treatment with estrogens and to undergo orchiectomy. The patient accepted the estrogens and refused to undergo orchiectomy. His postoperative course was basically uneventful and he was discharged in satisfactory condition on February 29th, 1980. He was given prescription for DES to take 3 mg daily. He was told to return to the office at the end of one week for followup evaluation and treatment as appropriate.

BAH/lep   CC: Dr. B.A. H████
DD: 3-31-80

405

Patient #42

Patient #42 is a 74-year-old man from California who has now survived nine years since his diagnosis of prostatic carcinoma.

Patient #42 has a long history of recurrent skin cancer, but otherwise he had been in good health when in April 1978 his physician noted an enlarged, tender prostate during a routine physical exam. Patient #42 was referred to a local urologist, who admitted him to the San Francisco Public Health Hospital on May 24, 1978 for a needle biopsy of his prostate. He was discharged before the diagnosis had been finalized, but when subsequent evaluation of the biopsy specimen confirmed adenocarcinoma, Patient #42 was re-admitted to the hospital on May 30, 1978.

At that time, a bone scan revealed an abnormality in the right eighth rib believed consistent with metastatic disease. Furthermore, a routine chest X-ray documented an infiltrate in the lower region of the left lung thought to be a possible additional area of metastases. This lesion had been present, but unnoticed, on an X-ray study from the previous hospitalization.

The patient's physicians recommended exploratory surgery, to determine the extent of disease, along with a course of radiation to the prostate. But Patient #42, already familiar with nutritional approaches to cancer, refused further testing and treatment. The attending physician wrote in his notes:

> He [Patient #42] declined all medical intervention [sic]. He appeared to
> be aware at the time of discharge of the consequences of his not receiving
> therapy for adenocarcinoma of the prostate.

Patient #42 was discharged from the hospital on June 14, 1978, but was re-admitted on June 25 for excision of two superficial skin cancers. During this third hospitalization, a repeat chest X-ray again revealed the suspicious region in the left lung, described in the records:

> the infiltrate [lesion] had not cleared and the possibility of an underlying
> neoplasm could not be excluded.

After leaving the hospital on June 29, 1978, Patient #42 consulted Dr. Kelley and began the full regimen shortly thereafter. Within weeks, he noticed an improvement in his general health and when last contacted nearly nine years after his diagnosis, Patient #42 still followed his nutritional protocol, and showed no sign of cancer. He reported—although I have no documentation to support this—that on a recent physical exam, his prostate was found to be completely normal.

In summary, Patient #42 was diagnosed by biopsy with prostate carcinoma that appeared to have metastasized, possibly to both bone and lung. Since he refused surgery, radiation, chemotherapy and hormones, it seems reasonable to attribute Patient #42's prolonged survival to the Kelley program.

Standard Form 515
Rev. Jan. 1957
Promulgated
By Bureau of the Budget
Circular A-32

☆ U.S. GOVERNMENT PRINTING OFFICE: 1970—409-099

CLINICAL RECORD	TISSUE EXAMINATION

SPECIMEN SUBMITTED BY *Dr B███*	DATE OBTAINED 5-24-78

SPECIMEN

Prostate bx Rt + Lt lobes.

BRIEF CLINICAL HISTORY (Include duration of lesion and rapidity of growth, if a neoplasm)

Firm Lt lobe. ?/o CA

PREOPERATIVE DIAGNOSIS

"

OPERATIVE FINDINGS

"

POSTOPERATIVE DIAGNOSIS

"

SIGNATURE AND TITLE VK ███

PATHOLOGICAL REPORT

NAME OF LABORATORY	ACCESSION NO(S). S78-1411

(Gross description, histologic examination and diagnoses)

GROSS

Specimen is received in fixative in two parts and are grossly similar consisting of delicate threads of prostatic tissue measuring up to 2 cms. in length and 1 mm. in diameter. Part 1 is labeled right lobe of prostate and Part 2 is labeled left lobe of prostate. The entire specimen is submitted.

DY:di
5/24/78

MICRO

Part 1. The biopsy of the right lobe of the prostate shows only hyperplastic change with both glands and stroma increased. No tumor is present.

Sections of the left lobe of the prostate biopsy consist of several fragments showing malignant change. The tumor is a very well differentiated adenocarcinoma forming regular glands. The tumor infiltrates into the adjacent stroma and quite frequently rests directly on smooth muscle fibers. No evidence of nerve involvement is seen.

DIAGNOSIS: 1. Prostate, right lobe, benign prostatic hyperplasia.
DY:rr   2.   left lobe, adenocarcinoma well differentiated infiltrating
5-25-78

(Continue on reverse side)

SIGNATURE OF PATHOLOGIST				DATE
DANIEL Y███, M.D. DEP. CH. OF PATHOLOGY				

	AGE	SEX	RACE	IDENTIFICATION NO.
Patient #42 ███				

PATIENT'S IDENTIFICATION (For typed or written entries give: Name—last, first, middle; grade; date; hospital or medical facility)

REGISTER NO. ███	WARD NO. O.P.D.

TISSUE EXAMINATION
Standard Form 515
515-105-06

19 1 78

408

GENERAL SERVICES ADMINISTRATION AND
INTERAGENCY COMMITTEE ON MEDICAL RECORDS
FPMR 101-11.806-8
OCTOBER 1975

CLINICAL RECORD	NARRATIVE SUMMARY

DATE OF ADMISSION 5/30/78	DATE OF DISCHARGE 6/14/78	NUMBER OF DAYS HOSPITALIZED

(Sign and date at end of narrative)

HISTORY: The patient is a 65-year-old white male, who is noted to have a nodular prostate with negative examination who had cystoscopy and prostate biopsy performed on 5/24/78, which revealed kissing lateral lobes, with moderate, coarse trabeculation of the bladder, and adenocarcinoma of the prostate on biopsy. Following his biopsy, he was begun on Septra prophylaxis, and developed a rash, indicating an allergy to Septra. He returned on 5/30/78 to this hospital. He was noted to be febrile. He was started on intravenous Ampicillin.

PHYSICAL EXAMINATION: At the time was unremarkable, save for a tender, swollen prostate on rectal examination at the time of admission.

LABORATORY DATA: When he was admitted revealed a white count of 12,400. Urinalysis: Hematuria and pyuria were present. chest x-ray was unremarkable. BUN was 9.0. Creatinine was 0.9. Liver function studies and acid phosphatase were within normal limits. Pro time was 11.5/11.5. Urine cultures showed no growths. EKG: Showed nonspecific ST-T changes.

HOSPITAL COURSE: Following biopsy, the patient underwent metastatic workup, which included bone scan, which had a suggestion of an osteoblastic lesion in the right 8th rib, posteriorly, but was otherwise unremarkable. This was not confirmed by x-rays in this area. Alkaline phosphatase, liver function studies were within normal limits. The patient was counseled as to the nature of his disease, and it was recommended to consider either surgical therapy or radiation therapy. The staging laparotomy was proposed as the initial surgical procedure, to evaluate the spread of his disease. He declined all medical intervention, and requested that his medical care be continued by his local physician. He appeared to be aware at the time of discharge of the consequences of his not receiving therapy for adenocarcinoma of the prostate. Additional chest x-ray at the time of discharge, 6/12/78, revealed a pneumonitis, which, in retrospect had been present on previous films. These had been read as normal. This may represent resolving acute disease or may possibly be an indication of metastatic disease. Further evaluation of this problem is indicated soon. (continued)

(Use additional sheets of this form (Standard Form 502) if more space is required)

SIGNATURE OF PHYSICIAN	DATE	IDENTIFICATION NO.	ORGANIZATION	
MICHAEL B▊▊, M.D.	6/26/78			AS

PATIENT'S IDENTIFICATION (For typed or written entries give: Name - last, first, middle; grade; date; hospital or medical facility)	REGISTER NO. ▊▊▊	WARD NO. 5E

Patient #42

PHS HOSPITAL, SAN FRANCISCO, CA 94118

NARRATIVE SUMMARY
Standard Form 502
502-112

409

GENERAL SERVICES ADMINISTRATION AND
INTERAGENCY COMMITTEE ON MEDICAL RECORDS
FPMR 101-11.806-8
OCTOBER 1975

CLINICAL RECORD	NARRATIVE SUMMARY	
DATE OF ADMISSION 5/30/78	DATE OF DISCHARGE 6/14/78	NUMBER OF DAYS HOSPITALIZED

(Sign and date at end of narrative)

page 2

DIAGNOSES:
1. Adenocarcinoma of prostate.
2. Pulmonary infiltrate, left lower lobe.
3. Stable angina.

OPERATIONS: None.

DISPOSITION:
1. The patient has been advised to receive appropriate medical therapy to be given by his local physician at the earliest possible date.
2. No activity limitations.
3. Admit to Plastic Surgery, 6/25/78, for removal of basal cell carcinoma of the nose, discovered during admission.

There are no medicines.

PROGNOSIS: Unknown at this time. *Pt advised to pursue further evaluation and treatment for prostate cancer and lung infiltrate.*

MB:bk
T 6/26/78

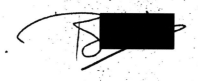

(Use additional sheets of this form (Standard Form 502) if more space is required)

SIGNATURE OF PHYSICIAN MICHAEL B████, M.D.	DATE 6/29/78	IDENTIFICATION NO.	ORGANIZATION	AS
PATIENT'S IDENTIFICATION (For typed or written entries give: Name - last, first, middle; grade; date; hospital or medical facility)		REGISTER NO. ████	WARD NO. 5E	

Patient #42

PHS HOSPITAL, SAN FRANCISCO, CALIFORNIA 94118

NARRATIVE SUMMARY
Standard Form 502
502-112

410

GENERAL SERVICES ADMINISTRATION AND
INTERAGENCY COMMITTEE ON MEDICAL RECORDS
FPMR 101-11.806-8
OCTOBER 1975

CLINICAL RECORD	NARRATIVE SUMMARY

DATE OF ADMISSION	DATE OF DISCHARGE	NUMBER OF DAYS HOSPITALIZED
6/25/78	6/29/78	

(Sign and date at end of narrative)

HISTORY: This 65 year old married white male American seaman was admitted for the treatment of skin lesions on the nasal tip and left cheek. Present illness: The patient has had two skin lesions, as noted above, which have not been particularly bothersome, save that the nasal tip lesion has bled and slightly increased in size over the past several weeks. He has had numerous skin neoplasms treated in the past by various mechanisms, including Liquid Nitrogen, Efudex, VMC, etc. He had a recent admission here on the Urology Service for work-up of a "malignant lump" on his prostate and was advised to have a surgical procedure, but elected not to have it at this facility, but to have it at his local hospital in Monterey, California, where his wife can assist in his postoperative care, and he is planning on being seen in consultation regarding this the last week in June. The patient is also noted to have a very slowly resolving pulmonary infiltrate in the left lower lobe and the possibility of neoplasm in this regard is also evident. The patient has had a relatively extensive work-up in the past while on the Urology Service in regards to his prostatic lesion, and metastatic carcinoma could not be completely ruled out. He has no bone pain as such, and he is re-admitted to the hospital at this time for the treatment of the nasal skin lesions, which are suspected of being basal cell epitheliomas. Past medical history, past family history and review of systems are essentially unchanged from his previous admission, the patient having been discharged from the hospital just 10 days ago. Current regular medications incluse Isordil, 5 mg., t.i.d. He is allergic to Sulfa drugs, but denies any history of hepatitis, jaundice or clotting defects and has not been a regular user of salicylates.

PHYSICAL EXAMINATION: The patient appeared to be a well developed, well nourished, white male who was alert, oriented, cooperative and in no acute distress. Lungs were clear to auscultation bilaterally. Cardiovascular examination was within normal limits as well. The pertinent physical findings revealed an 8 x 10 mm. elevated skin lesion, just to the left of the nasal tip, with several small telangiectatic vessels over its surface and with a tendency to have a rolled edge. There are also small, slightly ulcerated, skin lesions on the lower aspect of the left lower lids, in the upper left cheek area. The later lesion, which measured approximately 3 x 4 mm., did not appear to be tender and had no evidence of inflammation. No palpable adenopathy was noted in the cervical

CONTINUED

(Use additional sheets of this form (Standard Form 502) if more space is required)

SIGNATURE OF PHYSICIAN	DATE	IDENTIFICATION NO.	ORGANIZATION
JAMES H. K███, M.D.	6/28/78		AS

PATIENT'S IDENTIFICATION *(For typed or written entries give: Name - last, first, middle; grade; date; hospital or medical facility)*	REGISTER NO.	WARD NO.
Patient #42 PHS HOSPITAL, SAN FRANCISCO, CA 94118		3W

NARRATIVE SUMMARY
Standard Form 502
502-112

411

CLINICAL RECORD	NARRATIVE SUMMARY

DATE OF ADMISSION	DATE OF DISCHARGE	NUMBER OF DAYS HOSPITALIZED
6/25/78	6/29/78	

Page 2   *(Sign and date at end of narrative)*

area. Repeat rectal examination was not carried out at this time, in anticipation of an acid phosphatase determination by the Laboratory the day after admission.

LABORATORY DATA: The admission chest x-ray revealed some slight improvement since the original examination on 5/30, but the infiltrate had not cleared, and the possibility of an underlying neoplasm could not be excluded. BUN was 11 mg.%, creatinine 0.9 mg.%, uric acid 4.5 mg.%. Alkaline phosphatase 66 Centi units; acid phosphatase 55 Centi units; SGOT 87 Centi units. CBC, urinalysis and VDRL were within normal limits.

HOSPITAL COURSE: The patient was taken to the Operating Room on 6/26/78, where under local anesthesia he underwent removal of the left cheek lesion, with a transposition skin flap for closure of the defect, as well as excision of the basal cell epithelioma on the left nasal tip, with a left nasolabial flap as the method of closure for this defect. These areas healed quite well postoperatively, and at the time of discharge all areas were free of gross evidence of infection and appeared to be healing well. He was instructed to have the sutures removed on July 3 by his local surgeon, since he will be out of the city at that time. He is to be followed in Monterey, California by a local physician there in regard to further evaluation of his pulmonary infiltrate and his adenocarcinoma of the prostate. He was discharged, improved, ambulatory, taking a regular diet and afebrile on 6/29/78, on no new medications, save for topical Maxitrol Ophthalmic Ointment.

DIAGNOSIS:
1. Adenocarcinoma, prostate.
2. Left lower lobe pulmonary infiltrate, etiology undetermined.
3. Basal cell epitheliomata, left nasal tip and left cheek.

OPERATIONS:
1. Excision, basal cell epithelioma, left nasal tip, with left nasolabial flap.
2. Excision, basal cell epithelioma, left cheek, with transposition skin flap, 6/26/78 (on both procedures).

sheets of this form (Standard Form 502) if more space is required)

SIGNATURE OF PHYSICIAN	DATE	IDENTIFICATION NO.	ORGANIZATION
JAMES H. K████, M.D.	6/28/78		AS

PATIENT'S IDENTIFICATION (For typed or written entries give: Name - last, first, middle; grade; date; hospital or medical facility)	REGISTER NO.	WARD NO.
Patient #42 ████	████	3W

PHS HOSPITAL, SAN FRANCISCO, CA 94118

NARRATIVE SUMMARY
Standard Form 502
502-112

412

Patient #43

Patient #43 is an 81-year-old chiropractor from Arizona, alive 11 years since his diagnosis of metastatic prostatic carcinoma.

In November 1975, Patient #43 first experienced pain in the region of the right shoulder blade that worsened over a several-week period. After consulting his primary doctor, he was referred to an orthopedist. X-ray studies revealed compression fractures in the seventh and eighth thoracic vertebrae, believed to be the result of osteoporosis. At that point, the physician prescribed a number of supportive braces, but informed Patient #43 that nothing more could be done from an orthopedic perspective.

Over the following months, the shoulder pain gradually worsened. Finally, in the spring of 1976, Patient #43 consulted a second physician who discovered, after routine testing, an elevated level of the enzyme alkaline phosphatase—a finding at times associated with bone disease.

Patient #43 was admitted to Nebraska Methodist Hospital on June 2, 1976 for further evaluation. There, laboratory studies revealed an alkaline phosphatase of over 350 (normal less than 180) and an acid phosphatase of 302 (normal 0–10) with a prostatic fraction of 269, results strongly suggesting prostate cancer.

Patient #43 then underwent a needle biopsy of his prostate, which confirmed adenocarcinoma in all specimens. At that point, the bone lesions were thought to be definitely metastatic in origin, and subsequently Patient #43 underwent bilateral orchiectomy (removal of both testes), to reduce his testosterone levels. During the procedure, the surgeon discovered tumor extending into the bladder and subsequent diagnostic studies, including a bone scan, confirmed extensive, stage D-2 metastatic disease, clearly summarized in the records:

> Chest x-ray revealed extensive skeletal metastasis . . . Bone scan revealed multiple areas of increased uptake [areas of disease] throughout the skeleton.

While still hospitalized, Patient #43 began oral estrogen therapy and a course of radiation to his spine for pain relief. After his discharge on June 26, 1976, he continued the radiation as an outpatient, but despite the treatment, Patient #43 failed to improve. Then during the second week of July 1976, when his mental status suddenly deteriorated, in a confused, disoriented state, he was readmitted to Nebraska Methodist.

413

A thorough evaluation revealed the cancer was growing unchecked, as described in the hospital records:

> Chest x-ray revealed wide spread lytic and blastic lesions suggestive of prostatic carcinoma. There has been interval development of bilateral pleural effusions along with some increased markings suggestive of lymphatic metastases since the film of 6-3-76. Films of the thoraco-lumbar spine showed diffuse involvement with metastatic carcinoma with compression of T-7, T-8 [thoracic vertebrae] and slight compression of L-1 [lumbar vertebra] . . . Pathologic rib fractures were described. These were felt related to metastatic disease. X-ray of the pelvis revealed metastatic bony involvement. Films of the sacrum and coccyx again revealed again [sic] metastatic bony involvement . . . Chest x-ray of 7-27 revealed increase in the bilateral pleural fluid. Films of the left hip dated 7-31 revealed no evidence of fracture. Diffuse skeletal metastases were seen. Brain scan was normal. However, an abnormally positive skull or spine lesions [were noted] on the previous bone scan.

Patient #43 completed a second course of "palliative megavoltage external radiation to the lumbar spine." Eventually, after more than five weeks in the hospital, his pain and mental status improved sufficiently so that he could return home. Nevertheless, when discharged on August 26, 1976 Patient #43's physicians warned he most probably would not live out the year.

In desperation, Patient #43 decided to investigate unconventional approaches to cancer. In September 1976, he learned of Dr. Kelley, and shortly thereafter began the full nutritional program, at the same time discontinuing hormone medication.

Within several months, all of Patient #43's symptoms—his bone pain, fatigue, lethargy and malaise—resolved, and he says within two years he felt better than at any time in his life. Today, 11 years after his diagnosis, Patient #43 still follows the Kelley program, reporting excellent health with no sign of his once extensive disease. At age 81, he works part-time as a chiropractor and plays violin in a ragtime band.

Patient #43 is another unusual patient. He was initially diagnosed with widely metastatic prostatic cancer that failed to respond to orchiectomy, radiation, and

414

a course of estrogen therapy. His condition improved only after he abandoned conventional treatment and began the Kelley program. It seems logical, therefore, to attribute his prolonged survival and current good health to his nutritional protocol.

nebraska methodist hospital
8303 dodge street
omaha, nebraska 68114

CC: Back pain primarily in the right shoulder.

HPI: Since November of 1975 the patient has complained of right scapular pain, x-rays taken at that time revealed a compression fracture of the T-7 through tT-8 vertebrae according to the patient. He denies any incident of trauma. Patient consulted several doctors and had been wearing a number of supporative devices to help with the pain, which would exaberate on movement of the upper extremities. These devices range from a rib belt to a steel brace. However, patient suffered much soreness in the anterior ribs and as intermittently use the braces because of the soreness. Approximately 2 months ago the patient saw and endocrinologist by the name Dr. L___ in Arizona and the doctor notified the patient that he had an elevated alkaline phosphatase value being approximately 202. Dr. L___ then told _____, the patient, that he should have a urologist see him. Dr. L___ did do a prostate exam and on examination that the prostate was stony hard however he did not find any gross lesion. He however felt that the patient's symptoms may be secondary to CA of the prostate. At the time of Dr. L___'s exam and now the patient has had no GU symptoms. According to the patient, the right scapular pain would at times radiate to the left scapula and sometimes involve the muscles of the upper extremities. He was taking Tandaril loo mg. for the pain but he denies any relief. In addition yesterday the patient did use Darvon and he claims this has been of no help either.

PMH: Operations: T & A 1925, appendectomy 1926.
     Illnesses: Patient's childhood illnesses were unremarkable. In adult life he suffered
                    from asthma severely. He did live on a farm, moved to Arizona prim arily
                    because of his asthma and there he has had no problems and has taken no
                    meds.
     Allergies: Patient has no known drug or food allergies.
     Medications: Other than the medication Tandaril for pain and the Darvon unremarkable.

RCS: HEENT: Negative.
     Skin: Negative.
     CV: Negative. He denies any chest pains.
     Resp: Negative.
     GI: Occasional constipation which he relieves with laxative.
     GU: Negative other than that stated in the HPI.
     MS: Unremaarkable except for the in the HPI.
     Neuro: Negative.

FH: Patient's father died at the age of 70 of cancer of the pancreas. Patient has a 67 year old sister who is still alive and has diabetes. Patient has never had a ny children.

SH: This patient is a retired chiropractor presently lives in Arizona. He has never smoked and is.a social drinker.

PHYSICAL EXAMINATION:
     General: 70 year old white male, 5'4", 141 lbs. Patient was most cooperative,
                    very accurate historian and no acute distress.

HISTORY & PHYSICAL   HISTORY & PHYSICAL   HISTORY & PHYSICAL   HISTORY & PHYSICAL

416

PATIENT NAME: Patient #43

HOSPITAL NUMBER: PAGE 2

PHYSICIAN:

nebraska methodist hospital
8303 dodge street
omaha, nebraska 68114

Vital signs:	ORal temp. 98.2, pulse 62, resp. 16 and regular, BP 164/90 from left arm.
Skin:	Patient had numerous senile keratosis of the anterior chest and the posterior chest wall. He also had febrile areas that were slightly raised and erythematous but with scaling. These areas were not tender and seemed to be case of seborrheic dermatitis. Skin turgor was normal.
HEENT:	Normal cephalic and without bruits. Eyes clear sclera bilaterally and normal eyegrounds. PERRLA and normal EOMS. Nostrils is unremarkable. Throat revealed slightly hyperemic pharyngeal area, midline uvula, and no gross lesions.
Neck:	Not supple. There was some tenderness in the left supraclavicular area, however there were no nodes or masses found. Patient did have somewhat restricted range of movement, and movement would cause exacerbation of his back pain. Thyroid was not palpable. Trachea was midline. Carotids were 2+ on the left side and 1+ on the right side without bruits.
Chest:	Patient had rather barrel shaped chest. The lung fields were clear to A and P. There were no wheezes or rales or rhonchi. Axillary nodes were negative and there were no masses found in the chest wall. There was some slight tenderness around the 3rd-5th anterior ribs on the right side.
Heart:	Patient had a normal sinus rhythm. PMI was in the 5th intercostal space in the left midclavicular line, there were no murmurs or gallops or rubs.
Abdomen:	There is a scar in the lower right quadrant from his appendectomy. The abdomen was rather tender to palpation, he claims he was vomiting several times this morning and that his reason for the abdominal tenderness. There was no organomegaly or masses felt. There was no evidence of diastasis of the rectus muscle. Patient did seem to have some left CVA tenderness however.
Genitalia:	Normal uncircumsized male.
Rectal:	Patient had normal external sphincter tone, with no evidence of external hemorrhoids. Examination of the prostate revealed a rather stony hard prostate without any gross nodules. It could not be perceived if the patient's prostate was enlarged.
Extrem:	Radial was 2+/4 and equal, femoral pulse 1+/4 and equal, dorsalis pedis not perceived. Patient had normal muscle strength in all extremities. However he seemed to have some limited range of movement in the upper extremities particularly on elevating the hands above the head. There was no evidence of cyanosis, clubbing or edema.
Neuro:	Cranial nerves 2 thorugh 12 were grossly intact. DTRs were 2+/4 and equal. Patient had no obvious sensory loss. On the shin to heel test patient had some gross tremor but no pass pointing on the finger to nose test. He had no pathological reflexes such as Babinski or Hoffmann. Gait was rather stiff but steady.

IMPRESSION: Upper right back pain with history of compression fracture of T7 through T-8 possibly secondary to metastatic carcinoma of the prostate.
Stony hard prostate. High BP.

ES/kw 23-89
6-4-76

ERROL S_____, M4

RONALD W_____, M. D.

HISTORY & PHYSICAL   HISTORY & PHYSICAL   HISTORY & PHYSICAL   HISTORY & PHYSICAL

417

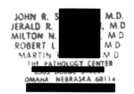

JOHN R. S█████ M.D.
JERALD R. █████ M.D.
MILTON N. █████ M.D.
ROBERT L █████ M.D
MARTIN █████ M.D
THE PATHOLOGY CENTER
█████████
OMAHA NEBRASKA 68114

Patient #43

6-9-75

█████ N 70 615 -1

Perineal prostatic biopsy. "F"
Right testicle.
Left testicle.

Hal W█████, M.D.

cc: R. W█████, M.D.

Omaha, NE

CLINICAL DIAGNOSIS AND HISTORY

Question of carcinoma of prostate.

GROSS DESCRIPTION

The first part, labeled "perineal prostatic needle biopsy", and previously submitted for frozen section with the diagnosis of adenocarcinoma, consists of two firm, gray-tan cylinders of fibrous-appearing tissue, the larger measuring 1.8 x 0.2 cm.

The second part, labeled "left testicle", consists of a soft, smooth, glistening gray-white, 4.5 x 3.2 x 2.8 cm. testicle together with coverings and a 2 cm. segment of spermatic cord with aggregate weight of 38 grams. Sectioning reveals a glistening, homogeneous, soft, tan cut surface from which seminiferous tubules string. Sectioning reveals no obvious lesions.

The third part, labeled "right testicle", consists of an entirely similar-appearing, 4.5 x 3.4 x 2.2 cm. testicle, coverings and section of vas and spermatic cord measuring 1.3 cm. The tunica is smooth and glistening. Sectioning the testis reveals a similar pattern to that noted above. No gross lesions are noted.

MICROSCOPIC DIAGNOSIS

Adenocarcinoma, perineal prostatic needle biopsy.
Oligospermia, mild, right and left testes.

do

ML:pl

418

PATIENT NAME: Patient #43

HOSPITAL NUMBER:

PHYSICIAN: A. F█████, M. D.

nebraska methodist hospital
8303 dodge street
omaha, nebraska 68114

ADMITTED: 6-2-76

DISCHARGED: 6-26-76

FINAL DIAGNOSIS: Adenocarcinoma of the prostate.

SECONDARY DX: Wide spread bony metastasis.

OPERATION: Prostate needle biopsy and bilateral orchiectomy on 6-8-76.
Biopsy of skin lesions of the back 6-23-76.

History: The patient is a 70 year old white male who has noted back pain since November of 1975.
He was treated symptomatically for his complaint. He also developed some pain in his anterior
ribs. About 2 months prior to admission the patient was seen by a physician for evaluation of
his problems. He was found to have a markedly elevated alkaline phosphatase. The patient is
now referred to NMH for evaluation and treatment. On physical examination the lungs were clear
to auscultation. There was no evidence of any peripheral adenopathy. No abdominal organomegaly
or masses were palpated. On rectal examination the prostate was hard without nodularity.
Several reddish, scalling, sharply circumscribed lesions were present on the lower back and
right upper chest.

X-ray and lab data: Perineal needle biopsy of the prostate revealed adenocarcinoma. Skin
biopsy of back lesions revealed basal cell carcinoma. CBC of 6-4-76 revealed white count of
6,500, hmg. 12.1, hmt. 37. Platelets were normal. BUN 26, glucose 100, TSP 6.3, albumin 3.9,
calcium 8.7, phosphorus 3.3, cholesterol 205, uric acid 5.5, creatinine 1.1, total bilirubin
0.6, alkaline phosphatase over 350, SGOT 10. Acid phosphatase 202, normal being 0-10, oros-
tatic fraction was 269 normal being 0-4. Chest x-ray revealed extensive skeletal metastasis.
IVP revealed prostatic enlargement. Irritability of the calyces consistent with pyelitis was
noted. Some nephrolithiasis on the left was seen. An old calcified infarct in the spleen was
present. Considerable osteoporosis of the lumbar spine was noted. Right retrograde pyelogram
revealed the upper pole calyces of the right kidney to be incompletely filled. The collecting
system and ureter showed no intrinsic abnormalities. No calculi are seen along the right
ureter. Bone scan revealed multiple areas of increased uptake throughout the skeleton.

Hospital course: During his hospitalization the patient was evaluated regarding the extent
of his disease. On 6-8-76 the patient was taken to the operating room where a perineal needle
biopsy of the prostate and a bilateral orchiectomy were performed. He was subsequently started
on Stilphostrol therapy. Megavoltage external radiation to the dorsal spine for relief of pain
was initiated. Circumscribed skin lesions of the back were biopsied and found to be basal
cell carcinoma. The diagnosis and treatment of these lesions were under the supervision of
Dr. F████████. Patient tolerated his treatment moderately well. He did have some nausea
which was treated with antimedication.

Disposition and instructions to patient:
At the time of discharge from the hospital the patient was improved. He will continue to take
his

419

PATIENT NAME:

HOSPITAL NUMBER:

PHYSICIAN

    A. F████, M. D.

   Admitted: 7-12-76

   Discharged: 8-26-76

nebraska methodist hospital.
8303 dodge street
omaha, nebraska 68114

FINAL DIAGNOSIS: Adenocarcinoma of the prostate with wide spread bony metastases.

SECONDARY DX: None.

OPERATIONS: None.

Patient is a 70 year old white male with a known diagnosis of adenocarcinoma of the prostate with wide spread metastases. Patient is presently undergoing a course of palliative external radiation to the dorsal spine on an outpatient basis. He has been doing well but during the past few days the patient has had trouble speaking especially with articulation of words. He has also had some photophobia along with dizziness. According to his wife the patient may be acting somewhat depressed. He is being admitted to the hospital for futher evaluation and treatment. On physical examination patient appeared to be somewhat lethargic and drowsy. There was no evidence of any peripheral adenopathy. Auscultation of the lungs reveals bronchial sounds on expiration. No abdominal organomegaly or masses were palpated. Prostate gland is slightly enlarged and hard.

X-ray and lab data: CBC of 7-12-76 reveals a white count of 4,700, hmg. 10.3, hmt. 31. Platelets were normal. Blood chemistry of 7-12 revealed sodium 136, potassium 4.7, chloride 106, CO2 29, BUN 18, glucose 88, TSP 5.7, albumin 3.3, calcium 7.9, phosphorus 3.9, cholesterol 149, uric acid 4.0, creatinine 0.7, total bilirubin 0.3, alkaline phosphatase over 350, SGOT 15. Protein electrophoresis appeared to be within normal limits. Acid phosphatase was within normal limits. Chest x-ray revealed wide spread lytic and blastic lesions suggestive of prostatic carcinoma. There has been interval developement of bilateral pleural effusions along with some increased markings suggestive of lymphatic metastases since the film of 6-3-76. Films of the thoraco-lumbar spine showed diffuse involvement with metastastic carcinoma with compression of T-7, T-8 and slight compression of L1. Degenerative changes at the lumbosacral level were noted. Patho-logic rib fractures were described. These were felt related to metastatic disease. X-ray of the pelvis revealed metastatic bony involvement. Films of the sacrum and coccyx again revealed again metatstatic bony involvement. Chest x-ray of 7-22 revealed increased infiltrative changes in the left base and increased pleural fluid in the right base. Chest x-ray of 7-27 revealed increase in the bilateral pleural fluid. Films of the left hip dated 7-31 revealed no evidence of fracture. Diffuse skeletal metastases were seen. Brain scan was normal. However an abnormally positive skull or spine lesions on the previous bone scan.

Hospital course: During his hospitalization the patient was srated on palliative megavoltage external radiation to the lumbar spine. The aim of this external radiation was the relief of pain secondary to bony metastases. A work up was undertaken to determine the cause of his dizziness. The brain scan was normal. Surgical curettement of several basal cell carcinomas of his lower back was performed. He was treated with diuretic medication and was noted to have less pitting edema of his legs. The curetted lesions of the lower back healed well. Patient did have some problem with nausea during the course of his treatment but this was symptomatically cntrolled with antimedic medication.

Disposition and instruments to patient: At time of dismissal from the hospital the patient appeared to be generally improved. We will continue to follow him on an outpatient basis for

DISCHARGE SUMMARY   DISCHARGE SUMMARY   DISCHARGE SUMMARY   DISCHARGE SUMMARY

420

nebraska methodist hospital
8303 dodge street
omaha, nebraska 68114

further evaluation and treatment of his disease.

AF/kw 207-187
11-11-76

Albert F█████, M. D.

421

RECTAL CANCER

Rectal cancer is an aggressive malignancy, responsible for 8,000 deaths in 1987. Despite advances in diagnosis, the five-year survival rate for this disease is still only 40%. When localized, rectal cancer can be cured with surgery and adjuvant radiation, but few patients with metastatic disease survive five years.

Patient #44

Patient #44 is a 62-year-old woman from Iowa who has survived more than five years since diagnosed with metastatic rectal carcinoma.

In late 1981, Patient #44 noted a change in her bowel habits, with onset of constipation associated with the passage of occasional blood-tinged, ribbon-like stools. Concurrently, her appetite diminished, and over a three month period, she lost ten pounds. When her symptoms persisted, Patient #44 consulted her local physician, who referred her to a proctologist. On January 25, 1982, sigmoidoscopy (examination of the rectum and lower colon with a flexible tube) revealed an ulcerated lesion in the lower rectum, with biopsies indicating rectal adenocarcinoma.

Patient #44 was then admitted to the University of Iowa Hospital on February 8, 1982 for further evaluation. Review of the previous biopsy slides confirmed "invasive moderately well differentiated adenocarcinoma," and on February 10, 1982, Patient #44 underwent surgery for resection of the tumor obstructing the sigmoid colon and upper rectum. Of 32 adjacent lymph nodes removed, 18 were positive for cancer—a very ominous sign.

After surgery, Patient #44's physicians informed her that the cancer would most likely metastasize and prove terminal, even with aggressive radiation and chemotherapy. Despite the poor prognosis, they nonetheless strongly recommended she proceed with adjuvant systemic treatment, but Patient #44, who already knew of Dr. Kelley's work, refused further conventional approaches. Instead, after leaving the hospital on February 20, 1982, she began the full Kelley program under the supervision of a counselor trained in the method.

Over a period of several months, Patient #44 reports she gradually regained her strength, energy, and sense of well being. Subsequently, she remained in excellent health until late 1986, nearly five years after her diagnosis, when she experienced nausea, anorexia, and indigestion that worsened throughout early 1987. Finally, on April 21, 1987, she was admitted to Des Moines General Hospital for emergency surgery and correction of what proved to be an acute intestinal obstruction, resulting from scar tissue forming after her original operation in 1982. However, she appeared to be completely free of cancer, and when last contacted, Patient #44 was recuperating from her recent ordeal, determined to continue her nutritional regimen.

The prognosis for rectal cancer, once metastatic to multiple regional lymph nodes, is dismal. Sugarbaker reports that lymph node involvement represents the single most important prognostic variable for colorectal cancer, with the chance for long-term survival diminishing significantly as the number of affected nodes increases.[1]

Copeland and his colleagues described a 10% five-year survival rate in 110 patients with colorectal cancer presenting initially with at least five cancerous lymph nodes.[2] In addition to surgery, most of these patients were aggressively treated with either chemotherapy or radiation, or both. In view of the 18 positive nodes discovered at the time of this patient's initial diagnosis, her continued cancer-free survival, now in excess of five years, represents an unusual outcome for such extensive disease.

REFERENCES

1. DeVita, VT, et al. *Cancer Principles & Practice of Oncology*. Philadelphia; J.B. Lippincott Company, 1982, page 672.

2. Copeland, EM, et al. "Prognostic Factors in Carcinoma of the Colon and Rectum." *American Journal of Surgery* 1968; 116:875–880.

UNIVERSITY OF IOWA HOSPITALS AND CLINICS

Iowa City, Iowa

COPY

(This carbon copy of correspondence regarding the patient to be filed in the patient's record UNDER other forms of Section B of the appropriate admission. Xerox, Verifax or Thermofax copies can be made from this sheet.)

February 22, 1982

Re: Patient #44

C. W. M███████, Jr., M.D.
███████
Toledo, Iowa 52342

Dear Doctor M█████:

███████ was admitted to the Surgery Service on February 8, 1982. She is a 57-year-old female with a three month history of ribbon-like and blood tinged stools and progressive constipation. She complained of a ten pound weight loss. Proctosigmoidoscopy performed locally revealed a sigmoid mass. Biopsy of this mass revealed moderately well differentiated adenocarcinoma. She was admitted at this time for surgical therapy of the sigmoid lesion.

Following admission proctosigmoidoscopy was performed. A friable mass was seen at the 9 o'clock position 10 to 12 cm beyond the anal verge. Review of the pathology slides from the previous biopsy confirmed the diagnosis of moderately well differentiated adenocarcinoma. Intravenous pyelogram was normal. Preoperative laboratory data including liver function tests were normal. Chest x-ray and EKG were normal.

On February 10 ███████ underwent anterior resection of the sigmoid mass with primary anastomosis of the colon. Pathologic examination of the tissue revealed invasive moderately well differentiated adenocarcinoma extending through the muscle to the serosa. Eighteen of 32 nodes were positive for tumor. ███████ tolerated the procedure well and had an uneventful postoperative course.

At the time of discharge on the tenth postoperative day she was afebrile and tolerating a regular diet well. The wound which was closed by delayed primary technique was healing well. Discharge medications included iron sulfate, 300 mg, p.o., t.i.d.; Colace, 100 mg, p.o., t.i.d.; and Demerol, 50 mg, p.o., q4h, p.r.n. She is to return to the Surgery Clinic in one month for routine followup. CEA level was pending at the time of discharge.

Sincerely,

Brance E. M█████, M.D.
Resident

Adel A█████, M.D.
Associate Professor of Surgery

BEM:sb

426

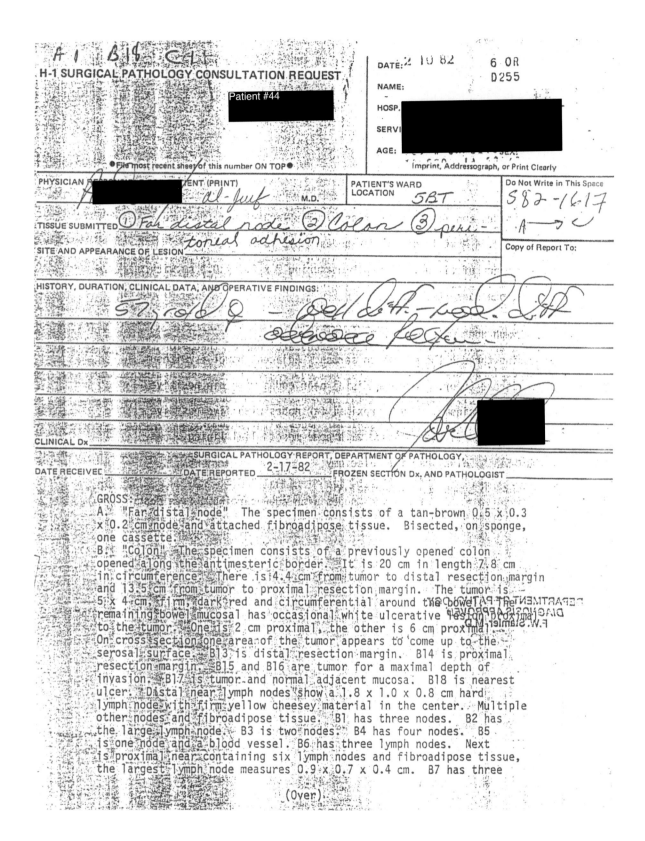

A 1 B18 C4

Patient #44

DATE: 2 10 82   6 OR
                  D 255
NAME:
HOSP.
SERVI
AGE: SEX:
● File most recent sheet of this number ON TOP ●   Imprint, Addressograph, or Print Clearly

PHYSICIAN R_____ENT (PRINT)   al-Juf   M.D.
PATIENT'S WARD LOCATION   5BT
Do Not Write in This Space
S 82-16-17
A → C

TISSUE SUBMITTED ① For distal node ② Colon ③ peri-
                 toneal adhesion

SITE AND APPEARANCE OF LESION

Copy of Report To:

HISTORY, DURATION, CLINICAL DATA, AND OPERATIVE FINDINGS:
57 y old ♀ — well diff. node. Lt.
                    obstare lesion.

CLINICAL Dx

SURGICAL PATHOLOGY REPORT, DEPARTMENT OF PATHOLOGY,
DATE RECEIVED _____ DATE REPORTED 2-17-82 _____ FROZEN SECTION Dx, AND PATHOLOGIST _____

GROSS:

A. "Far distal node" The specimen consists of a tan-brown 0.5 x 0.3
x 0.2 cm node and attached fibroadipose tissue. Bisected, on sponge,
one cassette.

B. "Colon" The specimen consists of a previously opened colon
opened along the antimesteric border. It is 20 cm in length 7.8 cm
in circumference. There is 4.4 cm from tumor to distal resection margin
and 13.5 cm from tumor to proximal resection margin. The tumor is
5 x 4 cm, firm, dark red and circumferential around the bowel. The
remaining bowel mucosal has occasional white ulcerative lesion proximal
to the tumor. One is 2 cm proximal, the other is 6 cm proximal.
On cross section one area of the tumor appears to come up to the
serosal surface. B13 is distal resection margin. B14 is proximal
resection margin. B15 and B16 are tumor for a maximal depth of
invasion. B17 is tumor and normal adjacent mucosa. B18 is nearest
ulcer. Distal near lymph nodes show a 1.8 x 1.0 x 0.8 cm hard
lymph node with firm yellow cheesey material in the center. Multiple
other nodes and fibroadipose tissue. B1 has three nodes. B2 has
the large lymph node. B3 is two nodes. B4 has four nodes. B5
is one node and a blood vessel. B6 has three lymph nodes. Next
is proximal near containing six lymph nodes and fibroadipose tissue,
the largest lymph node measures 0.9 x 0.7 x 0.4 cm. B7 has three

(Over).

427

nodes. B8 has three lymph nodes. Next is proximal far containing
lymph nodes and fibroadipose tissue. The largest node measures
1.7 x 0.8 x 0.5 cm. B9 has three nodes. B10 has two nodes. B11
two nodes. Next is distal far nodes. B12 four nodes.
C. "Peritoneal adhesion" The specimen consists of a white glossy,
fatty piece of tissue. The bulk measuring 2 x 2.5 x 0.3 cm with
a 0.1 cm in diameter, 6 cm long stringy attachment. All, in lens
paper, one cassette. JR

MICRO:
A. Lymph node with prominent germinal centers.
B. Moderately well differentiated adenocarcinoma of the colon
invading through the muscle to serosa. Adjacent bowel is without
diagnostic abnormality. The proximal and distal resection margins
are without tumor. Fourteen distal near nodes with nin positive
for adenocarcinoma. Six proximal near nodes with four positive
for adenocarcinoma. Seven proximal far nodes with five positive
for adenocarcinoma. Four distal far nodes without tumor.
C. Edematous fibrosis tissue with some mesothelial lining.

DIAGNOSIS: Colon, partial colectomy:
          Invasive moderately-well differentiated adenocarcinoma.
          Lymph nodes, pericolonic:
          18 of 32 lymph nodes with adenocarcinoma (see description).
          Peritoneum, excision:
          Consistent with peritoneal adhesion.

FWS/kjv   John R_____, M.D.

DEPARTMENT OF PATHOLOGY
DIAGNOSIS APPROVED
F.W. S_____ M.D.

Report Read by Responsible Physician

Signed

428

Patient #45

Patient #45 is a 47-year-old man from Pennsylvania alive nearly ten years since his diagnosis of locally metastatic rectosigmoid cancer.

In early 1977, Patient #45 experienced episodic abdominal pain, associated with constipation and a gradual ten-pound weight loss. During a six month period, as his condition worsened, on multiple occasions Patient #45 consulted his primary physician, who dismissed the symptoms as insignificant and recommended no testing.

Finally, in September 1977, after passing a large amount of blood with his stool, Patient #45 was referred to a proctologist. When a sigmoidoscopic examination revealed a large rectal tumor, Patient #45 was admitted to Lancaster General Hospital in Lancaster, Pennsylvania on September 26, 1977. Three days later, he underwent surgery for resection of the lesion along with his upper rectum and the lower, descending portion of his large intestine.

The pathology report describes an ulcerated, poorly differentiated adenocarcinoma growing through the bowel wall, with all seven lymph nodes examined positive for cancer. Postoperatively, Patient #45's doctors informed him the disease most likely would recur and prove terminal despite any therapy, but nonetheless recommended a course of the chemotherapeutic drug 5-fluorouracil, which he began while still hospitalized.

After returning home in mid-October 1977, Patient #45 continued the treatment as an outpatient, but since his prognosis seemed so dismal, he began investigating alternative approaches to cancer. After learning of Dr. Kelley, Patient #45 consulted with him in late December 1977 and shortly after began the nutritional regimen, at the same time refusing to proceed with any additional chemotherapy.

While pursuing his unconventional treatment, Patient #45 gained weight and enjoyed an improvement in his general health. He also mentioned to me that a case of chronic psoriasis, which had resisted the usual treatments, resolved.

Patient #45 eventually followed his nutritional protocol for three and a half years, before tapering down to a maintenance regimen which he still follows. At present, nearly ten years after his diagnosis, he is in excellent health with no sign of cancer.

Pathologists describe several characteristics of colorectal cancer, all identified in Patient #45's case, that predict a poor outcome. As a start, poorly differentiated adenocarcinoma is considered the most aggressive of the colorectal malignancies. Ulcerating tumors and tumors that encircle the bowel wall have a particularly dismal prognosis, and the seven positive lymph nodes reported in this patient predict no better than a 10% chance for five-year survival.

Patient #45 received a three-month course of 5-fluorouracil chemotherapy, but this drug, when given post-surgically, has never been shown to extend life in patients with rectal cancer. As Sugarbaker writes: "There is no evidence that single agent [one drug] chemotherapy significantly improves the survival of treated patients."[1]

I would not consider Patient #45 an extraordinary case since he had no evidence of active disease at the time he began the Kelley regimen. Nonetheless, he has experienced continuing good health and prolonged survival that is unusual considering his original diagnosis with involvement of multiple lymph nodes. He, like Patient #44, has beaten formidable odds.

REFERENCE

1. DeVita, VT, et al. *Cancer Principles & Practice of Oncology*. Philadelphia; J.B. Lippincott Company, 1982, page 690.

LAB NO.
S-77-11,819

HOSP NO.
▮▮▮▮▮

(PATIENT) NAME	SURGEON	DATE	ROOM NO.
Patient #45 ▮▮▮▮▮	Dr. Peter P. P▮▮▮▮	September 29, 1977	IMCU
New Holland, Pennsylvania 17557	AGE 37 years	DURATION OF SYMPTOMS	

OPERATION

RESECTION RECTOSIGMOID - CECOSTOMY - APPENDECTOMY.

ORGANS SENT FOR EXAMINATION

Rectosigmoid - Appendix.

HISTORY

PHYSICAL FINDINGS

FINDINGS AT OPERATION

Carcinoma, rectosigmoid.

DIAGNOSIS

Carcinoma, rectosigmoid.

PREVIOUS SURGERY

S-72-3,077 Pilonidal cyst.

SIGNED Dr. Peter P. P▮▮▮▮

GROSS DESCRIPTION

I. A 10cm. segment of colon. At a distance of 2cms. from one excised margin there is a 5cm. encircling mass. The neoplasm is pink. Ends of the excised specimen. 2SS.

II. The lesion. 2SS.

III. Regional lymph nodes. 7SS.

IV. Appendix which has a length of 7cms. ISS.

jh/
cal

Ward M. O'▮▮▮▮, M.D.
qPathologist

HISTOLOGICAL EXAMINATION

DIAGNOSIS:

I. The ends of the excised specimen are free of neoplasm.

II. Ulcerated adenocarcinoma arising in the colonic mucosa and infiltrating into the wall. The neoplasm is poorly differentiated.

III. Seven (7) regional lymph nodes isolated and examined contain metastatic carcinoma.

IV. Recurrent appendicitis and peri-appendicitis. No recent severe attack.

cal

1

Ward M. O▮▮▮▮, M.D.

PATHOLOGIST

431

Office Hours By Appointment:
1:30 - 3 — Mon., Tues, Thurs., Fri.
7 - 8 — Tues. And Fri.

Phone: 392-4700
Area Code: 717

PETER P█████ M.D., LTD.
████████████

LANCASTER, PA. 17602

Oct. 14, 1977

Dr. JOhn R███
Easthrook Family Health Center
███████
Ronks, Pa. 17572

Re: Patient #45

A 9/26 D 10/14

Dear Doctors:

████████, on whom I performed a Sigmoid-colon resection, Cecostomy, and appendectomy (carcinoma of rectosigmoid with lymph node metastases) on 9/29/77 at the Lancaster General Hospital, has had a good postoperative course and was discharged today.

Laboratory Data:
9/27/77: Hct. 43 vol.% Hgb. 14.7 grams
WBC 6,400   Urinalysis: 3-5 WBC; more than 100 RBC.   Serology: Negative.
Bl. Type: Group A Rh positive.
10/12/77 Hct. 55.% vol.% Hgb. 12.1 grams
WBC 5,500
EKG: Normal tracing.
Chest X-ray: Normal.
INFUSION Urogram: Within normal limits.
Liver Scan: No indication of metastatic disease.

I asked ████████ to see you on 10/20/77 (the remaining sutures can be removed at that time) and me in 1 month for his postoperative check-up.

RENAL CELL (KIDNEY) CARCINOMA

Kidney cancer killed 9,400 Americans in 1987. If diagnosed early, the disease can be cured by surgery, but once metastatic, it usually proves rapidly fatal. At present, 50% of all patients with renal cell carcinoma live five years.

Patient #46

Patient #46 died at age 64 from lung cancer, nearly eight years after being diagnosed with metastatic renal cell carcinoma.

Despite a long history of heavy cigarette use, Patient #46 had enjoyed good health when in April 1978 he first experienced chronic fevers associated with pain in the right side of his back. Patient #46 consulted his physician, who suspected a kidney infection. When he failed to improve after a course of antibiotics, Patient #46 was admitted to Heights Hospital in Houston on May 5, 1978 for further evaluation.

After renal dye studies revealed an obstruction of the right ureter, Patient #46 underwent exploratory surgery on May 10, 1978. During the procedure, his right kidney was found encased in a mass of scar-like tissue, believed due to retroperitoneal fibrosis, a rare disease of unknown cause.

The hospital summary describes the findings as follows:

> The entire kidney, renal pelvis and upper third of the right ureter were literally encased in a dense fibrotic covering with multiple blood vessels.

The surgeon made no attempt to dissect away the abnormal tissue, but did install a ureteral stent to bypass the area of blockage.

After recovering from his ordeal, Patient #46, still in pain, was discharged from the hospital on May 25, 1978, only to return a week later for removal of the stent. Although his physicians could not locate the device, Patient #46 improved sufficiently so that he left the hospital with no plans for any additional testing.

But when his urinary symptoms recurred, Patient #46 was re-admitted to Heights Hospital on June 17, 1978. X-ray studies of the abdomen revealed leakage of urine where the ureteral stent had previously been inserted. Additional testing documented deterioration in kidney function, as well as an occlusion in the iliac veins (the large veins draining the pelvic cavity).

Patient #46 returned to surgery on June 27, 1978, at which time the right kidney was removed—along with a large, previously undiagnosed tumor. The discharge note describes the operation as "a very, very difficult case with extensive fibrosis obliterating all the retroperitoneal structures."

The records describe locally advanced, stage III renal cell carcinoma, but nonetheless, postoperatively Patient #46 was initially assumed to be cured. However, several days later, after Patient #46 developed severe swelling in both legs, a staff oncologist recommended chemotherapy be instituted immediately. The doctor wrote:

> Because of the patient's 25% five-year survival at best with a stage III
> renal carcinoma post-nephrectomy [kidney removal], I feel it advisable
> to treat [Patient #46] with adjuvant chemotherapy.

Subsequently, after leaving the hospital on July 21, 1978, Patient #46 began a course of treatment with vinblastine and CCNU, two potent chemotherapeutic agents, along with Depo-Provera, a synthetic progesterone often given to patients with renal cell carcinoma.

Despite the therapy, in early fall Patient #46 developed severe lower back pain, believed to be the result of new onset bony metastases. In November 1978, after he had completed four months of chemotherapy, a CT scan revealed a new large tumor on the right side of the abdomen beneath the liver, as well as evidence of malignant disease in multiple abdominal lymph nodes and in multiple vertebral bodies. The records summarize these findings:

> retroperitoneal adenopathy with infrahepatic mass with destruction of
> L-2 [a lumbar vertebra] on the right side.

Patient #46 subsequently completed a course of 3,000 rads of radiation therapy to his spine for pain control. Nevertheless, during the final weeks of 1978 his pain worsened, his general health including his appetite deteriorated, and his weight dropped from 175 to 138 pounds.

In desperation, Patient #46 decided to investigate unconventional cancer therapies, learned of Dr. Kelley and in January 1979 began the full nutritional regimen. At that time, by his own description to me, he appeared to be acutely, terminally ill.

Patient #46 did continue chemotherapy along with his nutritional program, and with this combined approach gradually regained his strength, appetite, and weight. A CT scan on May 24, 1979 revealed that the abdominal and pelvic tumors had regressed significantly, as documented in the official report:

> there has been a tremendous decrease in the size of the intracaval (vena
> cava) neoplasm, obviously. The liver, left kidney, pancreas and other vi-
> sualized upper abdominal organs appear normal. There is no evidence of
> enlargement of retroperitoneal lymph nodes.

In June 1979, Patient #46 completed the drug regimen, and thereafter followed the Kelley regimen as his only therapy. Over the next year, Patient #46 improved sufficiently in terms of his general health so that he could return to work full time. A CT scan from October 1982—when Patient #46 was hospitalized because of a ruptured gallbladder—confirmed that the previously noted metastatic disease had completely regressed.

Patient #46 followed the full Kelley program for about five years, until late 1983, during which time he enjoyed excellent health. He then became careless, straying from the prescribed diet, even resuming his cigarette habit. In November 1984, after nearly six cancer-free years, Patient #46 was diagnosed with primary squamous cell carcinoma of the lung, attributed to his long history of smoking. He decided at that point to refuse all conventional therapy, and in January, 1985, began a nutritional program in Dallas promoted as the "Kelley Program," though not authorized by Dr. Kelley.

After two months on this regimen, Patient #46 had significantly deteriorated, to the point he required hospitalization in Dallas. He was then flown by private jet to Methodist Hospital in Houston where he completed a series of radiation treatments. After stabilizing for a time, he died in January 1986, never having resumed the authentic Kelley program.

The prognosis for patients with metastatic renal cell carcinoma is dismal, even with aggressive treatment. Paulson reports a median survival of only 7.1 months in a group of such patients receiving intensive chemotherapy.[1]

Obviously, Patient #46's long-term survival is unusual. He was diagnosed with widely disseminated kidney cancer that resisted radiation, chemotherapy, and a trial of the hormone Depo-Provera. Furthermore, he improved significantly only after beginning the Kelley program.

When I discussed Patient #46's unfortunate demise with Dr. Kelley, he repeated what he has said many times before; the many imitation "Kelley Programs" currently available are ineffective at best and often dangerous.

REFERENCE

1. DeVita, VT, et al. *Cancer Principles & Practice of Oncology*. Philadelphia; J.B. Lippincott Company, 1982, page 741.

DISCHARGE SUMMARY

ADMITTED: 5-5-78

DISCHARGED: 5-27-78

FINAL DIAGNOSIS: Retroperitoneal fibrosis with upper ureteral obstruction and urinary tract infection.

OPERATION PERFORMED: By Dr. B██ on 5-10-78 - Panendocystourethroscopy, bilateral retrograde pyeloureterograms.
By Dr. B██ on 5-15-78 - Exploration of the right kidney and right ureter with ureterolysis and removal of surrounding fibrotic tissue and release of obstruction of upper ureter. Exploration of the upper ureter.

COMPLICATIONS: None.

A 57 year old white male has been followed by me previously with very obscure, cloudy previous history. This has been over the last 5 or 6 weeks and mainly is centered around fever and a backache. The backache was noted in the right CVA radiating down to the anterior abdomen and down to the testicle. This is a very vague history. In addition, he has run fever and has progressively become weaker. I saw him as an out-patient and felt that he had a low grade urinary tract infection. Began treating this, however he continued to have difficulty and was admitted by Dr. B██ and Dr. S██. After admission SMAC-20 showed minor variations, all of them within acceptable limits. Repeat SMAC-20 again showed minor variations consistent with his post-operative state and intravenous fluids were given. Acid Phosphatase was reported 0.60 with a prostatic fraction of 0.4 and totally normal. Hemoglobin reported at 12.2 gms% with 36.5 vol% hematocrit, 5,800 white count. Urine culture was negative. Workup including Latex test as well as febrile agglutins were negative. Repeat urine culture negative. CEA 4.1 nanograms per m/l. EKG was within normal limits. X-ray studies revealed a normal chest X-ray. Left knee, abdominal series, skull series and paranasal sinuses were all within normal limits with the exception of osteoma within the floor of the right frontal sinus. A drip infusion IVP showed delayed function of the right kidney with suggestion of upper ureteral obstruction. Retrograde pyelogram on this side showed blunting of the minor calyces and concentric narrowing of the proximal right ureter or structure.

On 5-10-78 patient was taken to the operating room. Cystoscopy was carried out at which time the findings of the retrograde pyelogram were done. It was very obscure and diffi-cult to ascertain what was going on at the time of the first retrograde pyelography but the patient continued to have pain and the upper ureter was finally explored on 5-15-78. At that time the entire kidney, renal pelvis and upper third of the right ureter were literally encased in a dense fibrotic covering with multiple blood vessels. He bled fairly heavily and the only diagnosis evident at that time was probably retroperitoneal fibrosis and upper ureteral stricture. Ureterolysis was done.

(continued)

437

Patient was discharged home with the idea that repeat X-rays would be carried out and if he did not receive any benefit from the ureterolysis then further renal evaluation should be carried out. I plan to see him in the office in two weeks to repeat his pyelogram and followup X-rays as needed.

John M. B█████, M.D.

JMB:jwa
08228
08258

438

HEIGHTS HOSPITAL
DEPARTMENT OF LABORATORIES
SURGICAL PATHOLOGY

No. Patient #46   **Date**   6-27-78

Name   **Case No.** ▮▮▮▮ Rm. 311W

Dr. B▮▮   **Sex**   Male

Age   57

Tissue   Right kidney

Clinical Diagnosis   Acute urinary tract infection

GROSS: The specimen consists of a kidney which is received without the capsule and previously sections to the midline. The specimen weighs 285 grams and measures 13 X 8 X 6 cm. in greatest dimensions. There is a tumor mass located approximately 2 cm. from one pole and 7 cm. from the other which measures up to 4.5 cm. in diameter. This mass appears to have yellowish-reddish tumor tissue. The tumor is located immediately beneath the cortex. The cortex at the side of the tumor is markedly atrophic. Elsewhere, the kidney has grossly normal appearance. The cortex is up to 1 cm. in thickness and the medulla is up to 2 cm. in thickness. The collecting system appears to be unremarkable except at the site of the tumor it is markedly compressed. On cut sections throughout the hilus of the kidney there is thrombosis of the renal vein. The renal artery appears to be unremarkable. The ureter measures up to 2 cm. in length and also appears to be unremarkable.

In a separate container, multiple fragments of adipose tissue that appear to correspond to the capsule of the kidney are received. These fragments show extensive areas of hemorrhage. On cut sections areas suggesting fat necrosis are seen. Sections are submitted.

MICROSCOPIC: Histologic sections of the tumor show a clear cell carcinoma which is immediately beneath the external surface of the kidney. The sections from the tumor also show invasion of the blood vessels.

Sections taken elsewhere from the kidney show a diffuse acute inflammatory infiltrate within the stroma. Sections taken from the renal vein show invasion of the vein lumen with complete thrombosis by tumor. Sections taken from the ureter show mild chronic inflammation. Sections taken from the perirenal fat show multiple areas of fat necrosis.

DIAGNOSIS: KIDNEY, RIGHT NEPHRECTOMY - RENAL CELL CARCINOMA.
RENAL VEIN WITH TUMOR THROMBOSIS.
ACUTE AND CHRONIC PILONEPHRITIS.
PERIRENAL FAT, EXCISION - FAT NECROSIS.

Signed _____ M.D.
Humberto A. L▮▮, M.D.   HL/nb   6/28/78

"RYLEE" F. No. 076

439

DISCHARGE SUMMARY

CHISHOLM, [Patient #46]

ADMITTED: 6-17-78

DISCHARGED: 7-21-78

FINAL DIAGNOSIS: Renal cell carcinoma of the kidney, Stage III.

OPERATION PERFORMED: By Dr. B███ on 6-27-78 - Panendocystourethroscopy, bilateral retrograde pyeloureterograms and difficult right nephrectomy.

COMPLICATIONS: Venacava thrombosis presumably from tumor.

A 57 year old white male re-admitted after being initially evaluated about six weeks ago for what appeared to be an upper third ureteral obstruction on the right side. Patient has continued to have pain, fever and was re-admitted for further evaluation. The recent C&P done a week or so ago revealed extravasation of contrast media from previous ureterotomy and it was felt he had a large urinoma with collection of urine from the ureterotomy. Catheters were left up at that time and he was placed on antibiotics only to return with pain in the right flank as well as fever and chills. It was felt that patient was having non-function of the kidney to a great degree associated with urine extravasation and he was re-admitted for nephrectomy. After admission EKG was within normal limits. Chest X-ray unremarkable. Drip IVP showed probably some contrast medium into the extra-ureteral cavity which had previously been noted on a retrograde pyelogram. Retrograde pyelogram again showed a collection of the contrast media at the site of the previous ureterotomy. Pelvic ultra sound revealed no pelvic masses. An upper GI done post-operatively as well as a small bowel showed some delay in the gastric emptying but no other ulceration. An inferior venacavagram showed complete occlusion of inferior venacava in the right iliac veins as well as occlusion of the proximal portion of the left common iliac vein. Followup chest X-ray post-op as well as liver scan was within normal limits. SMAC-20 during this long hospitalization varied somewhat but was thought to be adequate and acceptable and within normal limits. Alkaline Phosphatase on 7-13-78 was noted to be 305. Renal function remained normal.

On 6-27-78 patient was taken to the operating room where a right nephrectomy was carried out which was a very, very difficult case with extensive fibrosis obliterating all the retroperitoneal structures. Lower pole tumor of the right kidney was noted incidently after removing the kidney and had previously been unsuspected. This appeared to be grossly tumor and subsequently was reported as renal cell carcinoma of the right kidney with renal vein thrombosis and acute and chronic pyelonephritis. His post-operative course was complicated by swelling of the extremities, especially on the right and a venacavagram supported the diagnosis of occlusion probably from combination of tumor and blood clot. Dr. Mylie E. D███ saw him in consultation and felt that conservative treatment was indicated and this was carried out. At time of discharge his leg was still swollen and he is under the care of Dr. T███████ for chemotherapy for presumably the metastatic clear cell carcinoma of the kidney.

John M. B███, M.D.

JMB:jwa
08228
08258

440

HEIGHTS HOSPITAL
HOUSTON, TEXAS

is a 57-year old gentleman who was admitted to Heights Hospital on 6/17/78. This is a patient of Dr. J. M. B█████ who was operated on six weeks prior to admission for what appeared to be an upper-third ureteral obstruction on the right side. The obstruction at that time was found to be all extrinsic, and was felt to be due to extensive retroperitoneal fibrosis. The collecting system showed no evidence of any mass lesion. Post-operatively the patient continued to have difficulty with flank pain, and a subsequent cystoscopy and pyelography showed extravasation of contrast media from the previous ureterotomy into the flank. The patient also had a long-term history of persistent fever and chills. An IVP was done, showing a poorly functioning kidney on the right side, but no displacement or distortion of the collecting system. Because the patient did not appear to have an adequately functioning right kidney, a nephrectomy was performed on 6/17/78 by Dr. B████. At the time of surgery, there was extensive fibrosis up and down the ureter, obliterating all retroperitoneal structures. In addition, a tumor was seen in the lower pole of the right kidney. The tumor did not appear to impinge or press on the collecting system. Pre-operative ultrasound examination of the kidney failed to disclose any evidence of the lesion. An extensive dissection was done, and the kidney was removed. The pathology report revealed a 4.5-cm. in diameter mass lesion in the lower pole of the right kidney. Histologic study showed a clear-cell carcinoma which was immediately beneath the external surface of the kidney. Sections from the tumor also showed invasion of the blood vessels. Sections taken from the renal veins showed invasion of the vein lumen with complete thrombosis by tumor. Consequently the patient had a Stage III renal adenocarcinoma with gross invasion of the renal vein. Post-operatively the patient did relatively well, but developed progressive lower leg edema, especially on the right side. A venogram was performed on 7/11/78, showing complete occlusion of the inferior vena cava and apparently the right iliac veins, and the proximal portion of the left iliac vein apparently is occluded also. Surgical consultation was sought, and it was decided that an inferior vena caval thrombectomy was not indicated. Since that time the patient's lower leg edema has gradually improved. A liver scan and chest X-ray both show no evidence of metastatic disease. Peripheral blood counts are normal, with a hemoglobin of 10.3, white blood cell count 7,500, with 71% neutrophils, and platelet count of 415,000. The SMA analysis is normal except for an alkaline phosphatase value elevated at 305 units, and an LDH value elevated at 239 units. The patient's albumin is 2.6 grams.

ASSESSMENT: Clear-cell carcinoma of the kidney, Stage III, Status post-nephrectomy with post-operative thrombosis and complete occlusion of the inferior vena cava.

M.D.

Dr. T. Z. L███████
Referred by Dr. J. M. B██████   CONSULTANT: T. F. T█████████ M.D.

Name of Patient		Date	Room No.	Hospital No.
████████████		7/17/78	311W	████████

CONSULTATION SHEET
ORIGINAL COPY FOR HOSPITAL RECORD

441

(continuation)

RECOMMENDATIONS: Because of the patient's 25% five-year survival at best with a Stage III renal carcinoma post-nephrectomy, I feel it advisable to treat Mr. Patient #46 with adjuvant chemotherapy. In spite of the fact that traditionally this tumor has been resistant to chemotherapy, there have been recent reports of a recovery of a combination of Velban and CCNU. Also, from a theoretical point of view, it makes more sense to treat this man at the present time, when he has minimal tumor burden, rather than wait till he has gross macroscopic disease which would be relatively insensitive to chemotherapy. I have discussed the rationale, potential side affects and potential benefits of therapy with ▮▮▮▮▮▮. If he is in agreement with this plan, his therapy will be instituted in the near future. He will receive Velban intravenously every other week, and CCNU orally every six to eight weeks. The therapeutic plan will be to continue chemotherapy for a period of one year, at which time it would be permanently discontinued if there was no evidence of recurrent hypernephroma.

Thank you for allowing me to see this interesting patient.

TFT:bt

07178
07178

Dr. T. Z. L▮▮▮▮▮				M.D.
Referred by Dr. J. M▮▮3▮▮▮	CONSULTANT: T. F. T▮▮▮▮▮▮, M.D.			
Name of Patient		Date 7/17/78	Room No. 311W	Hospital No.

CONSULTATION SHEET
ORIGINAL COPY FOR HOSPITAL RECORD

442

████████ 5-24-79 Dr. T████████

COMPUTED TOMOGRAPHY (ABDOMEN): Scans were made from the upper third of the liver thru the umbilicus. The right kidney is surgically absent as previously noted. In reviewing the previous scans in Nov. and Dec. of 1978, I believe it is now apparent that the mass described in the right subhepatic area and inferior vena cava grossly dilated by tumor. The previous scans show calcification around the periphery of the mass. The vena cava is now of normal size. There are still some calcifications in the right side of the inferior vena cava. The patient refused contrast material injections, so I cannot determine whether the vena cava is obstructed or how much residual tumor, if any is in the vena cava. However, there has been a tremendous decrease in the size of the intracaval neoplasm, obviously. The liver, left kidney, pancreas and other visualized upper abdominal organs appear normal. There is no evidence of enlargement of retroperitoneal lymph nodes. It is possible that the densities under the right crux of the diaphragm previously interpreted as enlarged lymph nodes were due to enlargement of azygos veins secondary to an obstructed inferior vena cava. In any case, these densities are no longer present.

J-XO-65-2540-4 PT. MEMORIAL HOSPITAL SYSTEM, DEPARTMENT OF RADIOLOGY

sjc

R. E. W████, M.D.

6\4

DISCHARGE SUMMARY

Patient #46

ADMITTED: 10/28/82
DISCHARGED: 11/8/82

FINAL DIAGNOSIS: 1. Ruptured gallbladder and cholecystitis.
                    2. History of carcinoma of the kidney.

SUMMARY: This is the case of a 61 year old gentleman with a history of renal cell
carcinoma dating back to 1978 who was admitted to Heights Hospital on 10/28 for fever
and chills, up to 104.00 degrees. Three to four days prior to admission the patient
began to develop spiking fevers up to 104.00 degrees, accompanied by chills. He was
taking oral Amoxicillin with no effect. He complained of abdominal discomfort and
nausea. He denied any dysuria, but did complain of some cough with clear sputum
production.

PAST MEDICAL HISTORY: In June, 1978, the patient was admitted to Heights Hospital
and had an obstructed of the upper third of his right ureter. At that time he had a
long history of persistent fever and chills. An IVP was done which showed a poorly
functioning right kidney. A nephrectomy was performed in June, 1978 by Dr. B████
At the time of surgery there was extensive fibrosis up and down the ureter oblitering
all retroperitoneal structures. In addition, tumor was seen in the lower pole of
the right kidney. There was a renal cell cracinoma which was a clear-cell carcinoma
pathologically. There was invasion of the blood vessels, invasion of the renal vein
with complete thrombosis by tumor. Post-operatively the patient developed lower leg
edema. A vemogram done in July showed complete occlusion of the inferior vena cava
which gradually showed some improvement. He was commenced on chemotherapy with Velban
and CCNU, receiving this from July, 1978 until July, 1979. At that time a C.T. scan
and chest X-ray showed no evidence of recurrent disease, and his chemotherapy was
discontinued. During that one-year period he also received Depo Provera approximately
1 gram per month. In November, 1978, a C.T. scan showed retroperitoneal adenopathy
with an infrahepatic mass with destruction of L-2 on the right side. The patient was
sent to Methodist Hospital and received irradiation therapy to the lumbar spine,
3,000 RADS over 3 1/2 weeks from November to December, 1978, with improvement in his
back pain. Since 1979 he has been followed, with no specific medications except
Dilaudid 2 mg. two or three times a day for persistent right lower quadrant pain,
judged to be incisional. A CAT scan of the abdomen was done on 10/4/82 which showed
the right kidney to be resected. There was no retroperitoneal mass or lymphadenopathy and
no abnormality of the liver noted. The gallbladder at that time was outlined and its
wall was thickened with possibly some calcium within the wall.

Physical examination revealed a tosic-appearing elderly gentleman who appeared
acutely ill. Temperature was 102.5 degrees, pulse 92 per minute and regular, respiratory rate 30 per minute and regular, blood pressure 120/70. Height was 5 feet, 8
inches, weight 168 pounds. There was no scleral icterus. There was mild pallor to
the skin and mucous membranes. There was no detectable lymphadenopathy. The oral
cavity revealed no erythema or exudates. There was no nuchal rigidity. Chest
examination revealed clear breath sounds bilaterally. Cardiac exam revealed a regular
rhythm of 92 per minute with no gallop. Abdominal examination revealed definite
right upper quadrant tenderness with the liver edge being palpable 2 fingerbreadths
below the right costal margin. It was firm, somewhat nodular and tender. The gallbladder was not obviously palpable. There was no definite left upper quadrant tenderness. There was a right flank incision from the patient's previous nephrectomy. Bowel
sounds were normally active. There was no rebound tenderness. Extremity examination
showed no pedal edema or calf tenderness. Neurological examination showed some
obtundation, but no focal signs.

(CONTINUED ON PAGE 2)

444

The patient was admitted to the hospital and placed on antibiotics with Claforan and Amikacin. He was seen by Dr. S███ who felt that the patient had acute cholecystitis. Chest X-ray was negative. KUB was unremarkable.

Laboratory analysis showed a normal BUN and creatinine. Serum electrolytes showed a low sodium and chloride, but were otherwise normal. Total protein and albumin were 5.6 and 2.6 respectively. Bilirubin was normal; alkaline phosphatase was normal; however, the GGT and SGOT were both elevated, and the LDH was elevated. Peripheral hemogram showed a hemoglobin of 12.7, white blood cell count 10,900 with 67% neutrophils and 18% BAND cells. Platelet count was 192,000. A C.E.A. determination was 2.0. Amylase and lipase were both normal. Blood cultures revealed no growth.

The patient was taken to surgery on 10/30/82 by Dr. S███. After the peritoneal cavity was entered, an acute inflammatory mass was identified in the right upper quadrant; the mass was made up of gastric wall, duodenum, greater omentum and gallbladder. By blunt dissection a large area of purulent material was unroofed and aspirated, and a specimen taken for culture. The gallbladder was perforated and decompressed. By blunt dissection the junction of the common and cystic duct was identified. A stone was impacted in the cystic duct and was removed. The cystic duct itself was ligated near its junction with the common duct, as was the cystic artery. The gallbladder was dissected free from the liver by blunt dissection. A sump drain was placed in the foramin of Winslow and brought out through an inferior stab wound incision. Exploration revealed previous evidence of right nephrectomy, but no evidence of recurrent disease. 1 gram of Kanamycin was placed in the sub-hepatic space on the right and the peritoneum was closed. The patient tolerated the procedure well. Pathology showed gallbladder--severe, acute and chronic cholecystitis with hemorrhagic necrosis and cholelithiasis.

Post-operatively the patient did well and was discharged from the hospital on 11/8. He will see both Dr. S███ and myself in the office for follow-up.

T. F. Te█████, M.D.

TFT:bt
04103
05043

DIPLOMATES, ~~RICAN~~ BOARD OF PATHOLOGY
V. Q. T█████ M.D.   J.S. L█████ M.D.   M.J. W█ █████ M.D.
T.M. J█████ M.D.   J.A. S█████ M.D.

SURGICAL PATHOLOGY REPORT

Patient:	Patient #46	Tissue No:	Age: 64
Physician:	Dr. J. T███ ~~Tannen~~ Date of Surgery: B-85-0706 Not given		Sex: 11
Specimen:	Sputum #3; Date Reported:	Clinical Information:	

DIAGNOSIS: bronchial washings   3/19/85
left upper lobe; slides #1-#3

GROSS DESCRIPTION:

Part (A) is 30 ccs of light green tinted sputum.

Part (B) is 16 ccs of thick red bronchial washing fluid from the left upper lobe.

Part (C) is 3 prepared slides from the left upper lobe.

MICROSCOPIC EXAMINATION:

The cell block and cytology sample in the first specimen are highly suspicious for squamous cell carcinoma. Small hyper-keratotic cells with misshapened pyknotic nuclei are present. Some of these cells have a tadpole configuration. These cells are most obvious on the cytology sample, with smaller numbers of cells found on the cell block.

The second sample has a hemorrhagic background. There are a few cells which are suspicious for squamous cell carcinoma. These are much less numerous than those found on the first sample.

The brush smears have neutrophils, respiratory epithelial cells and histiocytes as well as a few hyperkeratotic squamous cells suspicious for squamous cell carcinoma.

PATHOLOGICAL FINDINGS:

PARTS (A) THROUGH (C),   CELL BLOCK AND CYTOLOGY AND BRUSH
SMEAR SAMPLES FROM LEFT UPPER LOBE,
HIGHLY SUSPICIOUS FOR SQUAMOUS
CELL CARCINOMA.

JSL:Mel

J. Sloan L█████, M.D.

446

STOMACH CANCER

Stomach cancer can be cured by surgery if localized at the time of diagnosis, but once metastatic, the disease resists conventional treatments such as chemotherapy and radiation. In 1987, this malignancy killed 14,200 Americans, with estimates of five-year survival notoriously low, ranging from 12–15%.

Patient #47

Patient #47 is a 47-year-old woman from New Jersey alive ten years since her diagnosis of metastatic stomach carcinoma.

Before her bout with cancer, Patient #47 had a long history of general poor health, particularly chronic digestive problems. In 1974, she first experienced episodes of severe abdominal pain usually occurring between meals, and relieved by eating. Over the following three years, her symptoms gradually worsened, although she was not formally evaluated until the spring of 1977. At that time, a barium swallow revealed a gastric tumor, described in an official report as a "suspicious lesion in the fundus and cardia of the stomach."

Patient #47 then underwent endoscopy and biopsy of the suspect tissue, which proved to be gastric adenocarcinoma. Subsequently, Patient #47 was admitted to Patterson General Hospital on April 17, 1977 for a radical subtotal gastrectomy (resection of most of the stomach). At the time of surgery, the tumor had already metastasized into regional lymph nodes and the omentum, the thick fibrous sheath that covers the abdominal organs. The discharge summary describes the findings as: "Adenocarcinoma of the stomach with metastasis to the gastrocolic nodes and omentum."

Postoperatively, Patient #47's physicians informed her she most likely would not live a year, even with aggressive chemotherapy. With her options minimal, her doctors referred her to Memorial Sloan-Kettering Cancer Center in New York for possible experimental treatment. But Patient #47, who already knew of Dr. Kelley's work, decided to refuse any drug approach, standard or experimental. Instead, in late April 1977, after leaving the hospital, she consulted with Dr. Kelley and began the full nutritional program that same month.

Patient #47 followed her regimen for five years and presently, ten years after her original diagnosis, she reports excellent health with no sign of her once metastatic disease. According to Patient #47, her doctors are "dumbfounded" by her prolonged survival.

Patient #47, diagnosed with metastatic stomach cancer, is indeed a remarkable case. The five-year survival rate for patients with metastatic stomach cancer approaches 0%—even with aggressive therapy. Patient #47 received neither chemotherapy nor radiation after her surgery, but chose to follow only the Kelley program.

Greater Paterson General Hospital
DISCHARGE SUMMARY

DISCHARGE SUMMARIES MUST INCLUDE:
PERTINENT HISTORY
PERTINENT PHYSICAL FINDINGS
PERTINENT LABORATORY, X-RAY AND PATHOLOGICAL FINDINGS
HOSPITAL COURSE (MUST INCLUDE CONSULTATIONS AND
CONDITION ON DISCHARGE)
DISCHARGE RECOMMENDATIONS (MUST INCLUDE MEDICATION,
ACTIVITY LIMITATIONS, FOLLOW UP IF REQUIRED, AND BY WHOM)
FINAL DIAGNOSIS, SECONDARY DIAGNOSIS, COMPLICATIONS, OPERATIONS, PROCEDURES AND TRANSFUSIONS

ADMISSION DATE: 4-17-77
DISCHARGE DATE: 5-1-77
PHYSICIAN: John J. C██████████, M.D.

The patient was admitted with a history of pain in the abdomen since 1974.
It was usually present with hunger and relieved by eating. The patient
continued to have pain and was hospitalized in Rutherford, New Jersey. A
GI series showed a suspicious lesion in the fundus and cardia of the stomach.
A gastroscopy was performed and the biopsy showed suspicious cells. The
patient was re-x-rayed at Paterson General Hospital where she was thought
to have a benign myoma with ulceration. Past history includes tubal ligation
and dilatation and curettage one year ago. There are no known allergies.

Physical examination was essentially normal.

The x-rays showed a negative gallbladder. The flat and erect of the abdomen
were negative. The pathological report at Passaic General Hospital done by
the Passaic General Hospital, dated 3-30-77, #B38948, states, "Tissue consistent with gastric polypoid tissue containing foci suspicious for malignancy." Chest x-ray was negative. EKG was negative. The question of further
diagnostic workup was discussed with Dr. L████ and he advised none at this
time. The admitting laboratory workup showed a negative VDRL, normal urine.
CBC was normal. SMA 20 was normal.

The patient was operated on 4-18-77 at which time adenocarcinoma of the
stomach with metastasis to the gastrocolic nodes was found. A radical
subtotal was performed. The patient made a good recovery. She is extremely
apprehensive and arrangements will be made with Dr. L████ for consultation
at Memorial Hospital. The patient also wishes consultation with Dr. Kelly
from the State of Washington. This, too, will be arranged if the patient
so desires.

FINAL DIAGNOSIS: Adenocarcinoma of the stomach with metastasis
                     to the gastrocolic nodes and omentum.

OPERATION: Radical subtotal gastrectomy.

cc: Dr. A. L████

I HAVE READ AND APPROVED THIS COMPLETE MEDICAL RECORD

TL097 #2-6
DATE _Dictated: 4-30-77_

SIGNED _John J. C██████████, M.D._

DISCHARGE SUMMARY   7-2397(3)

449

PRESENTATION OF FIFTY CASE HISTORIES

TESTICULAR CANCER

Testicular cancers account for only 1% of all malignancies, but are nonetheless a leading cause of tumor death among young men in the second and third decade of life.

Overall, testicular cancer claimed 400 lives in 1987. Although the disease can be very aggressive, unlike most solid tumors this malignancy responds well to conventional approaches even when metastatic. With standard treatment including chemotherapy the prognosis is good, with more than 80% of all patients living five years after their initial presentation.

Patient #48

Patient #48 is a 33-year-old man from California who has survived six years since his diagnosis of metastatic testicular cancer.

During the spring of 1981, Patient #48's left testicle gradually enlarged over a period of several weeks. In mid-June 1981 he consulted his primary physician who, immediately suspecting cancer, admitted Patient #48 to Long Beach Community Hospital for further evaluation.

A CT scan of the chest showed no abnormalities, but a CT study of the abdomen revealed enlarged lymph nodes along the vena cava and aorta, as well as a 5 by 5 by 2 cm mass in the retroperitoneal (posterior abdominal) region, all consistent with metastatic disease.

On June 23, 1981, Patient #48 underwent resection of his left testicle with its tumor, identified as a malignant teratoma, "intermediate type." At that point, a staff oncologist recommended intensive chemotherapy, but Patient #48, who already knew of Dr. Kelley, decided to refuse all conventional treatment. His doctor wrote in the records:

> After weighing these alternatives the patient has decided that he does not wish to undergo chemotherapy at this time but wishes to undergo alternative cancer therapy with enemas and diet. The patient realizes that I do not think that this therapy is effective and maybe make [sic] his future therapy more difficult because of progressive tumor growth in the interval . . .

In July 1981, Patient #48 began the full Kelley program, and within weeks, noted an improvement in his general health. After seven months on his protocol, Patient #48 returned to his oncologist for a follow-up examination. At that time, a repeat CT scan showed no sign of the previously observed retroperitoneal mass or enlarged lymph nodes. The physician wrote in a letter on February 2, 1982:

> When examined today, he has no evidence of disease on recent physical examination, laboratory studies, chest x-ray or CT scan of the abdomen.

At present, six years after his diagnosis, Patient #48 still follows the full Kelley program, is in excellent health, and remains cancer-free.

Aggressive multi-agent chemotherapy can cure most cases of testicular cancer, but untreated, the disease is quickly fatal. Even as recently as the late 1960s, before the advent of effective drug regimens, fewer than 10% of patients survived five years.[1]

In summary, Patient #48 was diagnosed with metastatic testicular cancer, as documented by CT scan. After his initial surgery, his extensive disease regressed completely while he pursued only the Kelley program.

REFERENCE

1. DeVita, VT, et al. *Cancer Principles & Practice of Oncology*. Philadelphia; J.B. Lippincott, 1982, page 820.

LONG BEACH COMMUNITY HOSPITAL

1720 Termino Avenue, P.O. Box 2587, Long Beach, California 90801 (213) 597-6655

CHIEF COMPLAINT: Teratocarcinoma of the testes.

HPI: The patient is a 27 year old Caucasian male who for the past 2 months noted a painful swelling of the left testes. Today, 6-23-81, the patient underwent an inguinal orchiectomy and frozen section pathology revealed a teratocarcinoma.

In addition, the patient has had a CT scan of the chest which was negative and CT scan of the abdomen which revealed a 5 x 5 x 2 cm mass of nodes in the retro-peritoneum.

The patient is generally asymptomatic. He denies any breast tenderness or swelling, dyspnea, cough, sputum, headaches, double vision, blurring of vision, nausea, vomiting, diarrhea or constipation.

PAST MEDICAL HISTORY: No significant medical illnesses.

ALLERGIES: None.

OPERATIONS: No previous operations until today when he had an inguinal orchiectomy.

MEDICATIONS: None.

FAMILY HISTORY: Unremarkable.

PHYSICAL EXAMINATION

The patient is a well-developed, well-nourished, cooperative oriented Caucasian male who was seen initially preoperatively and again postoperatively.

The pulse was 80 and respirations were 16, blood pressure 120/68.

SKIN: Warm and dry without lesion.

HEENT: Sclerae and conjunctivae benign, EOMI. ENT negative.

NECK: Supple.

LYMPHATICS: No significant lymphadenopathy.

LUNGS: Clear to percussion and auscultation.

BREASTS: Without gynecomastia.

HEART: There is a regular sinus rhythm without murmur, gallop or rub.

ABDOMEN: With hepatosplenomegaly, masses or tenderness.

GENITALIA: Today the patient had an inguinal orchiectomy. Yesterday when the testes were examined, the right testes was normal and the left testes was 2-3 time normal in size and was extremely hard and minimally tender and somewhat

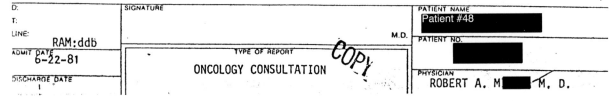

D:	SIGNATURE	PATIENT NAME
T:		Patient #48
LINE: RAM:ddb		M.D. PATIENT NO.
ADMIT DATE 6-22-81	TYPE OF REPORT ONCOLOGY CONSULTATION COPY	
DISCHARGE DATE		PHYSICIAN ROBERT A. M▮▮▮ M. D.

454

irregular in shape.

EXTREMITIES: Without cyanosis, clubbing or edema.

NEUROLOGICAL: Grossly intact.

IMPRESSION: 1) Teratocarcinoma of the testes,
                                  metastatic to the retroperitoneal
                                  lymph nodes as shown by CT scan
                                  of the abdomen with no evidence of
                                  metastases to the lung, STAGE II-B
                                  with bulky intra-abdominal disease.

DISCUSSION: I had a long discussion with the patient and his wife concerning
his diagnosis, prognosis and therapeutic alternatives. At the present time
I recommmended cheomtherapy with Cisplatinum, Velban, Bleomycin. This will be
continued for approximately 3 months and then the patient will be re-Staged
with CT scan and ultrasound of the abdomen and his hormonal   will
be followed. And consideration will be made at that time for possible exporatory
laparotomy and possible retroperitoneal lymphadenectomy or removal of any potential
residual disease.

The toxicity of chemotherapy was explained in detail including nausea, vomiting,
anorexia, weight loss, alopecia, pulmonary and renal toxicities.

The patient asked questions concerning non-standard forms of cancer therapy.
He explained that a best-friend of his has run a helath food store and has
"cured cancer" with Chinese herbs. I explained to him that I knew of no
potential benefit proven from this therapy, nor did I know whether it would
interfere with the chemotherapy or possibly adding to toxicity of lowering the
effectiveness of the chemotherapy.

Hopefully the patient will accept chemotherapy, but I am not sure at this time.
He and his wife are going to think about the therapeutic alternatives and contact
me early next week.

Thank you for allowing me to participate in the care of you fine patient.

CC: N, C██████████ M, D,

6-23-81	SIGNATURE		PATIENT NAME
6-23-81			Patient #48
NE: RAM:ddb		*COPY* M.D.	PATIENT NO.
JMIT DATE		TYPE OF REPORT	
		ONCOLOGY CONSULTATION	PHYSICIAN
ISCHARGE DATE			

455

Patient's Name	Patient #48	Age	27	Hospital No.	
Doctor	C	Room	303	Date Rec'd.	6-23-81
				Lab. No.	S-1969-81

SPECIMEN: "Left Testicle"
"Right Vas" (A)

The specimen consists of a testicle, its tunics and an attached segment of spermatic cord. The testicle measures 5 x 4.5 x 4.5 cm. in greatest dimensions. The attached spermatic cord measures 9 x 1 x 0.7 cm. The testicle is hemisectioned. It is extensively replaced by a multinodular extensively cartilaginous tumor. The largest nodule is almost entirely grossly cartilaginous. This nodule measures 4.5 cm. in greatest dimensions. It is glistening and grey to grey-white. Adjacent to it is a soft elevated oval tan nodule 3 x 1.5 x 1 cm. in greatest dimensions. The entire tumor is grossly confined by the tunica albuginea. It does not extend into it or through it. The epididymis is uninvolved. There is no gross tumor in the spermatic cord. A frozen section through the least cartilaginous portion of the tumor is performed and reported as: "Teratoma will need multiple microscopics to determine various other elements." An estimated 2 gram sample of the tumor is submitted for chemosensitivity studies. Photographs of the specimen are taken.

RS

1969-81

A - A formalin fixed grey segment of tissue measures 3 x 1 mm.

1969-81

MICROSCOPIC:

A - Cross sections of a vas deferens are present.
1969-81

Multiple sections of the testicular tumor show teratomatous elements that are both mature and immature. They include areas that are histologically benign and malignant. There are areas of adenocarcinoma (embryonal carcinoma). The teratomatous components include abundant squamous epithelium and areas forming keratin with cyst formation. Abundant well differentiated cartilage with focal transformation into bone, spindle shaped cells in areas recognized as smooth muscle tissue, glands lined by columnar epithelium and areas of mucin secretion, collagenous connective tissue, fat, malignant columnar epithelial cells forming glands and malignant spindle shaped epithelial cells are identified. The tumor does not microscopically extend through the tunica albuginea. It does not involve the rete testis or the epididymis. Testicular tissue uninvolved by tumor shows little or no spermatogenesis. The testicular tubules are predominantly composed of Sertoli cells or spermatogonia. Interstitial cells of Leydig are not hyperplastic.

1969-81

Sections of spermatic cord show no tumor.

None of the sections of tumor show areas of seminoma or choriocarcinoma.

REMARKS:

_____ M.D.
PATHOLOGIST

HISTO-PATHOLOGICAL REPORT

456

Patient's Name	Patient #48	Age 27	Hospital No.	
Doctor	Ch	Room 303	Date Rec'd.	6-23-81
			Lab. No.	S-1969-81

PAGE 2 .

This type of teratoma is classified as follows:

1. Malignant teratoma intermediate (Testicular Tumor Panel, 1975).

2. Teratocarcinoma (Friedman and Moore, 1946).

3. Teratoma with embryonal carcinoma, Group IV (Dixon and Moore, 1952).

4. Teratoma with histologically malignant area and with embryonal carcinoma (Mostofi and Price, 1973).

5. Teratoma with malignant transformation and embryonal carcinoma (WHO 1975).

I prefer the Testicular Tumor Panel term of 1975.

DIAGNOSIS: (6-26-81)

RADICAL LEFT ORCHECTOMY SPECIMEN.

    A. MALIGNANT TERATOMA, INTERMEDIATE.

    B. NO GROSS OR MICROSCOPIC INVOLVEMENT OF TUNICA ALBUGINEA, RETE TESTIS EPIDIDYMIS OR SPERMATIC CORD.   78-9083   9073

_____ M.D.

PATHOLOGIST

HISTO-PATHOLOGICAL REPORT

457

Patient was admitted with increasing size mass in the left testicle. Also, on CAT scan was found to have what appears to be large, retroperitoneal nodes along the vena cava and aorta. On 6/23/8 he was taken to the Operating Room where a radical left orchiectomy, right vasectomy and insertio of a testicular prosthesis was performed. His postoperative course was uneventful. Wounds healing pro-priman. Patient is now being discharged to be followed in the office.

LABORATORY DATA: Hemogram and urinalysis within normal limits. We are awaiting the HGC, CEA and alpha fetoprotein. Also waiting a file report on the testicle, but it appears on frozen section to represent an adenocarcinoma.

Patient is now being discharge. He will be followed by Dr. M███ and myself, probably will receive chemotherapy prior to having a retroperitoneal node dissection.

Final dx — Malignant teratoma, intermediate

D:	6/24/81	SIGNATURE		PATIENT NAME	
T:	6/25/81				Patient #48
LINE:			M.D.	PATIENT NO.	
ADMIT DATE		TYPE OF REPORT			

458

INITIAL VISIT AND CONSULTATION
Dictated by
Robert A. M█████, M.D. - 06-23-81

JUL 2 1981

Lt:
it:
'/P:
also:

7-2-81: (DR M) ██████████████████████OV: I explained to patient
indications, complications and alternatives of therapy for
teratocarcinoma of the testes with extensive intraabdominal
metastases presently thought to be unresectable. After weighing
these alternatives the patient has decided that he does not wish
to undergo chemotherapy at this time but wishes to undergo
alternative cancer therapy with enemas and diet. The patient realizes
that I do not think that this therapy is effective and maybe make
his future therapy more difficult because of progressive tumor
growth in the interval between now and the time that chemotherapy would
be appropriately administered. However, patient wishes to take this
risk. We will therefore see him back in one month and   at that
time obtain a repeat chest x-ray and compare ultrasounds of the
abdomen and HCG beta subunit and alpha fetoprotein tests.

COPY TO. DR. C█████████.

7-9-81: (DR M) ████████████,OV: Patient has decided to take
a "nontoxic" form of therapy for his testicular carcinoma. He
is electing to take the program described by William Kelly, D.D.S.
which is a nutritional form of cancer therapy management. I
have explained to patient that I do not approve of this program
and am recommending that he consider chemotherapy instead but
being that he is an adult and has been presented with the options
of therapy and has elected to choose the nontoxic form of therapy
I realize that he can make this choice freely. I will, however,
continue to see patient intermittently and inform him as to his
progress relating to either improvement or progression of
metastatic disease and perform appropriate tests as is deemed
necessary. The patient will return in one month.

JUL 31 198

wt; 155
 # 70
p 124
P. 80

7-31-81: (DR M) ████████████,OV: Patient's chest x-ray shows no
evidence of metastases. His abdominal ultrasound is unchanged.
His HcG and alpha fetoprotein are both within normal limits. He
has been taking coffee enemas and has been on a fast followed by
a diet as a part of an unorthodox method of neutritional therapy for
cancer. I have advised him against this but he wishes to proceed
with this program until we have proven evidence of progression of
disease. He actually states he is feeling well. He has no
symptoms suggestive of metastases.
PHYSICAL EXAM: LUNGS: Clear.

BREASTS: Without gynecomastia.
ABDOMEN: Without hepatosplenomegaly.
GENITALIA: Without evidence of tumor.
EXTREMITIES: Without edema.

du 84

IMPRESSION: Teratocarcinoma of the testes with embryonal cell
carcinoma with evidence of metastatic disease to the retroperitoneum
on CT scan of the abdomen. Patient undergoing unorthodox method
of cancer therapy.
PLAN: We will continue to follow patient without initiating therapy
until he shows evidence of progression of disease. Meanwhile we

459

EB 8 1982 ~F.A.

EB 12 1932
rt 170
fp 130/80
ilse 64

2-12-82: (DR M) ███████████████ OV: Patient comes in for a routine two month follow up. He is feeling very well and is very active having no particular complaints. Recent CT scan of the abdomen performed at Long Beach Community Hospital was read as negative. They did not see the retroperitoneal mass that was seen at Los

Alamitos General Hospital CT scan approximately six months ago. We will obtain these films for review. Patient was told the results.
PHYSICAL EXAM: No evidence of recurrence of disease.
IMPRESSION: Teratocarcinoma of the testes with CT scan previously showing metastatic disease in the retroperitoneum, patient

refusing retroperitoneal dissection, now with CT scan apparently normal.
PLAN: We will obtain patient's prior CT scan and review both together. Meanwhile we will see patient intermittently as before.

460

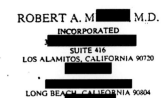
February 12, 1982

Re: Patient #48

To Whom It May Concern:

█████████ was diagnosed as having Terrato carcinoma of the testes, on 6-23-81, when he underwent a left inguinal orchiectomy. When examined today, he has no evidence of disease on recent physical examination, laboratory studies, chest x-ray, or CT scan of the abdomen.

Sincerely,

Robert A. M████, M.D.

461

Patient #49

Patient #49 is a 36-year-old man from Louisiana alive eight years since his diagnosis of metastatic testicular cancer.

In early 1979, Patient #49 noticed an enlarged left testicle. He consulted his family physician who on April 2, 1979, admitted him to Southern Baptist Hospital in New Orleans for evaluation. After a preliminary biopsy confirmed embryonal carcinoma, on April 4, 1979 Patient #49 underwent surgery for removal of his left testicle with its associated tumor, described in the records as an aggressive, "High grade malignancy."

Though a lymphangiogram the day after surgery revealed no evidence of metastases, the patient's surgeon nonetheless recommended a retroperitoneal (abdominal) lymph node dissection at a later date to determine conclusively the extent of disease.

Patient #49 was discharged from the hospital on April 6, 1979, then re-admitted on April 21, 1979 for the planned procedure. "Poorly differentiated embryonal carcinoma" was identified in six retroperitoneal lymph nodes and another 12 appeared cancerous on gross examination. In addition, according to the patient, X-ray studies demonstrated possible metastatic disease in his left lung and hip.

His doctors then proposed a course of multi-agent chemotherapy, to be administered on an outpatient basis. Initially, Patient #49 agreed to the plan, but after leaving the hospital on April 30, 1979, he decided to investigate alternative approaches to cancer. Within weeks, he learned of Dr. Kelley, decided to begin the nutritional program, and rejected all further conventional treatment.

At present, eight years since his diagnosis, Patient #49 still follows the Kelley regimen and is in excellent health, with no sign of his once extensive disease. Note that he has refused follow-up radiology studies, so I have no proof of tumor regression in his abdomen, lung or hip.

Nonetheless, Patient #49's long-term survival is unusual. He was diagnosed with metastatic testicular cancer, as documented by multiple lymph node biopsies and radiology studies. Since Patient #49 never received chemotherapy, it seems reasonable to credit the Kelley regimen with his long-term, disease-free survival.

DEPARTMENT OF PATHOLOGY

Name: Patient #49   Room: 5307-D   S -79-2229   Sex: M   Date: 4/4/79
Physician: Dr. C. E. C   Age: 29   Case No:
Clinical Diagnosis:

Tissue: LEFT TESTICLE

Gross Description:

The specimen was used for frozen section examination and interpreted as showing high grade malignancy with a definitive diagnosis deferred pending permanent section examination. The specimen consists of a structure recognizable as an adult testicle which measures 4 x 4 x 3.5 cm. in greatest overall dimensions. Attached to the specimen is an epididymis and a length of spermatic cord is attached which measures 10 cm. i length. The spermatic cord contains its usual structures. Multiple representative sections of the cord will be submitted. A firm nodule is palpated in the inferior portion of the testicle. This does not grossly penetrate the capsule. Upon cut section a grayish, lobular tumor mass is encountered which measures 2 x 2 x 2 cm. in greatest overall plane dimensions. This tumor mass is not encapsulated and is poorly demarcated from the surrounding tan testicular tissue. Focal areas of hemorrhagic necrosis are present in this tumor mass. Multiple representative sections will be submitted for microscopic examination.

JPJ/bj/caw

FROZEN SECTION INTERPRETATION: High grade malignancy, probably embryonal cell carcinoma.

JWS/caw

DIAGNOSIS: TESTES - EMBRYONAL CELL CARCINOMA SHOWING LYMPHATIC AND BLOOD VESSEL PERMEATION.

Note: The spermatic cord is free of tumor. Scattered syncytial giant cells are present within the tumor and there is focal intratubular atypical spermatocytic hyperplasia as well as Leydig cell hyperplasia.

The lesion was seen in consultation by R. J. R M.D., a copy of his consulatation is attached.

JPJ/caw
4/10/79

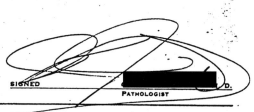

SIGNED   PATHOLOGIST   D.

Name: [Patient #49]   Room: 5321   S -79-2705   Date: 4/23/79

Physician: Dr. Charles C█   Surg: Drs C█ /.C█   Age: 28 Sex: M   Case No: █

Clinical Diagnosis:

Tissue: APPENDIX, LYMPH NODES

Gross Description: The specimen consists partially of several irregular segments of fatty appearing tissue incorporating lymph node structures. These together measure 11 x 6 x 2 cm. There is one irregular nodular mass within this fat measuring 4 x 3 x 2 cm. This appears to represent several adherent lymph nodes. On section they show a gray to gray-yellow surface with scattered areas of somewhat granular yellowish-brown tissue interspersed which appears to be metastatic tumor. There are 19 additional lymph nodes dissected from the specimen which vary from 3 mm. to about 1 cm. in diameter. About 12 of these are firmer than usual and could contain metastatic tumor. The appendix measures 11 x .6 cm. The serosa is smooth, grayish-pink. The lumen is patent and contains slightly firm, greenish-brown feces.

SRS:cw

DIAGNOSIS: POORLY DIFFERENTIATED EMBRYONAL CARCINOMA INVOLVING SIX (6) LYMPH NODES.

        Comment: Some foci show cells suggestive of trophoblasts, but definite diagnosis of choriocarcinoma cannot be made.

SRS:bj
4/26/79

SIGNED █ M. D.
PATHOLOGIST

SOUTHERN BAPTIST HOSPITAL   Surgical Pathological Report

464

ADMITTED: 4/21/79
DR. CHARLES C▮▮▮

Date of Discharge:	
	4/30/79
Reason for Admission:	Previously diagnosed embryonal cell carcinoma of left testicle.

Pertinent Physical Symptoms
and Signs, Laboratory and
X-ray Findings:

This patient had a left orchiectomy approximately two weeks earlier.
The final pathological diagnosis was embryonal cell carcinoma. He
was readmitted for lymph node dissection. This was done and he was
found to have numerous large retroperitoneal lymph nodes in the region of the hilum of the left kidney, one of which was intimately
attached to the renal vein. These were all malignant. Postoperatively he did quite well. He is discharged on a regular diet, full ambul-
ation to be followed in the office and to be seen for chemotherapy
by Dr. Charles B▮▮▮▮▮

Clinical Course, Therapy,
Response and Complications:

Condition on
Discharge:

Treatment and Care
after Discharge:

Diet Instructions
Medication
Activity
Follow up care

Signature _____
DR. CHARLES C▮▮▮/mch   5/30/79

FORM 324-A. REV. 11-77. DO1190

465

UTERINE CANCER

In 1987, uterine cancer claimed 2,900 lives. When localized, in most cases the disease can be cured with hysterectomy but once metastatic, the prognosis remains very poor.

Currently, approximately 80% of women with uterine cancer survive five years.

Patient #50

Patient #50 is a 72-year-old woman from Washington State alive nearly 18 years since her initial diagnosis of uterine carcinoma.

Patient #50, prior to developing cancer, had been in good health most of her life, with a history of five successful pregnancies before an uncomplicated menopause at age 52, in 1966.

In mid-September 1969, Patient #50 first experienced episodes of vaginal bleeding that persisted over a six-week period. In late October 1969, she consulted her gynecologist, who performed an endometrial (uterine) biopsy revealing uterine adenocarcinoma. Subsequently, Patient #50 was admitted to Group Health Hospital in Seattle on November 5, 1969 for a dilatation and curettage. Review of tissue samples confirmed a grade III adenocarcinoma, the most aggressive form of the disease.

Her doctors suggested a course of radiation as initial treatment, to be followed by hysterectomy. Patient #50 agreed to the plan, and while still hospitalized completed the proposed radiation implant therapy, receiving a total of 5,120 rads directly into the uterus. After finishing the treatment, she was discharged in stable condition on November 7, 1969 and re-admitted a month later, on December 9, 1969, for a hysterectomy and oophorectomy (removal of her ovaries). When no evidence of metastatic disease could be found at surgery, she was assumed cured.

Over the following six years, Patient #50's general health, which previously had been quite good, began to deteriorate. She experienced gradually worsening fatigue, malaise, depression, and chronic lower abdominal pain. Multiple evaluations by several physicians uncovered no cause for her declining health, and according to Patient #50, one aggravated doctor told her she suffered nothing more than a "bad case of nerves."

In the late fall of 1975, Patient #50 returned to her physician once again when the abdominal pain became intolerable. This time, after detecting a solid mass in the left pelvic area, he admitted Patient #50 to Group Health on November 23, 1975 for further evaluation.

A consulting surgeon thought the mass most likely represented recurrent uterine cancer. In addition, a chest X-ray revealed evidence of metastatic disease in both lungs, described in the radiology report, as "several bilateral pulmonary nodules, which have appeared since the last examination measuring up to 1.3 cm. in diameter and most likely representing metastatic nodules."

On November 24, 1975, Patient #50 underwent surgery for resection of a large 5.5 by 4.5 by 3.0 cm pelvic tumor that extended into the regional tissues. As expected, the tumor was found consistent with recurrent "metastatic endometrial adenocarcinoma," and an X-ray performed after surgery once again documented the multiple lung lesions. A staff oncologist assigned to the case recommended she begin aggressive chemotherapy at once, but Patient #50 promptly declined the suggestion. However, she did agree to a course of 17-alpha-hydroxyprogesterone, a synthetic progesterone frequently prescribed patients diagnosed with metastatic uterine cancer.

Patient #50 was discharged from the hospital on December 1, 1975, in a very weakened condition. Subsequently, she seemed to worsen despite the hormone therapy, becoming increasingly fatigued and lethargic, and experiencing constant shortness of breath assumed due to the metastatic disease in her lungs. By March 1976, she was largely bedridden, apparently in a near-terminal state.

By chance, Patient #50 learned of Dr. Kelley and decided to proceed with his therapy. After discontinuing the progesterone, she consulted with Dr. Kelley and in early April 1976 began the full nutritional regimen. Although her physicians objected to such "quackery," within a year all her symptoms, including her respiratory distress, resolved.

Today, more than 11 years after her diagnosis of metastatic disease, Patient #50 still follows a "modified" Kelley regimen, remains in good health, and appears to be cancer-free. She told me that if she had the money, she would still use the full program, but her insurance company refuses to reimburse the cost of the supplements. Nevertheless, Patient #50 reports no medical problems other than an irregular heart rhythm, diagnosed in 1975 as atrial fibrillation, at the time she first developed evidence of metastatic cancer in her chest.

After Patient #50 began the Kelley protocol, she broke off contact with her physicians until November 1984, when she returned for evaluation of her heart rhythm. In a letter to a colleague, her primary doctor details a rather unusual response to seeing Patient #50 again:

> I almost dropped dead when she told me she wanted a chest x-ray. I think
> she wants to know what's going on regarding her heart . . .

Chest film—except for a rather large heart which shows no sign of de-compensation that I can see, chest film is normal. Rib detail film also looks normal—specifically, I did not see any evidence of metastatic disease on either film which is quite remarkable in view of the fact that 9 years ago she had metastatic disease . . .

Since fewer than 14% of all patients with metastatic uterine survive five years even if aggressively treated, Patient #50's long-term survival is most remarkable. In 1975, she developed recurrent uterine cancer in both her pelvis and her lungs. She refused all conventional therapy except for hydroxyprogesterone, which she used only briefly. Even if Patient #50 had continued the treatment as prescribed, hormonal therapy does not cure metastatic uterine disease.[1]

It seems appropriate to attribute the documented regression of this patient's can-cer, her good health, and her long-term survival to the Kelley program.

REFERENCE

1. DeVita, VT, et al. *Cancer Principles & Practice of Oncology*. Philadelphia; J.B. Lip-pincott Company, 1982, page 857.

DISCHARGE SUMMARY

Patient #50

HOSPITAL NO.

ATTENDING PHYSICIAN	DATE OF ADMISSION	DATE OF DISCHARGE
THOMAS R███ M.D.	11/23/75	12/1/75

Significant history and physical findings, significant x-ray and laboratory findings, course in hospital including summary of surgical procedures and findings, complications, if any, treatment, final diagnosis, disposition on discharge, prognosis with recommendations for follow-up, if any.

FINAL DIAGNOSIS:
Probable Recurrent Adenocarcinoma of the Uterus.

HISTORY:
This 61-year old lady who several years ago underwent, after diagnostically she was found to have adenocarcinoma of the uterus, treatment including radiation and hysterectomy with bilateral salpingo-oophorectomy. The patient has had gradually developing symptoms of left lower quadrant abdominal pains of a mild degree. Abdominal mass was found in the left false pelvis area. IVP and barium enema examinations were normal. Because of the presence of the mass, the patient was admitted to the hospital for exploration.

At the time of surgery, it was found that a localized recurrent adenocarcinoma was present subperitoneally, just anterior to descending colon. This/mass was locally resectable and was resected. No other intra-abdominal evidence of recurrent disease was present.

The patient had a benign postoperative course. The patient had a chest x-ray which revealed the possibility of multiple pulmonary metastasis and a shoulder x-ray for chronic shoulder pain which revealed osteoarthritis.

The patient underwent physical therapy treatments for the osteoarthritis. DR. T███ was consulted regarding the patient's recurrent disease and he suggested chemotherapy consultation which was obtained. Dr. T██, at present, is in the process of evaluating the patient's status regarding whether or not chemotherapy should be instituted at this time. The patient, as of this date, desires to be discharged. She is feeling quite comfortable and desires no pain medications. She is aware of the problem related to the possible pulmonary metastasis and the possibility of further tests at Dr. T██'s discretion. An appointment will be arranged for her to return to see Dr. T██ in his office regarding the chemotherapy program he may institute.

DATE

Signed

DICTATED STAT 12/1/75
CC: Dr. T███

THOMAS R███ M.D./12/1/75 dagf 10:30AM

CODE | FILM | SERVICES | CHARGE | PREVIOUS X RAY ☒ YES ☐ NO | DATE

TYPE OF EXAMINATION

HISTORY AND DIAGNOSIS

11/23/75 GTR CHEST: PA view compared to 6/12/75 shows several bilateral pulmonary nodules, which have appeared since the last examination measuring up to 1.3 cm. in diameter and most likely representing metastatic nodules. It is still not clear whether the shadow superimposed on the right hemidiaphragm is a pulmonary nodule, but it does appear slightly larger than on the last examination.
     IMRPESSION: Bilateral pulmonary nodules, probably representing metastases.
jp
11/25/75

472

PATIENT Patient #50   AGE **1914** DATE **Nov. 24, 1975**

ROOM **S 205**   HOSPITAL NO.   HOLOGY NO. **150996**

DOCTOR R   ORIGIN OF TISSUE: **A) Mass from Peritoneal Surface; B) Abd. Mass Tissue**

PREOPERATIVE DIAGNOSIS: ABDOMINAL MASS

EXAMINATION OF PATHOLOGICAL SPECIMEN

GROSS APPEARANCE:

A) The specimen consisted of an irregular mass 5.5 x 4.5 x 3.0 cm. Small amounts of
fat were attached externally. Areas of peritoneal tissue were composed partially
of surface with irregular areas of pale gray-tan neoplastic tissue. Sections showed
a neoplastic mass of tan hemorrhagic tissue with a faintly lobulated cut surface and
a small irregular cyst. Representative sections were taken.
B) The specimen consisted of an irregular mass of firm indurated tissue 2.0 cm in
diameter. Sectioned and all embedded.

MICROSCOPIC EXAMINATION:

A) Multiple sections of the large peritoneal mass show a malignant glandular pattern
with cribriforming consistent with an endometrial origin. Morphologically, the tumor
shows an identical pattern as that seen in previous endometrial specimens, case # 67587
and #67816. As in the previous material, small foci of squamoid differentiation are
present. The surrounding stroma appears severely desmoplastic and congested with small
foci of necrosis.
B) Sections are of dense fibrocollagenous tissue and fat containing small foci of
metastatic carcinoma. A cystic space is present lined by malignant epithelial cells
of the adenocarcinomatous type and within the surrounding tissue are small nodular foci
of the metastatic squamous component.

ANATOMIC DIAGNOSIS:

A & B) METASTATIC ENDOMETRIAL ADENOCARCINOMA WITH SQUAMOUS FOCI (ADENOACANTHOMA),
SUB-PERITONEAL TISSUE, ABDOMINAL WALL.

F.S.
PAS-1
C-6
pb

_____ M.D.
                    PATHOLOGIST

R. K

473

November 16, 1984

I almost dropped dead when she told me she wanted a chest
x-ray. I think she wants to know what's going on regarding
her heart. Is still fibrillating. undergoing hair analysis
by someone who is telling her all the minerals she is low in
- manganese, copper; etc.

I told her I thought it somewhat unlikely that the results of
x-rays would make any difference in how we treated her but,
since I can't see that it will do her any harm I told her if
she wanted the x-rays, we'd get them. Has a rather prominent
flaring of rib cage at left anterolateral costal margin.

Chest film - except for a rather large heart which shows no
sign of decompensation that I can see, chest film is normal.
Rib detail film also looks normal - specifically, I did not
see any evidence of metastatic disease on either film which
is quite remarkable in view of the fact that 9 years ago she
had metastatic disease in both abdomen and lungs as nearly as
I can tell from he record. Had pelvic radiation followed by
total hysterectomy in 1970 and apparently had a recurrence of
the diease some 5 years later.

C███ G. N██████ M.D.

474

CHAPTER XI

—◆—

Pancreatic Cancer Study

Since the five-year survival rate for pancreatic cancer is, in conventional oncology, less than 5%, at Dr. Good's suggestion I decided to look more closely at Dr. Kelley's experience with this particular malignancy.

I first searched through Dr. Kelley's files, pulling the charts of all patients diagnosed with pancreatic cancer who had pursued his therapy between 1974 and 1982. Such cases were easy enough to recognize, since Dr. Kelley always wrote medical histories on his charts.

I eventually identified 22 patients who, at least according to Dr. Kelley's notes, had presented with pancreatic cancer during the specified time frame. With their records in hand, I began tracking each one down.

I learned that 17 of these patients had died. For twelve in this group, I was able to contact surviving next of kin—spouses, children, siblings, etc. In each case, family members willingly talked with me about their deceased relative, and his or her experiences with the Kelley program.

For five of the deceased patients, I never located any living family member, though I did interview at length the attending physician initially in charge of each case.

Finally, for all but one of the dead patients, I obtained complete medical records confirming the diagnosis, extent of disease, and previous treatment, as well as official death certificates. In one case, though I had in my possession the original biopsy report, initial radiographic studies, and the death certificate, I could never locate any records documenting the conventional treatment pursued prior to the consultation with Dr. Kelley.

A second group of five patients were alive when I began my investigation. One eventually died, although not from cancer, before completion of my study. I have discussed these five cases in detail in the previous "50 Cases" section, under the heading "Pancreatic Cancer."

The data base used to evaluate Dr. Kelley's pancreatic patients, updated as of May 1987, can be summarized as follows:

Living Patients (4)

Data Base	# Patients
Interviews with Patient	4
Medical Records	

Deceased Patients (18)

Data Base	# Patients
Interviews with Family	12
Medical Records	
Death Certificates	

Data Base	# Patients
Interview with Physician	5
Medical Records	
Death Certificate	

Data Base	
Interview with Patient (Died during study)	1
Interview with Family	
Medical Records	

Once I had identified these pancreatic cases, I determined compliance, that is, how rigorously each patient followed his or her prescribed nutritional regimen, using information from several sources to assess this factor. First of all, during my interviews with living patients, or with the family members and physicians of those who had died, I always asked in detail about compliance.

Dr. Kelley's files provided another source of data, since on most charts he himself chronicled each patient's adherence to the regimen. In addition, several of these patients had written to Dr. Kelley in the past, discussing their compliance. These documents, along with the patient records, were made available to me.

Prior to 1976, Dr. Kelley recommended supplements produced by several different companies, during which time he kept records of each patient's purchase orders. This information had helped him, and now helped me, determine if the patients who consulted him at that time were really buying the required quantities of nutrients and enzymes.

After 1976, Dr. Kelley assigned production of his supplements to a single manufacturer. At my request, company employees searched their files and sent me copies of relevant invoices for those of the 22 pancreatic cases who had ordered supplements from them.

I determined that 10 of the 22 patients had consulted Dr. Kelley only once, and had never followed the prescribed program, not even for a single day. All had died.

Seven patients pursued their nutritional regimen only partially and sporadically, for periods of time ranging from four weeks to 13 months. These patients, too, had all died, and none had complied with the Kelley program during the three months prior to death.

Patients failed to follow the regimen, or followed it incompletely, for a number of reasons. One patient, who succumbed the day after visiting Dr. Kelley, was too sick to begin. Another, whose disease had already bankrupted him by the time he consulted with Dr. Kelley, could not afford the ongoing cost of the supplements. Several patients gave up on the regimen because their physicians strongly opposed Dr. Kelley's approach and several found the lifestyle changes, the diet and detoxification routines too unappealing.

The reasons for non-compliance can be summarized as follows:

477

Reason for Non-Compliance	# Patients
Too sick	1
Couldn't afford	1
Too much trouble or physician opposition	10
Reason unknown	5

Five of the 22 patients followed the full regimen as prescribed, and for periods ranging from two to 10 years. Each experienced a significant response, based on either documented tumor regression or unusual long-term survival. Four of this group are still alive as of spring of 1987.

The data on compliance can be summarized as follows:

Extent of Compliance	# Patients	Status
Never followed	10	All dead
Followed partially	7	All dead
Followed completely	5	4 alive
		1 dead

In the next section, I briefly describe each of the 22 pancreatic cases, organized into three categories: the first group includes those who never followed the program, the second, those who complied with the prescribed nutritional regimen partially, and the third consists of the five patients who pursued the full program for significant periods of time.

In each case, I have calculated what I call "survival time." I measure this from the day of the first consultation with Dr. Kelley, until the day of death—or to the present (May 1987), for those still alive. For each of the three categories, I arrange the cases in order of this survival time, starting with the shortest-lived patient first.

Group I:

Patients Who Never Followed the Kelley Program

1. *Patient SK*

Official Diagnosis: Metastatic carcinoma of the pancreas

Date of Diagnosis: June 1976

Hospital: Gresham Hospital, Gresham, Oregon

Conventional Therapy: Chemotherapy

Date First Seen by Dr. Kelley: August 20, 1976

Date of Death: August 21, 1976

Survival Time: One day

2. *Patient SG*

Official Diagnosis: Metastatic carcinoma of the pancreas

Date of Diagnosis: December 1973

Hospital: Fairview General Hospital, Cleveland, Ohio

Conventional Therapy: Palliative surgery

Date First Seen by Dr. Kelley: May 31, 1974

Date of Death: July 9, 1974

Survival Time: 39 days

3. *Patient KT*

Official Diagnosis: Metastatic carcinoma of the pancreas

Date of Diagnosis: November 1975

Hospital: Mayo Clinic, Rochester, Minnesota

Conventional Therapy: Chemotherapy, radiation

Date First Seen by Dr. Kelley: October 20, 1976

Date of Death: December 1, 1976

Survival Time: 42 days

4. *Patient IU*

Official Diagnosis: Metastatic carcinoma of the pancreas

Date of Diagnosis: April 1976

Hospital: St. Anthony's Hospital, Denver, Colorado

Conventional Therapy: Palliative surgery

Date First Seen by Dr. Kelley: May 20, 1976

Date of Death: July 10, 1976

Survival Time: 51 days

481

5. *Patient MQ*

Official Diagnosis: Metastatic carcinoma of the pancreas

Date of Diagnosis: November 1979

Hospital: Virginia Mason, Seattle, Washington

Conventional Therapy: None

Date First Seen by Dr. Kelley: November 27, 1979

Date of Death: January 28, 1980

Survival Time: 62 days

6. *Patient IE*

Official Diagnosis: Metastatic carcinoma of the pancreas

Date of Diagnosis: May 1978

Hospital: Scott and White Clinic, Temple, Texas

Conventional Therapy: Chemotherapy, radiation

Date First Seen by Dr. Kelley: July 6, 1978

Date of Death: September 11, 1978

Survival Time: 67 days

7. *Patient FN*

Official Diagnosis: Metastatic carcinoma of the pancreas

Date of Diagnosis: February 1974

Hospital: Jackson Hospital and Clinic, Montgomery, Alabama

Conventional Therapy: Surgery, chemotherapy

Date First Seen by Dr. Kelley: July 16, 1974

Date of Death: October 8, 1974

Survival Time: 84 days

8. *Patient MN*

Official Diagnosis: Metastatic carcinoma of the pancreas

Date of Diagnosis: October 1976

Hospital: Mercy Hospital, Iowa City, Iowa

Conventional Therapy: Palliative surgery

Date First Seen by Dr. Kelley: May 31, 1977

Date of Death: August 24, 1977

Survival Time: 85 days

9. *Patient HD*

Official Diagnosis: Metastatic carcinoma of the pancreas

Date of Diagnosis: May 1977

Hospital: St. Rita's Hospital, Luna, Ohio

Conventional Therapy: Palliative surgery

Date First Seen by Dr. Kelley: June 23, 1977

Date of Death: September 24, 1977

Survival Time: 93 days

10. *Patient DG*

Official Diagnosis: Metastatic carcinoma of the pancreas

Date of Diagnosis: July, 1977

Hospital: Sacred Heart Hospital, Spokane, Washington

Conventional Therapy: Surgery, radiation

Date First Seen by Dr. Kelley: December 16, 1977

Date of Death: March 29, 1978

Survival Time: 103 days

Summary of Data for Group I

Median survival: 67 days

Mean survival: 62.7 days

Group II:

Patients Who Followed the Program Partially

1. *Patient TS*

Official Diagnosis: Metastatic carcinoma of the pancreas

Date of Diagnosis: October 1979

Hospital: American River Hospital, Carmichael, California

Conventional Therapy: Palliative surgery, chemotherapy

Date First Seen by Dr. Kelley: December 6, 1979

Length of Time on Program: Four weeks

Date of Death: April 3, 1980

Survival Time: 119 days

2. *Patient KX*

Official Diagnosis: Metastatic carcinoma of the pancreas

Date of Diagnosis: July 1979

Hospital: The Medical Center, Biggar, Saskatchewan

Conventional Therapy: Palliative surgery, chemotherapy

Date First Seen by Dr. Kelley: October 16, 1979

Length of Time on Program: Six weeks

Date of Death: March 31, 1980

Survival Time: 167 days

3. *Patient XL*

Official Diagnosis: Metastatic carcinoma of the pancreas

Date of Diagnosis: September 1975

Hospital: Santa Barbara Cottage Hospital, Santa Barbara, California

Conventional Therapy: Palliative surgery, chemotherapy, radiation

Date First Seen by Dr. Kelley: February 23, 1976

Length of Time on Program: Eight weeks

Date of Death: September 21, 1976

Survival time: 211 days

4. *Patient DD*

Official Diagnosis: Metastatic carcinoma of the pancreas

Date of Diagnosis: August 1977

Hospital: Sequoia Hospital, Redwood City, California

Conventional Therapy: Chemotherapy, radiation

Date First Seen by Dr. Kelley: December 12, 1977

Length of Time on Program: Approximately fourteen weeks

Date of Death: August 2, 1978

Survival Time: 233 days

5. *Patient IL*

Official Diagnosis: Metastatic carcinoma of the pancreas

Date of Diagnosis: Approximately February 1975

Hospital: Community General Osteopathic Hospital, Harrisburg, Pennsylvania

Conventional Therapy: Unknown (record to date incomplete)

Date First Seen by Dr. Kelley: November 26, 1975

Length of Time on Kelley Program: Six months

Date of Death: November 1, 1976

Survival Time: 340 days

6. *Patient FO*

Official Diagnosis: Metastatic carcinoma of the pancreas

Date of Diagnosis: August 1976

Hospital: Virginia Mason, Seattle, Washington

Conventional Therapy: Palliative surgery, chemotherapy

Date First Seen by Dr. Kelley: October 14, 1976

Length of Time on Program: Approximately 10 months, partially

Date of Death: January 24, 1978

Survival Time: 467 days

7. *Patient GC*

Official Diagnosis: Metastatic carcinoma of the pancreas

Date of Diagnosis: July 1979

Hospital: Surrey Memorial Hospital, Surrey, B.C., Canada

Conventional Therapy: Palliative surgery, radiation

Date First Seen by Dr. Kelley: October 15, 1979

Length of Time on Program: Approximately 13 months, partially

Date of Death: May 16, 1982

Survival Time: 578 days

Summary of Data for Group II

Median survival: 233 days

Mean survival: 302.1 days

Group III:

Patients Who Followed the Full Program

1. *Patient #34*

Official Diagnosis: Metastatic adenocarcinoma of the pancreas

Date of Diagnosis: August 1982

Hospital: St. Elizabeth Hospital, Appleton, Wisconsin

Conventional Therapy: Exploratory surgery only

Date Began Kelley Program: December 1982

Length of Time on Program: Four years

Survival Time: 4.50 years, still alive

2. *Patient #35*

Official Diagnosis: Metastatic islet cell carcinoma

Date of Diagnosis: January 1981

Hospital: District One Hospital, Faribault, Minnesota

Conventional Therapy: Chemotherapy briefly, with no improvement

Date Began Kelley Program: June 1981

Length of Time on Program: 6 years, still follows

Survival Time: 6 years, still alive

3. *Patient #36*

Official Diagnosis: Metastatic adenocarcinoma of the pancreas

Date of Diagnosis: March 1978

Hospital: St. Barnabas Hospital, Bronx, New York

Conventional Therapy: Surgery, brief course of BCG immunotherapy

Date Began Kelley Program: April 1978

Length of Time on Program: Two years on full program, modified program since

Survival Time: 9 years, still alive

4. *Patient #37*

Official Diagnosis: Metastatic adenocarcinoma of the pancreas, carcinoid

Date of Diagnosis: June 1977

Hospital: Christian Hospital, St. Louis, Missouri

Conventional Therapy: Exploratory surgery only

Date Began Kelley Program: August 1977

Length of Time on Program: Five years on full program

Survival time: 9.75 years, still alive

5. *Patient #38*

Official Diagnosis: Inoperable adenocarcinoma of the pancreas (no biopsy)

Date of Diagnosis: August, 1974

Hospital: Halifax Hospital, Daytona Beach, Florida

Conventional Therapy: Exploratory surgery only

Date Began on Kelley Program: November 1974

Length of Time on Program: 10 years

Date of Death: April 12, 1986

Survival Time: 11.5 years, died of Alzheimer's Disease

Summary of Data for Group III:

Median survival: 9 years

Mean survival: 8.2 years

The Pancreatic Study: Conclusions

The survival times for the three groups can be summarized in chart form as follows:

Group	Median Survival	Mean Survival
I. Never Followed (10 patients)	67 days	62.7 days
II. Followed Partially (7 patients)	233 days	302.1 days
III. Followed Completely (5 patients)	9 years	8.2 years

As described, one extremely ill patient died the day after consulting Dr. Kelley. Otherwise, based on my evaluation of the medical records, I do not believe patients overall in one group were significantly sicker than those in any other group when first seen by Dr. Kelley.

Over the years of my investigation, Dr. Kelley repeatedly told me that cancer patients should follow the full program for at least several years to regain good health, and thereafter continue a maintenance protocol. Nevertheless, the mean survival time for those who pursued the program only partially, and usually briefly, is 4.8 times greater than the survival time of patients who never began the regimen.

Finally, the data allows an estimation, though admittedly informal, of Dr. Kelley's "success rate" with pancreatic cancer, considering only those five patients who complied with the full nutritional program as prescribed. In this group, 100% of patients responded. Though the numbers are small, nonetheless I think the data represents an impressive outcome for a terrible disease; I wonder if any oncologist in America could match these results.

CHAPTER XII

Conclusion

A study such as mine cannot, of course, prove conclusively that Dr. Kelley "cures" cancer, since the patients evaluated were not treated under controlled conditions prospectively in a formal academic clinical trial setting. Nevertheless, a large number of patients with appropriately diagnosed, obviously poor prognosis or terminal cancer have experienced impressive regression of disease and/or long-term survival while pursuing the Kelley regimen. I believe this finding alone warrants a full, fair, unbiased investigation of Dr. Kelley's methods.

I think, as a start, it would be constructive if oncologists and conventional cancer researchers approached Dr. Kelley with a spirit of cooperation and reconciliation, rather than with the usual disdain, hysteria, and anger. First of all, disdain, hysteria, and anger rarely, if ever, lead to the advancement of knowledge, which is, hopefully, what science is all about. Furthermore, I do not believe our success with cancer and other degenerative diseases is so extraordinary that we can afford to dismiss any promising therapy simply because it does not conform to our preconceived notion of what the truth should be.

I suppose it will be embarrassing, if this country orthodontist with no position, no funding, and no scientific staff has outsmarted the National Cancer Institute and the American Cancer Society and the rest of the academic research community. But whether we like it or not, Dr. Kelley may be right, in much of what he says. And if he is, unquestionably the course of medicine will be changed forever.

ABOUT THE AUTHOR

Nicholas J. Gonzalez, M.D. graduated from Brown University, Phi Beta Kappa, magna cum laude with a degree in English Literature. He worked as a journalist, first at Time Inc., before pursuing premedical studies at Columbia University. He received his medical degree from Cornell University Medical College in 1983. During a postgraduate immunology fellowship under Dr. Robert A. Good, considered the father of modern immunology, Dr. Gonzalez investigated the nutritional regimen developed by the dentist Dr. William Kelley and used in the treatment of advanced cancer. Dr. Gonzalez's research has been funded by The Procter & Gamble Company, Nestle, and the National Cancer Institute/National Institutes of Health. Since 1987, Dr. Gonzalez has been in private practice in New York City treating cancer and other degenerative diseases through individualized dietary and supplement protocols including pancreatic enzymes. For more information, see his website at www.dr-gonzalez.com.

For other books and lecture recordings by Dr. Gonzalez, please contact New Spring Press.

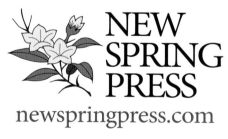

NEW SPRING PRESS

newspringpress.com

PO Box 200   New York, NY 10156